Perspectives in
Behavioral Medicine

QUALITY OF LIFE IN BEHAVIORAL MEDICINE RESEARCH

Perspectives in Behavioral Medicine
Sponsored by the Academy of Behavioral Medicine Research

Riley/Matarazzo/Baum: *The Aging Dimension*
Weiner/Baum: *Eating Regulation and Discontrol*
Stunkard/Baum: *Eating, Sleeping, and Sex*
Weiss/Fielding/Baum: *Health at Work*
Shapiro/Baum: *Behavioral Aspects of Cardiovascular Disease*
Schneiderman/McCabe/Baum: *Stress and Disease Processes*
Dimsdale/Baum: *Quality of Life in Behavioral Medicine Research*
Stein/Baum: *Chronic Diseases*

Perspectives in
Behavioral Medicine

QUALITY OF LIFE IN BEHAVIORAL MEDICINE RESEARCH

Edited by

Joel E. Dimsdale
University of California, San Diego

Andrew Baum
University of Pittsburgh

Routledge
Taylor & Francis Group
LONDON AND NEW YORK

First Published by
Lawrence Erlbaum Associates, Inc., Publishers

Published 2016 by Routledge
2 Park Square, Milton Park, Abingdon, Oxfordshire OX14 4RN
711 Third Avenue, New York, NY 10017

First issued in paperback 2016

Routledge is an imprint of the Taylor and Francis Group, an informa business

Cover design by Kate Dusza

Cover illustration: *Self-Portrait*
by Kathe Kollwitz. Courtesy,
Museum of Fine Arts, Boston.

Library of Congress Cataloging-in-Publication Data

Quality of life in behavioral medicine research / edited by Joel E.
Dimsdale, Andrew Baum.
p. cm.
Includes bibliographical references and index.
ISBN 0-8058-1653-4 (alk. paper)
1. Medicine and psychology—Congresses. 2. Quality of life—
Congresses. I. Dimsdale, Joel E., 1947- . II. Baum, Andrew.
[DNLM: 1. Quality of Life. 2. Chronic Disease—therapy.
3. Behavioral Medicine—United States. 4. Health Services Research—
United States. WT 500 Q11 1994]
R726.5.Q34 1994
615.5—dc20
DNLM/DLC
for Library of Congress 94-28512
CIP

ISBN 13: 978-1-138-98434-9 (pbk)
ISBN 13: 978-0-8058-1653-2 (hbk)

Publisher's Note
The publisher has gone to great lengths to ensure the quality of this reprint but points out that some imperfections in the original may be apparent.

This book is dedicated to our families,
who do so much to enhance our own quality of life.

Contents

Preface

Quality of life studies have burgeoned in the last decade. Such studies reveal vital new information about the costs and benefits of illness and various medical interventions. At the core of the quality of life perspective is the recognition that medical interventions have proximal and distal effects. Medicine has traditionally focused on proximal effects, such as the effects of the intervention on mortality. In addition, medicine has long been interested in major morbidity side effects of interventions, although this is a more complex matter for study. One person's "major morbidity" may be another's "acceptable side effect." It is increasingly difficult to quantify subtle morbidity or to reach consensus as to its seriousness. The "authority" of medicine as the judge of such morbidity is being increasingly challenged when the morbidity involves values and judgments of comparative worth. Is consensus possible about how to define quality of life effects of treatment? Is there a way of quantifying quality of life so that comparisons can be made across treatments? Given that all treatments have diverse side effects, is there a way of comparing "rotten apples" and "spoiled oranges" so that the patient/doctor/insurer can make a choice?

All of these questions were thrashed out at a spirited meeting sponsored by the Academy of Behavioral Medicine Research in June 1992. The meeting convened an unusual combination of university researchers, federal health policy regulators, and pharmaceutical industry researchers. This book represents a summary of this meeting and is the latest in a series of books sponsored by the Academy on major policy issues in behavioral medicine.

The book is divided into two sections. The first section examines quality of life from a regulatory perspective. The second reviews progress in this field as it relates to a number of illnesses.

The first section begins with Kaplan's discussion of studies from an econometric perspective. He suggests that quality of life studies must be at the core of any logical plan to allocate resources for health care. This perspective is controversial for two reasons. It forces us to recognize that we do not have enough resources to solve all health care problems, and it challenges us to rationally decide what treatments should be adopted, as opposed to having these decisions made in a haphazard manner. The second controversy stems from his approach of distilling quality of life into one variable. This approach seems opposed to common clinical perspectives, which consider side effects by organ system or functional domain as opposed to global systems.

The section continues with perspectives from Erickson, Wilson, and Shannon of the National Center for Health Statistics. One of the blueprints for federal planning on health is the document *Healthy People 2000,* which indicates numerous objectives for health promotion and disease prevention. Implicit in this document is a substantial emphasis on quality of life, and the National Center for Health Statistics is tracking progress on these objectives. University academics may be unaware of the volumes of data being obtained in this area as part of the National Health Interview Survey. Erickson and colleagues summarize some of these data concerning large-scale sampling of quality of life in the United States.

Schuttinga, from the Director's Office at the National Institutes of Health, then discusses policy aspects of quality of life assessment rather than substantive research per se. He notes that quality of life concerns have not yet played a major role in health-care regulation. With constrained budgets this field faces considerable obstacles and skepticism. Schuttinga argues that these sorts of conflict are endemic in policy planning in Washington, DC where an adversarial process characterizes federal planning. This dialectic process can be viewed alternately as either destructively contentious or as ensuring consensus and reasonable compromise. Although there is some resistance to quality of life research in Washington, DC because of a concern that such an approach provides soft data and encourages even greater health-care costs, there is also the recognition that many of the components of a quality of life assessment are crucial and straightforward. Schuttinga describes the activities of the National Institutes of Health in terms of inclusion of quality of life studies in clinical trials. He also discusses how various registries (such as that dealing with Medicare) may provide important data. He concludes with a warning that the field will be stunted unless investigators reach some agreement as to common measurement strategies for quality of life studies. Unless a standard is developed, he forecasts increasing reluctance of policy officials to commit to quality of life studies.

The section then presents an interesting chapter by Epstein and Lydick of Merck Pharmaceuticals, who discuss quality of life research from the perspective of drug development in the pharmaceutical industry. They point out that the type of illness being treated has a direct impact on the type of quality of life question to be addressed. Because of the uncertainty about questionnaires for measuring quality of life, the pharmaceutical industry is interested in encouraging some consensus. At the same time, if a given company has already invested considerable resources in developing a new quality of life inventory, it will be less willing to shelve that inventory and the hard-won data relying on it in favor of some new industrywide inventory. He also reminds us that the pharmaceutical industry is multinational, and that there are considerable problems with translation of these complex inventories from one culture to another.

In a companion chapter, Freeman from Sterling Winthrop Pharmaceuticals expands on similar points. In addition, he discusses the internal debates within the pharmaceutical industry about the costs and benefits of such quality of life studies. He mentions the potential ethical tensions between researcher and pharmaceutical industry in terms of dissemination of information. Such conflicts may involve data about the efficacy of a given drug, but also can involve data showing the utility of a given quality of life instrument developed under industry sponsorship. He also notes the perception within the pharmaceutical industry that various branches within the Food and Drug Administration (FDA) differ in their emphasis on the value of quality of life studies.

The second section considers in detail substantive studies on quality of life as pertaining to specific disease entities. We have included discussion of cancer, hypertension, acquired immune deficiency syndrome (AIDS), and diabetes because these illnesses touch so many people's lives.

Cancer studies are discussed in two chapters. Moinpour, Savage, Hayden, Sawyers, and Upchurch discuss quality of life studies in cancer clinical trials conducted by cooperative groups. The experience of one such cooperative group is discussed in detail in terms of constraints on conducting quality of life studies, the value of patient-completed versus proxy-completed quality of life inventories, and the respective advantages of generic versus disease-specific inventories. They also discuss the formidable problems with quality control procedures for such multisite studies; this issue is particularly important if quality of life is an add-on to clinical trials that emphasize drug effects on survival.

Ganz and Coscarelli describe a decade of work on quality of life after breast cancer treatment. They have developed a number of inventories targeting quality of life in this population. This area has historically been dominated by assumptions of the superiority of one type of treatment over another. Their work is important because it specifically compares the different rehabilitation problems of women receiving modified radical mastectomy with those receiving segmental mastectomy and radiation therapy. There is a wide variation in psychosocial adjustment to these procedures; it is hoped that the quality of life assessment techniques developed may better identify prospectively those patients in need of increased psychosocial intervention.

There are numerous studies relating to quality of life in hypertension. Such studies typically examine the neuropsychologic or mood effects of various antihypertensive treatments, but occasionally examine the effect of hypertension itself. Both hypertension itself and antihypertensive treatment have been associated with deficits in quality of life.

Elias, Elias, Cobb, D'Agostino, White, and Wolf report on an unusually rich database, the Framingham Heart Study. This communitywide prospective study, begun in 1948, involves biennial examinations of cardiovascular risk factors. Three studies of associations between blood pressure level and neuropsychological performance are reviewed. The first finds few significant relationships. The second and third find that unmedicated blood pressure levels are inversely associated with memory and learning when blood pressure was averaged over many examinations. In the third study, significant, although modest, relationships between blood pressure and cognitive functioning are observed for a sample never treated for hypertension. This is true even though blood pressure measurements preceded neuropsychological testing by 12 to 14 years. The chapter considers how different aspects of experimental design may account for the various findings.

Thyrum and Blumenthal review the literature on hypertension and neuropsychologic functioning. One commonly used approach employs a battery of neuropsychologic tests. Another approach employs measures of information processing. The authors note the disparities in the literature and emphasize the importance of considering possible confounders such as social class, duration of hypertension, and presence of related illnesses such as diabetes, which in their own right may have detrimental effects on cognition.

Shapiro, Muldoon, Waldstein, Jennings, and Manuck provide an overview of their studies on blood pressure and behavioral effects of antihypertensive medications. For more than 10 years this group has published intriguing data to suggest that hypertensives have subtle cognitive deficits that improve after the underlying hypertension is treated. This brief chapter discusses these findings as well as some of the problems in designing such studies. They present data on a study of six antihypertensive drugs. The drugs differed pharmacologically and had somewhat different impacts on cognition. The authors note that the patient is frequently unaware of the subtle effects of drug treatment, that these effects are best revealed on careful quality of life examination.

Rosen and Kostis examine quality of life effects of antihypertensive treatment on a broader array of variables—sleep, mood, and sexual functioning. Many of these drugs have adverse effects on these dimensions, but interestingly, the effects are not across-the-board. Given that many drugs have adverse effects in these areas, the authors argue for studies of nondrug treatment of hypertension. They also point out the dearth of studies comparing men and women in terms of side effects. Given the side effects on male sexual functioning, it is important that future studies specifically enroll women as well.

Shapiro, Hui, Oakley, Pasic, and Jamner specifically examine whether behavioral treatments for hypertension can improve quality of life. Employing a combined behavioral and drug intervention, they examine whether reductions in drug requirements are associated with changes in quality of life, and whether quality of life differs in patients treated with drugs alone versus patients treated with both drugs and a multimodal cognitive-behavioral intervention. The behavioral intervention was effective in reducing drug requirements. Despite the many assessments used, few quality of life effects were obtained, perhaps reflecting the fact that minimal drug requirements were established and stepdown of medication was individualized for each patient. Medication reduction was associated with reductions in patients' hostility and defensiveness.

Given the magnitude of the public health challenge of AIDS, it is encouraging that behavioral medicine researchers have been studying quality of life in this illness. Two chapters detail somewhat different approaches along these lines. Lutgendorf, Antoni, Schneiderman, Ironson, and Fletcher discuss extensively the different challenges raised at various phases of the illness, from diagnosis to early asymptomatic infection to emergence of symptoms and to progression of AIDS. They describe the important role of a cognitive-behavioral intervention to enhance coping and social support and thus improve the quality of life.

Cleary, Wilson, and Fowler take a different tack, discussing not so much interventions as much as a conceptual model or framework for quality of life studies of human immunodeficiency virus (HIV) infection. They note that few studies have examined the interrelationships between the various measures of quality of life. Such measures, when obtained in conjunction with disease-specific parameters, may improve detection of slowly progressing chronic symptoms. Using this approach, they examine if specific symptom profiles were associated with impaired functioning. Interestingly, fatigue is the strongest measure for activity limitations.

The book concludes with a discussion of quality of life issues in diabetes. Jacobson, de Groot, and Samson describe the complex medical course of this major illness and then present intriguing data about the costs and benefits of various sorts of newer treatments for diabetes. There is increasing evidence that intensive insulin treatment may delay progression of diabetes complications; however some have wondered whether these intensive treatments may have adverse psychosocial outcomes. In order to answer this crucial question, a measure of diabetes-related quality of life needed to be devised. This chapter describes the evolution of such a measure and gives a hint of the data that will be forthcoming.

The Academy of Behavioral Medicine Research sponsors this book in the hopes that it will kindle increased communication and discussion of quality of life. The topic is a core issue for behavioral medicine as a scholarly endeavor and has wide ramifications for public policy and the health-care industry.

ACKNOWLEDGMENTS

Numerous colleagues assisted in critiquing early drafts of these chapters. The editors would like to thank: W. Stewart Agras, M.D.; Ben Allmann, M.B., B.Ch., M.B.A., Michael A. Andrykowski, Ph.D.; Michael H. Criqui, Ph.D.; Sydney H. Croog, Ph.D.; Jimmie C.B. Holland, M.D.; Rolf G. Jacob, M.D.; Kathleen C. Light, Ph.D.; Matthew F. Muldoon, M.D.; Thomas Patterson, Ph.D.; Evan G. Pattishall, Jr.; Ph.D., M.D.; Raul C. Schiavi, M.D.; Richard S. Surwit, Ph.D.; Lydia P. Temoshok, Ph.D.; and Raymond J. Townsend, Pharm.D., FCCP. This book represents a summary of a meeting sponsored by the Academy of Behavioral Medicine Research. We would also like to thank Upjohn Pharmaceuticals for their help in defraying some of the costs of this conference.

Finally, the skilled editorial assistance of Ruth Newton, Ph.D. and Wendy Hunziker is gratefully acknowledged.

Joel E. Dimsdale

List of Contributors

MICHAEL H. ANTONI University of Miami, Department of Psychology.

JAMES A. BLUMENTHAL Duke University Medical Center, Department of Psychiatry.

JOEL E. DIMSDALE University of California, San Diego, Department of Psychiatry.

PAUL D. CLEARY Harvard Medical School, Department of Health Care Policy.

JANET COBB Boston University, Department of Mathematics.

ANNE COSCARELLI Jonsson Comprehensive Cancer Center and University of California, Los Angeles, School of Medicine.

RALPH D'AGOSTINO Boston University, Department of Mathematics.

MARY de GROOT Joslin Diabetes Center.

MERRILL F. ELIAS The University of Maine, Department of Psychology.

PENELOPE K. ELIAS The University of Maine, Department of Psychology.

ROBERT S. EPSTEIN Merck Research Laboratory.

PENNIFER ERICKSON U.S. Department of Health & Human Services, National Center for Health Statistics.

MARY ANN FLETCHER University of Miami, Department of Medicine.

FLOYD J. FOWLER, JR. University of Massachusetts, Boston, Center for Survey Research.

ROBERT A. FREEMAN Sterling Winthrop, Inc.

PATRICIA A. GANZ Jonsson Comprehensive Cancer Center and University of California, Los Angeles.

KATHERINE A. HAYDEN University of Arkansas for Medical Sciences.

KA KIT HUI University of California, Los Angeles, Department of Medicine.

GAIL IRONSON University of Miami, Department of Psychology.

ALAN M. JACOBSON Joslin Diabetes Center.

LARRY D. JAMNER University of California, Irvine, Department of Psychology and Social Behavior.

J. RICHARD JENNINGS University of Pittsburgh School of Medicine.

ROBERT M. KAPLAN University of California, San Diego, Department of Family & Preventive Medicine.

JOHN B. KOSTIS Robert Wood Johnson Medical School, University of Medicine and Dentistry of New Jersey, Department of Medicine.

SUSAN LUTGENDORF University of Miami, Department of Psychology.

EVA LYDICK Merck Research Laboratories.

STEVEN B. MANUCK University of Pittsburgh School of Medicine.

CAROL M. MOINPOUR Fred Hutchinson Cancer Research Center, Southwest Oncology Group Statistical Center.

MATTHEW F. MULDOON University of Pittsburgh School of Medicine.

MARK E. OAKLEY University of California, Los Angeles, Department of Psychiatry and Biobehavioral Sciences.

JAGODA PASIC University of California, Los Angeles, Department of Medicine.

RAYMOND C. ROSEN Robert Wood Johnson Medical School, University of Medicine and Dentistry of New Jersey, Department of Psychiatry.

MARGUERITE SAVAGE Veterans Affairs Medical Center, Baltimore.

JACQUELINE SAMSON Harvard Medical School, Department of Psychiatry.

JULIA SAWYERS Vanderbilt University, Owen Graduate School of Management.

NEIL SCHNEIDERMAN University of Miami, Department of Psychology.

JAMES A. SCHUTTINGA National Institutes of Health, Office of the Director.

ILDY SHANNON U.S. Department of Health & Human Services, National Center for Health Statistics.

ALVIN P. SHAPIRO University of Pittsburgh School of Medicine.

DAVID SHAPIRO University of California, Los Angeles, Department of Psychiatry and Biobehavioral Sciences.

ELIZABETH A. TOWNER THYRUM Duke University Medical Center, Department of Psychiatry.

CHRISTINE UPCHURCH Fred Hutchinson Cancer Research Center, Southwest Oncology Group.

SHARI R. WALDSTEIN University of Pittsburgh School of Medicine.

LON R. WHITE National Institute on Aging, Epidemiology, Demography, and Biometry Program.

IRA B. WILSON Tufts Medical School, Department of Medicine.

RONALD WILSON U.S. Department of Health & Human Services, National Center for Health Statistics.

PHILIP A. WOLF Boston University School of Medicine, Department of Neurology.

I QUALITY OF LIFE FROM A REGULATORY PERSPECTIVE

1 Quality of Life, Resource Allocation, and the U.S. Health-Care Crisis

Robert M. Kaplan
University of California, San Diego

The United States spent an estimated $838 billion for health care in 1992, and these expenditures are expected to be well over $1 trillion by 1995 and may be $2 trillion by the turn of the century. Economic forecasts suggest that the increasing proportion of the gross domestic product (GDP) devoted to health care may have serious consequences for the economic viability of the U.S. economy in the 21st century. Despite the enormous costs of our health-care system, the system is inequitable, denying access to between 32 and 38 million Americans who have no insurance coverage. Perhaps most disturbing is that we know remarkably little about the relationship between expenditures on health care and health outcomes.

In order to analyze these problems, we propose a General Health Policy Model (GHPM). The model provides the basis for an innovative experiment on expanded access to care and health-care resource allocation in one U.S. state. The model attempts to identify services that produce the greatest benefit within the constraints of resources. In order to accomplish this it is necessary to build a comprehensive theoretical model of health status that includes components for mortality, morbidity, utility (health value), and prognosis. Data sources for the model include life tables, data on health status from population surveys, and community preferences for health outcomes. One of the advantages of the GHPM is that it allows comparisons between health-care services that have different specific objectives. The major deficiency of the model is that there are currently too few data to estimate the benefits of most medical and preventive services.

Most people in the United States disagree about the solutions for most social problems. However, there is near consensus that the U.S. health-care system requires reform. Those calling for reform in the health-care system include peculiar bedfellows. They are Republicans and Democrats, conservatives and liberals, management and labor. Public opinion polls consistently demonstrate that only one quarter of the U.S. public has faith in the current system (Jajich-Toth & Roper, 1990). Health care was one of the major issues considered in the 1992 U.S. presidential election and the search for innovative solutions has become the first priority of the Clinton administration. In this chapter I review problems with the U.S. health-care system. Then a model for quantifying the costs and effects of care is presented. The model emphasizes the measurement of quality of life. Next, the chapter suggests how the model can be used to resolve some of the problems of the health-care system. A proposal to apply the model by the state of Oregon is reviewed. Finally, ethical challenges to the model are considered.

THE PROBLEM

There are three basic deficiencies in the U.S. health-care system (Relman, 1989). First, health care costs too much. Those who pay for health care, primarily large employers and governments, can no longer afford to continue to offer the same level of payment. A second problem is that the system is inequitable. Despite the fact that Americans spend more on health care as a proportion of the GDP than any other country, we still have between 32 and 38 million persons who have no insurance or inadequate resources to cover their medical care. The third, and perhaps most challenging problem, is that we have failed to be good consumers of health care. Theoretically, we purchase health care in order to obtain health. Yet we know very little about the relationship between health care and health outcomes. Many of the services we purchase may either be unnecessary or ineffective (Brook & Lohr, 1986). A simple mnemonic for these three problems is "The three As: Affordability, Access, and Accountability." Each of these issues is briefly summarized in the following sections.

Affordability: The Problem of Cost

In the United States, health-care costs have grown remarkably during the last 50 years (see Fig 1.1). In 1940, approximately $4 billion was spent on health care in the U.S. That annual expenditure had tripled by 1950. Since then, growth in health care expenditures has been astronomical. The 1992 expenditure of $838 billion was more than 200 times greater than the 1940 expenditure. Today the United States spends more in 2 days than it spent in

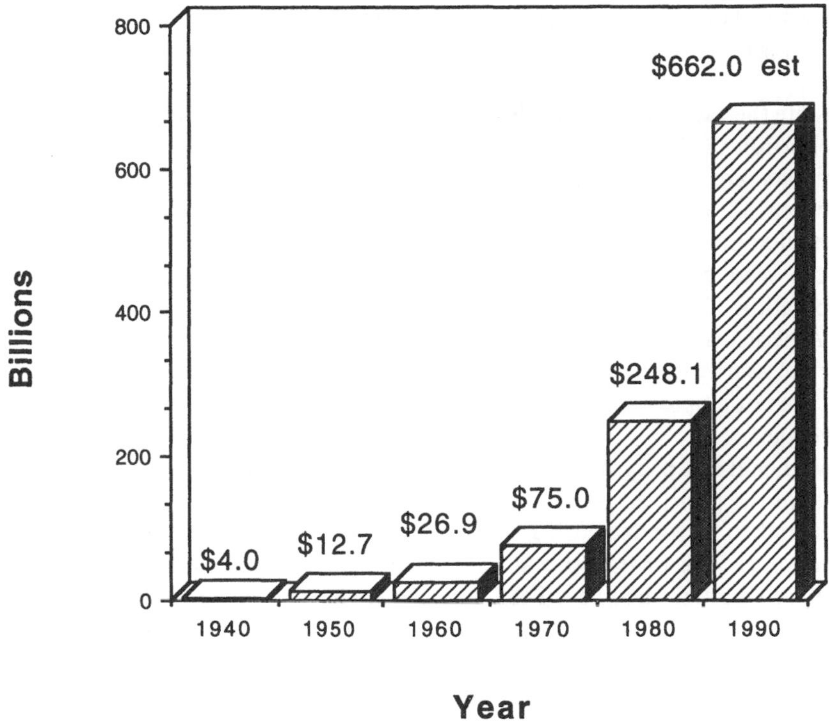

FIG.1.1. Increases in U.S. health-care costs between 1940 and 1990.

the entire year of 1940. This growth far exceeds what would be expected on the basis of inflation. The proportion of the GDP devoted to health care exceeds that in any Westernized country. In 1960, medical services accounted for only about 5% of the U.S. economic output. By 1992 this proportion had increased to nearly 14% (Vincenzino, 1993). At current growth rates, 1990 expenditures will double by 1995 and triple by the turn of the century.

High expenditures on health care have raised serious concerns about the likelihood that U.S. products can successfully compete with those offered by foreign competitors. For example, it has been estimated that the Chrysler Corporation spends about $700 (U.S.) per automobile on health care, whereas the comparable figure for Japanese auto makers is less than $300 (U.S.). Discrepancies in health insurance account for a major portion in the cost differences required to produce products in different countries. In 1986, Great Britain spent only about 6% of its GDP on health care. Japan spent less than 7%, and West Germany spent only about 8%.

Access: The Problem of the Uninsured or Underinsured

Despite the fact that U.S. health care is remarkably expensive, a substantial proportion of the U.S. population is excluded from the system. The exact numbers are difficult to estimate. However, most experts believe that between 32 and 38 million Americans have no health insurance at any particular point in time (Short, 1990; Short, Monheit, & Beauregard, 1989). Those who are uninsured are not a random sample from the general population. The only group that is really exempt is the elderly, for virtually all Americans older than 65 are covered under Medicare. The uninsured are not necessarily the unemployed. In fact, the majority of the uninsured work but are not employed in professions that provide adequate health insurance coverage.

Medicaid is a program administered by each U.S. state to provide health care for the poor, the blind, and the disabled. In recent years, Medicaid has been able to help a decreasing share of the poor. In most states the eligibility criterion is 50% of the federal poverty level. That makes a family of three with an annual income of $5,800 too rich to receive help. Medicaid recognizes certain specific categories. For example, Congressional action in the 1980s required Medicaid coverage for pregnant women. Governors of 49 states asked the U.S. Congress to cease requesting special coverages because states simply do not have the money to expand services. Yet current policies lead to the nonsensible actions. Because Medicaid provides coverage for pregnant women, many low-income women find that the only way to obtain health insurance is to become pregnant. Furthermore, most states allow low-income families support for dependent children. Yet the age criteria for coverage varies. A family may get coverage for young children but may be excluded as the children age through adolescence.

Medicaid also has become highly political. Governors or legislators attempting to win votes have sometimes committed money that encumbered large pieces of the expenditure pie. These decisions typically make access worse. For example, Illinois passed a 1985 bill that guaranteed reimbursement of up to $200,000 for any citizen who needed an organ transplant. At the same time, more than 60% of African-American children in Chicago's inner cities did not receive routine medical care and were not even immunized against common diseases such as polio. In 1990, Florida's Governor Martinez committed $100,000 to a heroic attempt to save the life of a single child who had nearly drowned in a swimming pool accident. All experts agreed that the case was futile. Although the governor received great acclaim for his compassion, thousands of Florida children were denied basic services through Florida's underfunded Medicaid program (Kitzhaber,

1990). When funds are directed toward rescue, prevention programs are typically the first victim of the revenue shortfall.

In summary, the current system has failed miserably in providing adequate access to health care. It is a widely held assumption that health care is a basic right rather than a luxury. Despite the willingness of the United States to spend more on health care than any other country in the world, we still have substantial proportions of our population who have no health insurance at all. The poor and members of certain ethnic and minority groups are disproportionately left with no insurance and no regular source of care. Although proposed solutions differ, few groups are willing to defend the current system.

Accountability: The Problem of Outcome

We invest in health care to gain improved health status. However, it has been difficult to demonstrate that investments in care result in better health outcomes. A recent interest in outcomes research grew out of the observations of small area variation. It has always been assumed that medical need is the primary reason for receiving medical care. Doctors perform procedures when people are sick. We would assume that the demand for medical services should be roughly the same among demographically homogeneous communities. Yet systematic studies show that there is substantial variation in the rate at which medical services are used in different places. The per capita cost of hospitalization in New Haven, Connecticut, for example, is about half of what it is in Boston, Massachusetts (Wennberg, 1990). In San Diego, about 8 of every 10 well-insured patients receive angiography following a myocardial infarction (MI) if they are treated in a private hospital. However, only 40% of the patients in the San Diego Veterans Administration Medical Center receive the procedure following a heart attack. In Vancouver, only 20% of post-MI patients get angiography, and only about 10% receive the procedure in Sweden (Nicod et al., 1991). This variation might be acceptable if we knew that more care led to better health. Yet we have little evidence that aggressive medical care results in better patient outcomes. Controlling for seriousness of heart attack (ejection fraction), the probability of surviving an MI is the same in San Diego, Vancouver, and Sweden. Life expectancy in New Haven is about the same as it is in Boston, even though Boston citizens are hospitalized significantly more often and at a higher cost.

A growing number of studies have questioned whether particular medical technologies achieve their intended goals. For example, Brook, Park, Chassin, Kosecoff, Keesey, and Solomon (1990) at the Rand Corporation studied carotid endarterectomies. When carefully reviewed, the RAND researchers found that between 25% and 33% of the surgeries probably should not have been done. In these cases the surgeries were unlikely to lead to better health outcomes and may have placed the patients at risk. Careful reviews of a wide variety of other procedures have suggested that the use of medical procedures in the United States is out of control (Hadorn & Brook, 1991). In many cases the procedures had no likelihood of making patients better, and in some cases aggressive medical care endangers patients.

The first section of this chapter can be summarized rather simply. The U.S. health-care system is in serious trouble. The problem with health care in the United States has at least three components. The health-care system is unaffordable, it excludes 32 to 38 million Americans, and we have little evidence that the system is making people healthier or that Americans are more satisfied with the care they receive than citizens in other countries that spend less on health care. Solutions to these problems require that we consider all three dimensions.

PROPOSED SOLUTIONS

There are plenty of proposed solutions to the troubling problems of U.S. health care. However, the proposals are often overly simplistic. Elsewhere I have reviewed suggestions that the problem can be resolved by limiting lawsuits, controlling physician groups, or doing away with health-care administrators (Kaplan, 1993) . All of these solutions are naive and unlikely to produce lasting benefits. Policy changes such as prospective payment or reimbursing physicians based on the resources required to produce a service may have an impact on health-care costs. However, they do not necessarily resolve the access problem and may do very little to improve health outcome. The last two sessions of Congress saw at least a dozen proposals on health-care reform. The proposals came from all aspects of the political spectrum. They included those from the far left and those from the far right, as well as a substantial number of proposals from the middle. The backing for these bills ranged from groups such as the American Medical Association and the American Hospital Association, to specific politicians, to political advocacy groups such as the American Heritage Foundation. Several of the proposals would enhance access. However, only a few of the proposals take on the issue of affordability, and none of the proposals specifically attempt to produce more health care for the invested dollar. We believe that a successful proposal must attack all three problems. In order to accomplish this, we have proposed a GHPM.

Mathematical models of decision making are now being proposed in a variety of health-care systems. The most important challenge in developing a formal model for resource allocation is in defining a common unit of health benefit that is based on quality and quantity of life. Typically, the value of each specific intervention in health care is determined by considering a measure specific to the intervention or the disease process. Treatments for hypertension, for example, are evaluated in terms of blood pressure, whereas those for diabetes are evaluated by blood glucose. Yet it is difficult to compare the relative value of investing in blood glucose versus blood pressure reduction. Traditional public health measures, such as life expectancy, are usually too crude to allow appropriate prioritization.

A General Health Policy Model

In order to understand health outcomes, it is necessary to build a comprehensive theoretical model of health status. This model includes several components. The major aspects of the model include mortality (death) and morbidity (health-related quality of life). Elsewhere, it has been suggested that diseases and disabilities are important for two reasons. First, illness may cause the life expectancy to be shortened. Second, illness may make life less desirable at times prior to death (health-related quality of life; Kaplan & Anderson, 1988a, 1988b).

Over the last two decades, a group of investigators at the University of California, San Diego, has developed the GHPM. Central to the GHPM is a general conceptualization of quality of life. The model separates aspects of health status and life quality into distinct components. These are life expectancy (mortality), functioning and symptoms (morbidity), preference for observed functional states (utility), and duration of stay in health states (prognosis).

Mortality

A model of health outcomes necessarily includes a component for mortality. Indeed, many public health statistics focus exclusively on mortality through estimations of crude mortality rates, age-adjusted mortality rates, and infant mortality rates. Death is an important outcome that must be included in any comprehensive conceptualization of health.

Morbidity

In addition to death, quality of life is also an important outcome. The GHPM considers functioning in three areas: mobility, physical activity, and social activity. Descriptions of the measures of these aspects of function are given in many different publications (Kaplan & Anderson, 1988a, 1988b). Most public health indicators are relatively insensitive to variations toward the well end of the continuum. Measures of infant mortality, to give an extreme example, ignore all individuals capable of reading this chapter because they have lived beyond 1 year following their births (we assume that no infants are reading the chapter). Disability measures often ignore those in relatively well states. For example, the RAND Health Insurance Study reported that about 80% of the general populations have no dysfunction. Thus, they would estimate that 80% of the population is well. Our method asks about symptoms or problems in addition to behavioral dysfunction (Kaplan, Bush, & Berry, 1976). In these studies, only about 12% of the general population report no symptoms on a particular day. In other words, health symptoms or problems are a very common aspect of the human experience. Some might argue that symptoms are unimportant because they are subjective and unobservable. However, symptoms are highly correlated with the demand for medical services, expenditures on health care, and motivations to alter lifestyles. Thus, we feel that the quantification of symptoms is very important.

Utility (Relative Importance)

Given that various components of morbidity and mortality can be tabulated, it is important to consider their relative importance. For example, it is possible to develop measures that detect very minor symptoms. Yet, that these symptoms are measurable does not necessarily mean they are important. A patient may experience side effects of a medication but be willing to tolerate them because the side effects are less important than the probable benefit that would be obtained if the medication is consumed. Not all outcomes are equally important. A treatment in which 20 of 100 patients die is not equivalent to one in which 20 of 100 patients develop nausea. An important component of the GHPM attempts to scale the various health outcomes according to their relative importance. This exercise adds the quality dimension to health status. In the preceding example, the relative importance of dying would be weighted more than developing nausea. The weighting is accomplished by rating all states on a quality continuum ranging from *dead* (0) to *optimum functioning* (1.0). These ratings are typically provided by independent judges who are representative of the general population. Using this system it is possible to express the relative importance of states in relation to the lifedeath continuum. A point halfway on the scale (0.5) is regarded as halfway between optimum function and death. The quality of life weighting system has been described in several different publications (Kaplan, Bush, & Berry, 1976, 1978, 1979).

Prognosis

Another dimension of health status is the duration of a condition. A headache that lasts 1 hour is not equivalent to a headache that lasts 1 month. A cough that lasts 3 days is not equivalent to a cough that lasts 3 years. In considering the severity of illness, duration of the problem is central. As basic as this concept is, most contemporary models of health outcome measurement completely disregard the duration component. In the GHPM, the term *prognosis* refers to the probability of transition among health states over the course of time. In addition to consideration of duration of problems, the model considers the point at which the problem begins. A person may have no symptoms or dysfunctions currently but may have a high probability of health problems in the future. The *prognosis* component of the model takes these transitions into consideration and applies a discount rate for events that occur in the future. Discount rates are used to value resources and health outcomes differently if the onset is delay as opposed to immediate. A headache that will begin a year from now may be less of a concern than a headache that will start immediately.

Quality of Well-being Scale. The Quality of Well-being (QWB) scale is one of several different approaches for obtaining quality-adjusted life years (Kaplan & Anderson, 1988b). Using this method, patients are classified according to objective levels of functioning. These levels are represented by scales of mobility, physical activity, and social activity. In addition to classification into these observable levels of function, individuals are also classified by the symptom or problem they found most undesirable. On any particular day, nearly 80% of the general population is optimally functional. However, fewer than half of the population experience no symptoms. Symptoms or problems may be severe, such as serious chest pain, or minor, such as taking medication or a prescribed diet for health reasons.

Human value studies have been conducted to place the observable states of health and functioning onto a preference continuum for the desirability of various conditions, giving a quality rating between *death (0)* and *completely well* (1.0). A quality-adjusted life year is defined as the equivalent of a completely well year of life, or a year of life free of any symptoms, problems, or health-related disabilities. The well-life expectancy is the current life expectancy adjusted for diminished quality of life associated with dysfunctional states and the durations of stay in each state. It is possible to consider mortality, morbidity, and the preference weights for the various observable states of function. The model quantifies the health activity or treatment program in terms of the quality-adjusted life years that it produces or saves.

The QWB scale has been applied in studies of patients with a variety of illnesses, including chronic obstructive pulmonary disease, congestive heart failure, arthritis, cystic fibrosis, asthma, depression, human immunodeficiency virus (HIV) infections, diabetes, and several others. Specific validity and reliability data are available in each disease area. In cystic fibrosis patients, for example, QWB scores have been shown to be positively correlated with pulmonary function and exercise tolerance, and negatively correlated with age. Furthermore, the QWB scale was able to track improvement over time in a 2-week intervention for treatment of pulmonary exacerbation, with changes in QWB statistically significantly correlated with changes in pulmonary function (Orenstein, Nixon, Ross, & Kaplan, 1989; Orenstein, Pattishall, Ross, & Kaplan, 1990).

A mathematical model integrates components of the model to express outcomes in a common measurement unit. Using information on current functioning and duration, it is possible to express the health outcomes in terms of equivalents of well-years of life, or as some have described them, Quality-Adjusted Life Years (QALYs). The model for point in time QWB is:

$$\begin{aligned} \text{QWB} = 1 \quad & (\text{observed morbidity} \times \text{morbidity weight}) \\ & (\text{observed physical activity} \times \text{physical activity weight}) \\ & (\text{observed social activity and social activity weight}) \\ & (\text{observed symptom/problem} \times \text{symptom/problem weight}). \end{aligned}$$

The net cost/utility ratio is defined as:

$$\frac{\text{net cost}}{\text{net QWB} \times \text{duration in years}} = \frac{\text{cost of treatment} - \text{cost of alternative}}{[\text{QWB}_2 - \text{QWB}_1] \times \text{duration in years}}$$

Where QWB_2 and QWB_1 are measures of quality of well-being taken after and before treatment.

Consider, for example, a person who is in an objective state of functioning that is rated by community peers as 0.5 on a 0 to 1 scale. If the person remains in that state for 1 year, he or she would have lost the equivalent of 1/2 year of life. Thus, a person limited in activities who requires a cane or walker to get around the community would be hypothetically rated at 0.5. If he or she remained in that state for an entire year, such individual would lose the equivalent of 1/2 year of life. However, a person who has the flu may also be rated as 0.5. In this case, the illness might only last 3 days, and the total loss in well-years might be $3/365 \times 0.5$, which is equal to 0.004 well-years. This may not appear as significant an outcome as the disabled person. But suppose that 5,000 people in a community get the flu. The well-years lost would then be $5,000 \times .004$, which is equal to 20 years. Now suppose that a vaccination has become available and that the threat of the flu can be eliminated by vaccinating the 25,000 people in the community. The cost of the vaccine is \$5 per person or \$125,000.

The cost/utility of the program would be:

$$\frac{\$125{,}000 \text{ (cost)}}{20 \text{ years (utility)}} = \$6{,}250/\text{well-year}$$

Table 1.1 summarizes the cost/utility for several programs that have been analyzed with the system.

TABLE 1.1
Summary of Cost/Well-Year Estimates for Selected Medical, Surgical, and Preventive Interventions[a]

Program	*Reference*	*Cost/ Well-Year*
Seat belt laws	Kaplan (1988)	0
Ante-partum and anti-D injection[b]	Torrance & Zipursky (1984)	1,543
Pneumonococcal vaccine for the elderly	OTA (1979)	1,765
Post-partum and anti-D injection[b]	Torrance & Zipursky (1977)	2,109
Coronary artery bypass surgery for left main coronary	Weinstein & Stason (1982)	4,922
Neonatal intensive care, 1,000–14,999 g	Boyle et al. (1983)	5,473
Smoking cessation counseling	Schulman et al. (1991)	6,463
T4 (thyroid) screening	Epstein et al. (1981)	7,595
PKU screening[c]	Bush et al. (1973)	8,498
Treatment of severe hypertension (diastolic > 105 mm Hg) in males age 40	Weinstein & Stason (1976)	10,896
Oral gold in rheumatoid arthritis	Thompson et al. (1987)	12,059
Dapsone for prophylaxis for PCP pneumonia[d]	Freedberg (1991)	13,400
Treatment of mild hypertension (diastolic 95–104 mm Hg) in males age 40	Weinstein & Stason (1976)	22,197
Oat bran for high cholesterol	Kinosian et al. (1988)	22,910
Rehabilitation in COPD[e]	Toevs et al. (1984)	28,320
Estrogen therapy for postmenopausal symptoms in women without a prior hysterectomy	Weinstein (1980)	32,057
Neonatal intensive care, 500–999 g	Boyle et al. (1983)	38,531
CABG (surgery) 2-vessel disease[f]	Weinstein & Stason (1982)	39,770
Hospital hemodialysis	Churchill et al. (1984)	40,200
Coronary artery bypass surgery for single-vessel disease with moderately severe occlusion	Weinstein & Stason (1982)	42,195
School tuberculin testing program	Bush et al. (1972)	43,250
Continuous ambulatory peritoneal dialysis	Churchill et al. (1984)	54,460
Cholestipol for high cholesterol	Kinosian et al. (1988)	92,467
Cholestyramine for high cholesterol	Kinosian et al. (1988)	153,105
Screening mammography	Eddy (1990)	167,850
Total hip replacement	Liang et al. (1986)	293,029
CABG (surgery) 1-vessel heart disease[f]	Weinstein & Stason (1982)	662,835
Aerosolized pentamidine for prophylaxis of PCP pneumonia[d]	Freedberg (1991)	756,000

Note. From Kaplan (1993). By permission of author.
[a]All estimates adjusted to 1991 U.S. dollars; [b]treatment for Rh immunization; [c]PKU, phenylketonuria; [d]PCP, pneumocystic carinii pneumonia; [e]COPD, chronic obstructive pulmonary disease; [f]CABG, coronary artery bypass graft.

How This Model Differs From Traditional Conceptualizations

The two major differences between the GHPM and other approaches to quality of life measurement are: (a) the attempt to express benefits and consequences of health in a common unit known as the well-year or QALY, and (b) emphasis on area under the curve rather than point-in-time measurement. A basic objective for most people is to function without symptoms as long as possible. Clearly, early death contradicts this objective. Illness and disability during the interval between birth and death also reduces the total potential health status during a lifetime. Many approaches to quality of life assessment consider only current functioning. We refer to these snapshots of life quality as *point-in-time measures*. The GHPM considers outcome throughout the life cycle. This is what we characterize as the *area under the curve*. The more wellness a person experiences throughout the life span, the greater is the area under the curve. Success of interventions is marked by expanded area.

The general nature of the model leads to some different conclusions than more traditional medical approaches. For example, the traditional medical model focuses on specific diseases and on pathophysiology. Characteristics of illness are quantified according to blood chemistry or in relation to problems in a specific organ system. Often, focus on disease specific outcome measures leads to different conclusions than those evaluated using a more general outcome measure. For example, studies on the reduction of blood cholesterol have demonstrated reductions in deaths due to coronary heart disease. However, the same studies have failed to demonstrate reductions in total deaths from all causes combined (Lipid Research Clinics, 1984). Most studies in which patients are assigned to cholesterol lowering through diet or medication or to a control group have revealed that reductions in cardiovascular mortality for those in the cholesterol lowering group are compensated for by increases in mortality from other causes (Kaplan, 1984, 1985). A meta-analysis of these studies has demonstrated that the average statistical difference for increase in deaths from nonillness causes (i.e., accidents, murders, etc.) is larger than the average statistical difference for reduction in cardiovascular deaths (Muldoon, Manuck, & Matthews, 1990).

Similar results have been reported for reductions in cardiovascular deaths attributable to taking aspirin. The disease-specific approach focuses on deaths due to MI because there is a biological model to describe why aspirin use should reduce heart attacks. Yet, in a controlled experiment in which subjects were randomly assigned to take aspirin or placebo, there was no difference in total deaths between the two groups (Muldoon et al., 1990). Aspirin may reduce the chances of dying from an MI, but it does not reduce the chance of dying (Steering Committee of the Physicians' Health Study Research Group, 1988, 1989). The traditional, diagnosis-specific, medical model argues that there is a benefit of aspirin because it reduces heart attack, but the GHPM argues that there is no benefit of aspirin because there is no change in the chances of dying from all causes (Kaplan, 1989).

This same line of reasoning applies to many other areas of health care. Many treatments produce benefits for a specific outcome, but induce side effects that are often neglected in the analysis. Estimates of the benefits of surgery must take into consideration the fact that surgery causes dysfunction through wounds that must heal prior to any realization of the treatment benefits. Furthermore, surgeries often create complications. The general approach to quality of life assessment attempts to gain a global picture of the net treatment benefits, taking into consideration both treatment benefits, side effects, and estimates of their relative importance. One application of the GHPM is in resource allocation. Quality of life measures and QALYs can be used to quantify the benefits of treatments. Combining this information with cost allows the construction of cost-effectiveness ratios. These ratios can be used to prioritize expenditures so that limited resources can be directed to gain benefit for the largest number of people. Several years ago Oregon proposed to apply these ideas to address some of the health policy problems they faced.

THE OREGON EXPERIMENT

In 1987 a young boy in Oregon developed acute leukemia, and his physicians decided that he needed a bone marrow transplant. At that time, the Oregon Medicaid program did not reimburse for transplants. The state legislature recognized that 34 transplants to Medicaid patients during the period of 1987 to 1989 used the same financial resources as prenatal care and delivery to 1,500 pregnant women. The legislature decided that they would use their limited resources to provide a small benefit to the large number of pregnant women instead of providing a larger benefit to a small number of beneficiaries. The family of the young leukemia sufferer protested this policy, but the boy died while the case was under appeal. After the case attracted substantial media attention, Oregon began to systematically explore alternative approaches to resource allocation.

The dilemma in Oregon is similar to the problem in essentially all other U.S. states. The costs of health care are expanding much more rapidly then are the budgets for Medicaid. The only alternative is to change eligibility criteria and remove some individuals from the Medicaid roles. Oregon also recognized that U.S. health care was not a two-tiered system, but rather a three-tiered system. The three-tiered system included people who had regular insurance and could pay for their care, people enrolled in Medicaid, and a growing third tier of people who had no health insurance at all. By 1993 this third tier represented about one fifth of the population of the state. In Oregon, that accounts for about 450,000 citizens. In addition, another 230,000 were underinsured. The trend indicated the number of uninsured and underinsured was steadily increasing. Collectively, Oregon citizens spent approximately $6 billion on health care in 1989, which is about three times what they spent in state income taxes.

Led by a grassroots citizens group known as Oregon Health Decisions, it was argued that Oregon (and most other states) were rationing health care. The problem was that rationing was implicit and not open to public scrutiny. Because of funding shortages, people were being rationed rather than services. In other words, many individuals in need of care received none because they were in the wrong category. A young woman employed as an hourly worker, for example, may be ineligible for health care, whereas an unemployed person on Medicaid would become eligible if she became pregnant. Thus, the system created incentives to become pregnant in order to have a regular source of health care. The system allowed health care under Medicaid for poor families with young children but disallowed coverage for poor families with older children. Oregon, like many other states, defined Medicaid eligibility for the Aid for Families with Dependent Children (AFDC) as 50% of the poverty line. That policy set the criterion income at about $5,700 per year for a family of three. A hard-working independent carpenter earning $11,000 might be completely excluded by the system even though he was at high risk for injury.

These arguments caught the attention of John Kitzhaber, the Physician President of the State Senate. Under Kitzhaber's leadership, Oregon passed three pieces of legislation to attack this problem. Here, I focus most specifically on Senate Bill 27. This bill created a health services commission to oversee the prioritization of health services. The commission mandated that health services be prioritized using something similar to the GHPM. The justification for the prioritization was to eliminate services that did not provide benefit. The process of creating the prioritized list was an extremely difficult one. The commission began by creating a prioritized list of all health services. However, it soon became apparent that this was a nearly impossible task. Thus, the commissioners began searching for a combination of conditions and treatments that could be lumped together. They referred to these as condition–treatment pairs. Examples of these condition–treatment pairs are shown in Table 1.2. For example, the problem of rectal prolapse is paired with the treatment partial colectomy, and osteoporosis is paired with medical treatment.

The commission obtained several sources of information. First, they held public hearings to learn about preferences for medical care in the Oregon

TABLE 1.2
Examples of Condition-Treatment Pairs

Condition	*Treatment*
Rectal prolapse	Partial colectomy
Osteoporosis	Medical therapy
Ophthalmic injury	Closure
Obesity	Nutritional and lifestyle counseling

communities. These meetings helped clarify how citizens viewed medical services. Various approaches to care were rated and discussed. On the basis of 48 town meetings, which were attended by more than 1,000 people, 13 community values emerged. These values included prevention, cost effectiveness, quality of life, ability to function, length of life, and so on. The major lesson from the community meetings was that citizens wanted primary care services. Furthermore, the people consistently stated that the state should forego expensive, heroic treatments for individuals or small groups in order to offer basic services for everyone.

In order to pay for preventive services, it was necessary to reduce spending elsewhere. A major portion of the commission's activity was to evaluate services using the QWB scale from the GHPM. The commissioners could not have possibly conducted clinical trials for each of the many condition–treatment pairs. Further, estimation of treatment benefit using the QWB could not have been left to laymen. So, the commission formed a medical committee that had expertise in essentially all specialty areas and had the participation of nearly all of the major provider groups in the state. Working together, the committee estimated the expected quality of life benefit from 709 condition–treatment pairs. The QWB also requires preference weights. These weights are not medical expert judgments, but should be obtained from community peers. The Oregon citizens were particularly concerned about using weights from California in order to assign priorities in their state. Thus, 1,001 Oregon citizens participated in a separate weighting experiment. The weights were obtained in a telephone survey that was conducted by Oregon State University.

In 1990, the commission released a draft of its first prioritized list. Unfortunately, many of the rankings seemed counterintuitive, and the approach drew serious criticism in the popular press. As a result, the system was reorganized according to three basic categories of care: essential, very important, and valuable to certain individuals. Within these major groupings there were 17 subcategories. The commission decided to place greatest emphasis on problems that were acute and fatal. In these cases treatment prevents death, and there is full recovery. Examples include appendectomy for appendicitis, nonsurgical treatment for whooping cough, and so on.

Other categories classified as essential included maternity care, treatment for conditions that prevent death but do not allow full recovery, preventive care for children, and so on. There were nine categories classified as essential (see Table 1.3). Listed as very important were treatments for nonfatal conditions that would return the individual to a previous state of health. Also included in this category were acute nonfatal, one-time treatments that might improve quality of life. These might be hip replacements, cornea transplants, and so on. At the bottom of the list were treatments for fatal or nonfatal conditions that did not improve quality of life or extend life. These might be progressive treatments for the end stages of diseases such as cancer and AIDS or care for conditions in which the treatments were known not to be effective. In the revised approach, the commission decided to ignore cost information and to allow their own subjective judgments to influence the rankings on the list. Table 1.4 summarizes the conditions selected from the top of the list, the middle of the list, and the bottom of the list. Unfortunately, the final exercise in Oregon resulted in many deviations from the GHPM. However, the exercise demonstrates an attempt to resolve the health-care crisis on the basis of health outcome. In the next section I consider several of the ethical issues raised by the Oregon experiment.

ETHICAL ISSUES RAISED BY THE OREGON EXPERIMENT

The Oregon experiment has been a target for many legal, social, and ethical critics. A few of these concerns are briefly reviewed here.

Community Preferences Disallowed

One of the most robust findings relevant to the GHPM is that preferences do not differ greatly across social or demographic groups. This is illustrated in Fig. 1.2, which compares arthritis patients to nonpatients, Fig. 1.3, which compares men to women, and Fig. 1.4, which compares medically insured to uninsured. In each case, these groups rated the same case descriptions and the points on the graphs are mean ratings of a particular item obtained from the two groups. In all cases, there is remarkable similarity between the preferences. Even using completely different methodologies, preferences obtained from citizens in Oregon are remarkably similar to those obtained from residents of California (Fig. 1.5). These findings have been replicated in several other studies.

TABLE 1.3
Every Person Is Entitled to Services Necessary for a Diagnosis

Category	*Services*
	Essential
Acute fatal	Treatment prevents death and allows full recovery: appendectomy for appendicitis; nonsurgical treatment for whooping cough; repair of deep, open wound in neck, nonsurgical treatment for infection of the heart muscle (myocarditis)
Maternity care	Includes most newborn disorders: obstetrical care for pregnancy; care of the newborn
Acute fatal	Treatment prevents death but does not allow full recovery: nonsurgical treatment for stroke; all treatment for burns; treatment for severe head injuries
Preventive child care	Includes immunizations and well-child exams
Chronic fatal	Treatment improves life span and quality of life: nonsurgical treatment for insulin-dependent diabetes medical and surgical treatment for treatable cancer of the uterus; medical treatment for asthma; HIV drug therapy
Reproductive services	Excludes maternity and infertility services; birth control and sterilization
Comfort care	Includes pain management and hospice care for the end stages of diseases such as cancer and AIDS
Preventive dental care	Includes exams; cleaning and fluoride treatments
Proven effective adult preventive care	Includes mammograms; blood pressure screening; Pap smears
	Very Important
Acute nonfatal	Treatment causes return to previous health: nonsurgical treatment for acute thyroiditis; medical treatment for vaginitis; fillings for cavities
Chronic nonfatal	One-time treatment improves quality of life: hip replacement; corneal transplants for cataracts; rheumatic fever
Acute nonfatal	Includes treatment without return to previous health: relocation of dislocated elbow, repair of cut to cornea
Chronic nonfatal	Repetitive treatment improves quality of life: nonsurgical treatment for rheumatoid arthritis; gout; migraine headaches
	Valuable to Certain Individuals
Acute Nonfatal	Treatment speeds recovery: medical treatment for viral sore throat; diaper rash
Infertility services	Includes medical treatment for infertility; in-vitro fertilization; artificial insemination
Less effective adult preventive care	Includes routine screening for those people not otherwise at risk, such as diabetes screening if the person is under 40 years old and not pregnant
Fatal or nonfatal	Treatment causes minimal or no improvement in quality of life: aggressive treatment for end stages of diseases such as cancer and AIDS; medical treatment for nongenital warts

Each health service on the list is presumed to include necessary ancillary services such as hospital care, prescription drugs, and medical equipment and supplies necessary for successful treatment

Note. From Oregon Health Services Commission, in the public domain.

TABLE 1.4
Examples of Condition—Treatment Pairs From Top, Middle, and Bottom of List

Top 10	
1.	Medical treatment for bacterial pneumonia
2.	Medical treatment of tuberculosis
3.	Medical or surgical treatment for peritonitis
4.	Removal for foreign body from pharynx, larynx, trachea bronchus and esophagus
5.	Appendectomy
6.	Repair of ruptured intestine
7.	Repair of hernia with obstruction and/or gangrene
8.	Medical therapy for croup syndrome
9.	Medical therapy for acute orbital cellulitis
10.	Surgery for ectopic pregnancy
Middle 10	
350.	Repair of open wounds
351.	Drainage and medical therapy for abscessed cysts of Bartholin's gland
352.	Medical therapy for polynodal cyst with abscess
353.	Medical therapy for acute thyroiditis
354.	Medical therapy for acute otitis media
355.	PE Tubes or T & A for chronic otitis media
356	Surgical treatment for cholesteatoma
357.	Medical therapy for sinusitis
358.	Medical therapy for acute conjunctivitis
359.	Medical therapy for spina bifida without hydrocephalus
Bottom 10	
700.	Mastopexy for gynecomastia
701.	Medical and surgical therapy for cyst of the kidney
702.	Medical therapy for end stage HIV disease (comfort care excluded—it is high on list)
703.	Surgery for chronic pancreatitis
704	Medical therapy for superficial wounds without infection
705.	Medical therapy for constitutional aplastic anemia
706.	Surgical treatment for prolapsed urethral mucosa
707.	Paracentesis of aqueous for central retinal artery occlusion
708.	Life support for extremely low birth weight (< 500 gm) and under-23-week gestation
709.	Life support for anencephalous

The Rule of Rescue

Hadorn (1991) expressed serious concerns about the original Oregon priority list. As an emergency room physician, Hadorn was also concerned because many technologies improve quality of life but do not rescue people from imminent death. The rule of rescue argues that there is a moral obligation to invest in rescue whenever saving a life is a possibility. Lifesaving procedures should always rank above those that can be delayed.

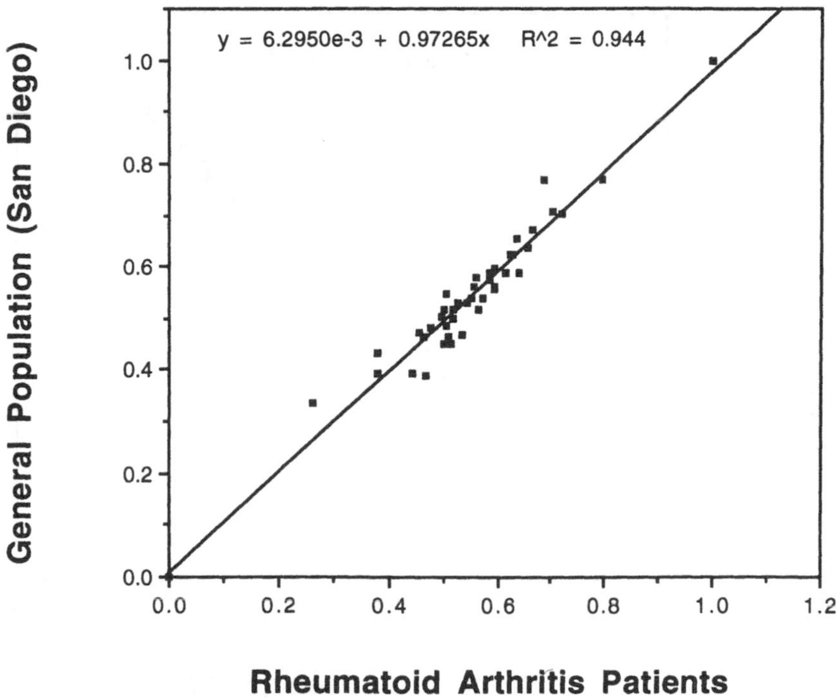

FIG. 1.2. Comparison of preference weights for arthritis patients and citizens for the San Diego community (adapted from Balaban et al., 1986).

In other words, we should not spend money on prevention if it detracts from the opportunity to rescue, even if the rescue effort is highly likely to fail.

According to the rule of rescue, the rankings provided by the Oregon Health Services Commission did not make intuitive sense. However, a review of Hadorn's statement suggests that there were problems with his analysis. For example, Hadorn reviewed the original version of the list and pointed out that tooth capping produced the same expected benefit as surgery for ectopic pregnancy. However, surgery for ectopic pregnancy saves lives in almost all cases. The reason that these two results were similar was that tooth capping provides a small benefit at a small cost, whereas surgery for ectopic pregnancy provides a big benefit at a big cost. The cost–utility ratio appears to be the same.

There were several problems with Hadorn's analysis. In particular, the cost of tooth capping was probably underestimated. He used a cost of $38, when the market price was over $500. Furthermore, Hadorn overestimated the benefit of treatment for tooth capping by assuming that without treatment people would be in continuing dental pain and that this pain

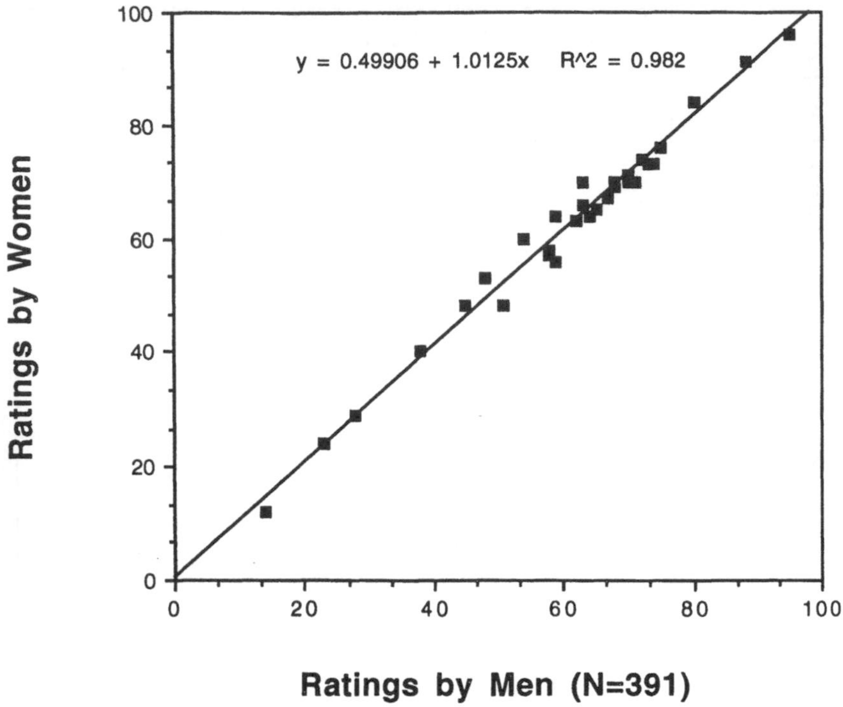

FIG. 1.3. Comparison of preference ratings for case descriptions by men and women in Oregon.

would be eliminated by the procedure. The problem that Hadorn identified was that there was a substantial number of errors in the early construction of the list. The list that Hadorn referred to was quickly and appropriately abandoned by the commissioners. The Oregon law does allow continual revisions of the list when new data become available. Through successive review and critiques, the list will be improved.

The Program Discriminates Against Children

A consumer group known as The Children's Defense Fund (CDF) attacked the Oregon program, asserting that it discriminated against children. In Oregon, poor women and children make up about 75% of Medicaid recipients. Furthermore, the blind and the disabled were excluded from the initial version of the proposal. Critics charge that the proposal was a way of denying health care to those who needed it most. Although these arguments are compelling, it is also important to consider the benefits the program provides for poor women and children. Currently, thousands of women and

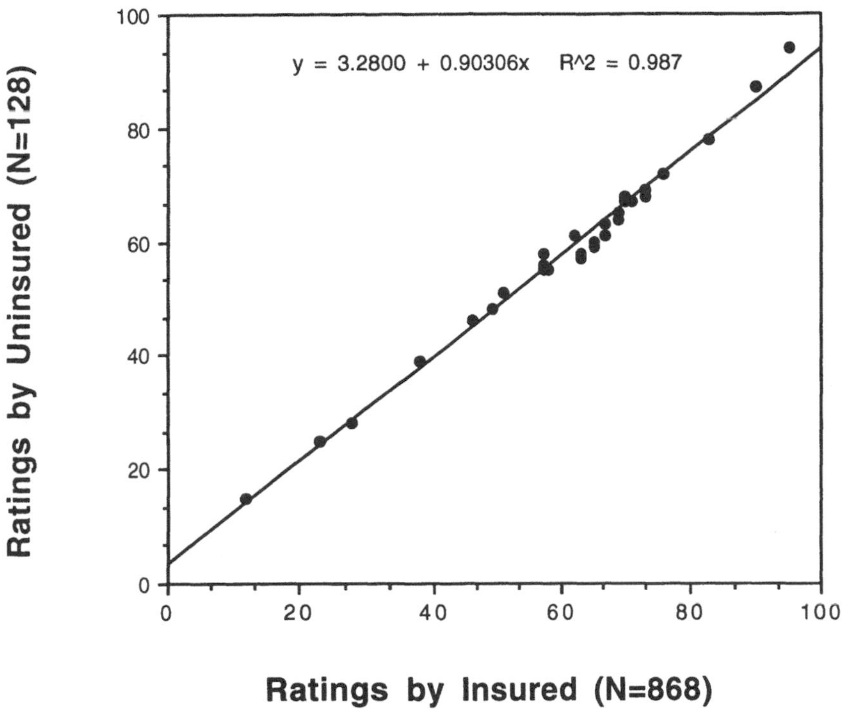

FIG. 1.4. Comparison of preference ratings for case descriptions by insured and uninsured citizens in Oregon.

children have no health-care coverage at all. The Oregon plan will make funding available to an estimated 60,000 children and women who now receive no care. The GHPM in no way discriminates against children. Usually services for children are well evaluated because they have the potential to produce many years of benefit. In fact, critics have suggested that the model is biased in favor of children. For example, prevention of a birth defect may produce large numbers of well-years over the course of the life span. Lasting treatment effects are counted over and over again as the person ages.

Legal Challenges

The CDF vowed to launch several legal challenges against the Oregon proposal. The CDF advocates programs for children through legal and political action. The major advocates are attorneys who express deep concerns about one essential component of the proposal. In order to have a prioritized list, is necessary to offer malpractice immunity for physicians

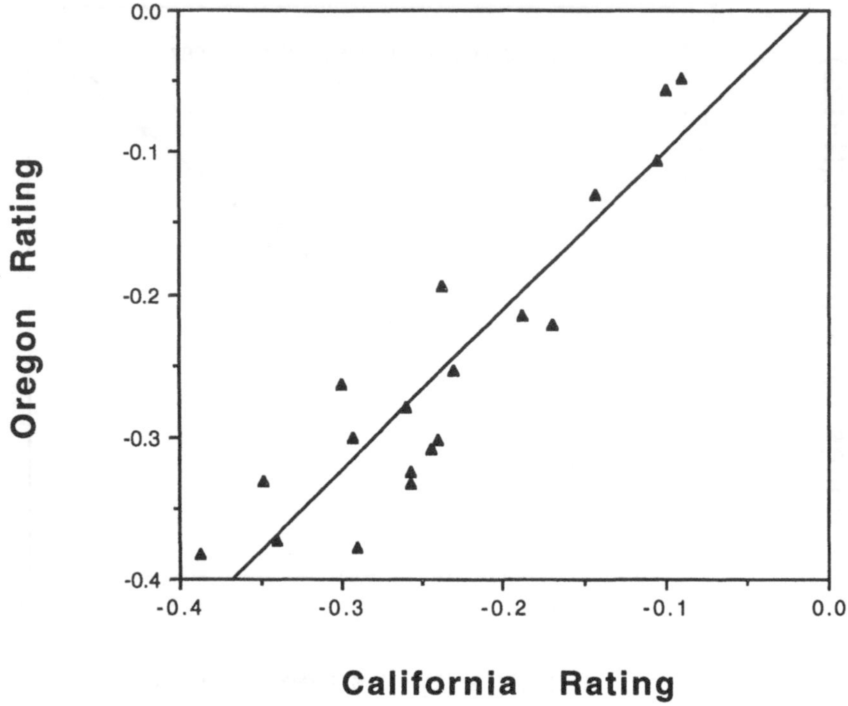

FIG. 1.5. Comparison of preferences obtained in 1975 from citizens in California with those obtained from Oregon citizens in 1990. Three outlier points are not shown.

who deny some low-priority services to patients. The CDF felt this was not acceptable.

In order to stop the experiment, the CDF argued that the Oregon plan creates a form of social experimentation in which women and children are forced to participate without consent. Furthermore, they suggested that the program was unconstitutional because it discriminated on the basis of race and gender. The U.S. Congress Office of Technology Assessment (OTA) retained legal counsel to evaluate these challenges. Although it is always difficult to predict with certainty how the court will receive particular challenges, the independent counsel suggested that the program did not violate equal protection clauses of the U.S. Constitution, nor did it require the approval of a human subjects committee. Perhaps the most peculiar aspect of the CDF arguments is the assertion that the program would be bad for the socially disadvantaged. The Oregon Medicaid program now denies access to substantial numbers of women and children. These people are unable to get any medical services. Many women who are not pregnant and who do not have children cannot gain access to medical care. Apparently this situation is acceptable to CDF. In order to protect the current system, they vowed to submit petitions that will interfere with any attempt to broaden coverage so that 60,000 currently uninsured women and children can receive needed medical care. The aspect of the Oregon plan that apparently was missed by CDF is that there is little evidence that the implementation of the plan will damage anyone. Indeed the funds to expand coverage or increase benefit would be captured through the elimination of services that provide little or no benefit.

FEDERAL DENIAL, REVISION, AND ACCEPTANCE OF OREGON PLAN

Although Oregon passed legislation to go forward with their experiment, their efforts required approval by the Department of Health and Human Services (DHHS). Medicaid is funded jointly by both the states and the federal government, and any alteration in standard policy requires approval by the federal government. When Oregon filed their petition for a waiver of traditional Medicaid policies, substantial public debate erupted. Although they had been promised a decision early in 1991, no formal action had been taken by the summer of 1992. Unexpectedly, DHHS rejected Oregon's application in August 1992, suggesting that the proposal violated the Americans with the Disability Act. The particular concern was that the preference survey for the quality of life dimension of the QWB "quantified stereotypic assumptions about persons with disability." The department suggested that people with disabilities would be systematically undervalued by the system.

The DHHS analysis assumed that people with disabilities would be discriminated against because treatment could not improve their chronic problems. However, this analysis is incorrect. The effectiveness of a treatment is based on the estimated course of illness with and without treatment. Treatment that makes life last longer, even without improvements in quality of life, will produce substantial benefits—for example, if a person has a chronic condition that places him or her in a state at .6 on a 0 to 1 scale and the treatment will maintain the person at this level, whereas withdrawal of the treatment will result in death. According to the QWB model, treatment will produce .6 (calculated as 0.6 - 0.0) each year the person is maintained in this state. The treatment that produces .6 years of life each year it is administered is a very powerful treatment in comparison to alternatives. Clearly, such important and powerful treatments would not be eliminated in the Oregon system. Targeted for elimination would be treatments that produce little or no benefit.

It is true that people with disabilities gain lower QWB scores than people without disabilities. Low scores suggest that resources should be used to aid these individuals. A low quality of life score is not a badge of disgrace, but rather an indication that health status is not optimal and an indication of where funds need to be targeted.

After the disappointing rejection by DHHS, Oregon revised and resubmitted their application. In November, 1992 they submitted a modified program, which changed the prioritization method to eliminate any consideration of quality of life. The new method ranked pairs of conditions and treatments in two stages. First, the treatments were subjectively ranked by effectiveness. The criteria for establishing effectiveness included preventing death, returning patients saved from death to an asymptomatic state, returning symptomatic patients to an asymptomatic state, and average cost of the procedure. Instead of using public preferences, conditions were ranked by medical experts, and the commissioners reordered the lists to be consistent with the values they perceived to be representative of Oregon citizens. By eliminating the quality of life portion of the model, Oregon answered some of the criticisms in the initial DHHS review. However, they created new problems because they eliminated the possibility of applying cost-effectiveness analysis in an objective manner. The Clinton administration has encouraged states to experiment with different approaches to Medicaid. In March 1993 the Clinton administration approved the revised plan, and it was implemented in February 1994.

WHERE DO WE GO FROM HERE?

This chapter has outlined a new paradigm for thinking about alternatives in health care. In short, it suggests that limited health-care resources be used to maximize health-related quality of life. Services that do not work should not be funded, and the savings should be used to extend basic health-care benefits to people currently uninsured. The proposed model is consistent with the thinking of several groups, including scholars in the United States (OTA, 1979; Russell, 1986; Weinstein & Stason, 1976, 1977), the United Kingdom (Drummond, Stoddard, & Torrance, 1987; Maynard, 1991; Williams, 1988), Canada (Torrance, 1986, 1987), and Australia (Richardson, 1991). Although the exact methodologies proposed by these different research groups vary slightly, the theory is nearly identical. Recently, Patrick and Erickson (1993) offered a detailed account of the methodological steps required to implement the system. Methods are now available to begin guiding policy decisions. However, our information base for the implementation of the model is still incomplete.

In addition to the financial problems in U.S. health care, there is a second crisis—the crisis of ignorance. Our understanding of the effects of contemporary health care on health outcomes is shameful. When new treatments are introduced, we typically know something about the biological theory, the mechanism of action, and the effect of treatment on some specific biological outcome. However, the effects of treatment on everyday functioning and the quality of life is rarely evaluated. When the Oregon Health Services Commission began to prioritize health services, they recognized that there was no good information to help them appraise the value of many current services. The U.S. Congress, in recognition of our ignorance about outcome, recently created the Agency for Health Care Policy and Research (AHCPR) to focus on medical outcome studies. A recent emphasis on outcomes by the FDA has stimulated the evaluation of health outcomes in the evaluation of pharmaceutical products. Furthermore, the U.S. National Heart Lung and Blood Institutes (NHLBI) now require quality of life assessment in clinical trials. Other National Institutes for Health (NIH) have also encouraged the measurement of health-related quality of life. New data are becoming available. Yet, it may be several decades before we have enough information to apply the model with great confidence. Nevertheless, many steps toward the implementation of the model can be taken even as we await new information.

CONCLUSIONS

The United States is facing a very serious crisis in health-care delivery. A GHPM can contribute to the resolution of these problems. When properly applied, the model uses the best scientific information on costs, risks, and benefits of treatment. The model is directed toward using available resources to produce the greatest benefit for the largest number of people. Ethical challenges to the model are important, but can be addressed. The greatest problem facing implementation of the model is lack of scientific data. We need considerably more research on the efficacy of clinical interventions. Until this information becomes available, we must recognize that the application of the model is an iterative process in which the best data available should be used. However, it is also important to recognize that we have limitations in our current understanding. Thus, evaluations must be continually modified as we learn more. Ultimately, policy science can contribute to the health and well-being of the population.

REFERENCES

Balaban, D. J., Sagi, P. C., Goldfarb, B. A., & Nettler, S. (1986). Weights for scoring the quality of well-being instrument among rheumatoid arthritics. *Medical Care*, *24*, 973–980.

Boyle, M. H., Torrance, G. W., Sinclair, J. C., & Horwood, S. P. (1983). Economic evaluation of neonatal intensive care of very-low-birth-weight infants. *New England Journal of Medicine, 308*(22), 1330-1337.

Brook, R. H., Kamberg, C. J., Mayer-Oakes. A., et al. (1990). Appropriateness of acute medical care for the elderly: An analysis of the literature. *Health Policy, 14*, 177-280.

Brook, R. H., & Lohr, K. (1986). Will we need to ration effective health care? *Issues in Science and Technology*, 68-77.

Brook, R. H., Park, R. E., Chassin, M. R., Kosecoff, J., Keesey, J., & Solomon, D. H. (1990). Carotid endarterectomy for elderly patients: Predicting complications. *Annals of Internal Medicine, 113*(10), 747-753.

Bush, J. W., Chen, M. M., & Patrick, D. L. (1973). Cost-effectiveness using a health status index: Analysis of the New York State PKU screening program. In R. Berg (Ed.), *Health Status Index* (pp. 172-208). Chicago: Hospital Research and Educational Trust.

Churchill, D. N., Lemon, B. C., Torrance, G. W. (1984). A cost-effectiveness analysis of continuous abulatory peritoneal dialysis and hospital hemodialysis. *Medical Decision Making*, 4(4), 489-500.

Drummond, M. F., Stoddard, G. L., & Torrance, G. W. (1987). *Methods for the economic evaluation of health care programmes.* Oxford, United Kingdom: Oxford University Press.

Eddy, D. M. (1989). Screening for breast cancer. *Annals of Internal Medicine, 111*, 389-390.

Epstein, K. A., Schneiderman, L. J., Bush, J. W., & Zettner WR (1981). The "Abnormal" screening of Thyroxine (T4): Analysis of physician response, outcome, cost and health effectiveness. *Journal of Chronic Disease, 34*, 175-190.

Freedberg, K. A., Tosteson, A. N., Cohen, C. J., Cotton, D. J. (1991). Primary prophylaxis for Pneumocystis carinii pneumonia in HIV-infected people with CD4 counts below 200/mm3: A cost-effectiveness analysis. *Journal of Acquired Immune Deficiency Syndromes, 4*(5), 521-531.

Hadorn, D. C. (1991). Setting health care priorities in Oregon: Cost-effectiveness meets the rule of rescue. *Journal of the American Medical Association, 265*, 2218-2225.

Hadorn, D. C., & Brook, R. H. (1991). The health care resource allocation debate. Refining our terms. *Journal of the American Medical Association, 266*, 3328-3331.

Jajich-Toth, C., & Roper, B. W. (1990). Americans' views on health care: A study in contradictions. *Health Affairs, 9*, 149-157.

Kaplan, R. M. (1984). The connection between clinical health promotion and health status: A critical review. *American Psychologist, 39*, 755-765.

Kaplan, R. M. (1985). Behavioral epidemiology, health promotion, and health services. *Medical Care, 23*, 564-583.

Kaplan, R. M. (1988). New health promotion indicators: The general health policy model. *Health Promotion, 3*(1) 35-49.

Kaplan, R. M. (1989). Models of health outcome for policy analysis. *Health Psychology, 8*, 723-735.

Kaplan, R. M. (1993). *The hippocratic predicament: affordability, access, and accountability in health care.* San Diego: Academic Press.

Kaplan, R. M., & Anderson, J. P. (1988a). A general health policy model: Update and applications. *Health Services Research, 23*, 203-235.

Kaplan, R. M., & Anderson, J. P. (1988b). The quality of well-being scale: Rationale for a single quality of life index. In S.R. Walker & R. Rosser (Eds.), *Quality of life assessment and applications* (pp. 51-77). London: MTP Press.

Kaplan, R. M., Bush, J . W., & Berry, C. C. (1976). Health status: Types of validity and the index of well-being. *Health Services Research, 11*, 478-507.

Kaplan, R. M., Bush, J. W., & Berry, C. C. (1978). The reliability, stability, and generalizability of a health status index. *American Statistical Association, Proceedings of the Social Status Section* , 704-709.

Kaplan, R. M., Bush, J. W., & Berry, C. C. (1979). Health status index: Category rating versus magnitude estimation for measuring levels of well-being. *Medical Care, 17,* 501–525.

Kinosian, B. P., & Eisenberg, J. M. (1988). Cutting into cholesterol. Cost-effective alternatives for treating hypercholesterolemia. *Journal of the American Medical Association, 259*(15), 2249–2254.

Kitzhaber, J. (1990). *The Oregon Basic Health Services Act.* Salem, OR: Oregon State Senate.

Liang, M. H., Cullen, K. E., Larson, M. G., et al. (1986). Cost-effectiveness of total joint arthroplasty in osteoarthritis. *Arthritis and Rheumatism,* 29, 937–943.

Lipid Research Clinics Coronary Prevention Trial Results. (1984). 1. Reduction in incidence in coronary heart disease. *Journal of the American Medical Association, 251,* 351–364.

Maynard, A. (1991). Economic issues in HIV management. In A. Maynard (Ed.), *Economic aspects of HIV management* (pp. 6–12). London: Colwood House Medical Publications.

Muldoon, M. F., Manuck, S. B., & Matthews, K. A. (1990). Lowering cholesterol concentrations and mortality: A quantitative review of primary prevention trials. *British Medical Journal, 323,* 1112–1119.

Nicod, P., Gilpin, E. A., Dittrich, H., Henning, H., Maisel, A., Blacky, A. R., Smith, S. C., Jr., Ricou, F., & Ross, J., Jr. (1991). Trends in use of coronary angiography in subacute phase of myocardial infarction. *Circulation, 84*(3), 1004–1115.

Office of Technology Assessment, United States Congress. (1979). *A review of selected federal vaccine and immunization policies: Based on case sudies of pneumococcal vaccine.* Washington, DC: U. S. Government Printing Office.

Orenstein, D. M., Nixon, P. A., Ross, E. A., & Kaplan, R. M. (1989). The quality of well-being in cystic fibrosis. *Chest, 95,* 344–347.

Orenstein, D. M., Pattishall, E. N., Ross, E. A., & Kaplan, R. M. (1990). Quality of well-being before and after antibiotic treatment of pulmonary exacerbation in cystic fibrosis. *Chest, 98,* 1081–1084.

Patrick, D. L. & Erickson, P. (1993). *Health status and health policy: Allocating resources to health care.* New York: Cambridge University Press.

Relman, A. (1989, July). Confronting the crisis in health care. *Technology Review,* 31–40.

Richardson, J. (1991). *Economic assessment in health care: Theory and practice.* Melbourne, Austrailia: Monash University, National Centre for Health Program Evaluation.

Russell, L. (1986). *Is prevention better than cure?* Washington, DC: The Brookings Institution.

Schulman, K. A., Lynn, L. A., Glick, H. A., & Eisenberg, J. M. (1991). Cost effectiveness of low-dose zidovudine therapy for asymptomatic patients with human immunodeficiency virus (HIV) infection. *Annals of Internal Medicine, 114*(9), 798–802.

Short, P. F. (1990). *National medical expenditure survey: Estimates of the uninsured population, calendar year 1987: Data summary 2.* Rockville, MD: National Center for Health Services Research and Health Care Technology Assessment.

Short, P. F., Monheit, A., & Beauregard, K. (1989). *National medical expenditure survey: A profile of uninsured Americans: Research findings 1.* Rockville, MD: National Center for Health Services Research and Health Care Technology Assessment.

Steering Committee of the Physicians' Health Study Research Group. (1988). Preliminary report: Findings from the aspirin component of the ongoing Physicians' Health Study. *New England Journal of Medicine, 318,* 262–264.

Steering Committee of the Physicians' Health Study Research Group. (1989). Final report on the aspirin component of the ongoing Physicians' Health Study. *New England Journal of Medicine, 321,* 129–135.

Thompson, M. S., Read, J. L., Hutchings, H. C., Patterson, M., & Harris, E. D., Jr. (1988). The cost-effective of Auranofin: Results of a randomized clinical trial. *Journal of Rheumatology, 15,* 35–42.

Toevs, C. D., Kaplan, R. M., & Atkins, C. J. (1984). The costs and effects of behavioral programs for chronic obstructive pulmonary disease. *Medical Care,* 22, 1088–1100.

Torrance, G. W. (1986). Measurement of health state utilities for economic appraisal: A review. *Journal of Health Economics, 5,* 1-7.

Torrance, G. W. (1987). Utility approach to measuring health-related quality of life. *Journal of Chronic Diseases, 40,* 593-600.

Torrance, G. W., & Zipursky, A. (1984). Cost-effectiveness of antepartum prevention of RH immunization. *Clinics in Perinatology,* 11(2), 267-268.

Vincenzino, J. V. (1993). Developments in medical care costs: An update. *Statistical Bulletin: Metropolitan Life,* 29-35.

Weinstein, M. C. (1980). Estrogen use in postmenopausal women—costs, risks, benefits. *New England Journal of Medicne,* 303, 308-316.

Weinstein, M. C., & Feinberg, H. V. (1980). *Clinical decision analysis.* Philadelphia: Saunders.

Weinstein, M. C., & Stason, W. B. (1976). *Hypertension: A policy perspective.* Cambridge, MA: Harvard University Press.

Weinstein, M. C., & Stason, W. B. (1977). Foundations of cost-effectiveness analysis for health and medical practice. *New England Journal of Medicine, 296,* 716-721.

Weinstein, M. C., & Stason, W. B. (1982). Cost-effectiveness of coronary artery bypass surgery. *Circulation, Suppl. 3,* 56-66.

Wennberg, J. (1990). Small area analysis and the medical care outcome problem. In L. Sechrest, E. Perrin, & J. Bunker (Eds.), *Research methodology: Strengthening causal interpretations of nonexperimental data* (USPHS/DHHS, Publication No. PHS 90-3454, pp. 177-206). Washington, DC: Agency for Health Care Policy and Research, Department of Health and Human Services.

Williams, A. (1988). The importance of quality of life in policy decisions. In S. Walker, & R. Rosser (Eds), *Quality of life: Assessment and application* (pp. 279-290). London: MTP Press.

2 Quality of Life from a Federal Regulatory Perspective

James A. Schuttinga
National Institutes of Health

Health-related quality of life (HQL) assessment, if designed and implemented correctly, provides an especially comprehensive and sensitive vehicle for communicating information on the burden of disease and the effectiveness of treatment. As a research methodology, it plays a supporting role in research and policy formulation. Although HQL assessment does not provide simple solutions to the problems plaguing the U.S. health-care system, it can contribute to the improved design and evaluation of the health-care delivery system. It can help to inform and refine the policy debate, influence priorities, and facilitate new approaches to research and regulation.

Health-related quality of life assessment measures the benefits of health research programs and the utility of specific treatments "in terms that matter most to the American people, such as the capacity to function in everyday life" (Ware, 1993, p. 53). In a workshop on HQL assessment sponsored by the National Institutes of Health (NIH; Furberg, Schuttinga, Shumaker, & Wenger, 1993), participants identified benefits of HQL assessment for clinical decision making and for research and offered guidance in the planning and implementation of HQL studies. Several specific advantages of HQL measures were cited:

- Increase comprehensiveness by bringing human values to the health-outcome equation.
- Have good predictive validity—that is, patients' perceived health status correlates well with future morbidity risk (low health status

implies use of more medical services) and future job performance (high health status implies high job performance).
- Show promise for increasing understanding of the dynamics of disease severity and quality of life.
- Provide a common denominator useful in comparing the burden of different diseases and benefits of alternative treatments.
- Provide a vehicle to address patient individuality in clinical decision making.

The focus of this chapter is on the policy aspects of HQL assessment rather than on research. However, the distinction is a bit artificial. Collectively, the individual biomedical research findings and clinical decisions do actively influence the quality of care provided, the resultant HQL, and the level of health expenditures.

To date, however, HQL assessment has not played a major role in the regulatory process despite the benefits identified by its advocates. The adoption of HQL assessment into the policy/regulatory process is undoubtedly inhibited because it is a complex research methodology that is still in its formative stage. Results are affected by how, when, where, by whom, and from whom the data are gathered. Thus, the design of the HQL assessment must be carefully integrated into the design of the larger study. Quality control of data collection and processing as well as statistical analysis of the findings are just as important for validity and interpretation of HQL results as they are for the clinical and biological outcomes.

Because of the complexity, there are many pitfalls in the design and implementation of HQL assessment that can adversely affect the reliability and interpretation of the results. Even experienced practitioners and advocates of HQL assessment may disagree on the appropriate strategy for a particular study.

The controversy surrounding the methodology and the interpretation of its results understandably inhibits senior policy officials, who are relatively unfamiliar with HQL assessment, from routinely including it as part of the policy/regulatory process. Also, because it is costly and time consuming to collect HQL data, it does not easily fit in projects with constrained budgets and short time horizons required by the political and administrative process.

The novelty and controversy surrounding HQL assessment may also engender skepticism by officials responsible for funding health research as well as those more directly concerned with the delivery and regulation of health care. This is especially true in the present climate of extremely tight research and evaluation budgets where a greater number of interesting research topics and methodologies are proposed than can be funded. With tight budgets, there is a tendency to dismiss new or unfamiliar topics and methodologies as too risky and to fund proposals that incorporate well-established research methods and address topics that are most likely to meet their stated objectives.

However, the nature of the policy process and the evolution of a number of patient care and consumer issues are converging to encourage more frequent adoption of HQL assessment in research and evaluation studies. This chapter briefly reviews those forces that increase the apparent need for HQL assessments and ease the perceived problems associated with the implementation of such studies.

THE REGULATORY PROCESS AND THE NEED FOR HQL ASSESSMENT

The first important influence is the adversarial nature of the health-care regulatory process. For this analysis, regulation includes everything that the government does to influence the production and distribution of goods and services in our economy. Although the focus here is on regulation of health care, it should be recognized that regulations specifically directed at aspects of health care (e.g., research, training and licensing personnel, funding and certification of facilities, and access of patients to health care) affect and are affected by policies directed at nonhealth aspects of the economy and the nation's welfare. As suggested by Phelps (1982), the government implements policy but it does not so much set policy as provide a forum or a vehicle for affected parties to express their interests, to combat and eventually to compromise. Health-care professional associations, provider organizations, insurance companies, advocates for victims of particular diseases, employers, and others who wish to control health-care costs compete for influence. That competition limits the power of any single person or group to set policy and eventually leads to a compromise among the groups. Each of the competing organizations is likely to discover aspects of the compromise policy that they did not intend or support.

The regulatory mechanisms or policies implemented by the government reflect that adversarial debate and compromise. Historically, the specific regulatory mechanism adopted has been a response to a perceived threat to the nation's health or to a deficiency in the health-care delivery system, combined with the perception that a solution is feasible and affordable. Apparently successful advocates may not so much assert their increasing power as simply provide voice for an idea whose time has come.

Examples of this process abound. In response to threats of infectious and communicable diseases, the federal government increased support for biomedical research and development. Early successes encouraged support for research on numerous additional diseases and afflictions. Today the federal obligations for health research exceed \$10.7 billion (NIH, 1992).

Again, when fraudulent claims and assorted quacks preyed on the public, the federal government established the Food and Drug Administration (FDA). State governments initiated numerous occupational and facility licensing laws and procedures to regulate the qualifications of providers allowed to practice medicine and provide health care.

When access to effective health care was deemed lacking the government took steps to increase the supply and distribution of services and to increase affordability of care. For some patients the government provides health care directly as through the military health-care system and the public health service. More often, however, the federal government has subsidized the construction of facilities and the training of health-care personnel. Income transfer programs increase the purchasing power of individuals and organizations to facilitate the purchase of health care as well as other goods and services. Access to health care is also improved by reducing the out-of-pocket costs of care through the provision of public health insurance—Medicare and Medicaid—and through tax subsidies for private health insurance premiums.

The adversarial nature of the policy process and the responsiveness to new threats and opportunities continue today and will influence the rate of adoption of HQL assessment. HQL will be used by an advocacy or interest group when it is found useful to document the adverse impact of a particular disease, the benefits of a new drug or device, or the benefits or costs of a proposed policy or program.

Currently, the major health policy debate centers on the dilemma of controlling the growth of health-care costs and at the same time increasing access. Per capita health expenditures were up from \$204 in 1965 to an estimated \$3,057 in 1992. As a share of gross domestic product (GDP), national health-care expenditures rose from 5.9% in 1965 to 13.4% in 1992. They are projected to reach 16.4% of GDP in the year 2000 (Sonnefeld, Wald, Lemieux, & McKusick, 1991).

Despite the federal provision and subsidy of insurance, it is estimated that 37 million people do not have health insurance (Foley, 1992) and, therefore, do not have access to the best health care. But the high cost of health insurance inhibits the expansion of public and private coverage. Many private companies are eliminating or reducing insurance for their employees as well.

Today's high costs are partly the result of previous federal interventions. The successful eradication or control of infectious and communicable diseases as well as other improvements in effectiveness and access to care have resulted in an aging population with more chronic conditions to manage. More recently, research and development achievements have contributed to the development of expensive technology for the diagnosis and management of these chronic conditions. The increased efficacy and safety of health care and the spread of public and private health insurance have increased the demand for health care. Availability of health insurance, which reduces or eliminates the share of costs paid by the patient at point of service, encourages the adoption and use of high-cost technologies that are not affordable for uninsured patients.

Because of rising health-care costs, cost containment has been a major issue for several years. Yet both federal and private industry constraints have not notably slowed the growth of total health-care expenditures. The perception is growing that the health cost and access problems are finally becoming so great that the operation of the health-care delivery system must be changed.

Despite high costs, the United States scores lower on such health status measures as life expectancy and infant mortality than do most other developed countries. Several studies have also documented the substantial difference in health status by ethnic group and the variation in patterns of care and cost per procedure by geographical area, gender, and race. The two- to threefold differences in hospital admission rates and rates of major surgical procedures cannot be satisfactorily explained by obvious differences in patient needs or in patient outcomes.

Thus, there is already concern with the quality and equity of health-care delivery. The threat to maintaining quality of care will increase with efforts to cut costs. Patient advocates and provider groups have begun to question whether the cost controls simply inhibit access and lower quality of care. New proposals to control costs will induce conflict because appropriate and inappropriate care is difficult to distinguish as the standards for judging are often subjective and differ with the setting and the characteristics of the patient.

Proposals for reform, whether they emphasize detailed regulations or embrace managed competition, must grapple with what should be included in a basic health plan and with how to define appropriate care and eliminate inappropriate care. Just how this will be done remains moot, but it will undoubtedly include establishment of practice guidelines based on available data as interpreted by experts. Development of such guidelines would clearly benefit from systematic information on medical outcomes that include HQL dimensions. Where HQL data are lacking, the initial guidelines will be based on less complete measures of outcomes and measures of process. Over time, the pressure (from dissatisfied patients and providers) will grow to include HQL assessment in studies to re-evaluate guidelines and benefit packages for insurance plans.

The success at eradicating many acute and life-threatening illnesses has resulted in a higher share of the health dollar being expended on the management of chronic conditions. Judgments regarding cost effectiveness of treatment for chronic conditions now require multidimensional, multilevel measures of HQL. The impact of chronic conditions and progress in treatment cannot be adequately captured by such traditional measures as mortality rates, incidence and prevalence, or measures of morbidity such as bed days or hospital days. Chronic conditions affect more than one dimension of health—functioning and pain, for example. These chronic conditions are not usually cured, nor are they totally debilitating. Rather, successful management means that health is partially restored or progressive debilitation is inhibited. Also, treatments for cancer, hypertension, and other chronic, non-life-threatening conditions frequently involve adverse side effects. Control of these side effects is an important component of the treatment, as the side effects may affect compliance, successful management of the principal condition, and the cost of treatment.

FEDERAL EXPERIENCE WITH HQL ASSESSMENT

This discussion has focused on forces encouraging the adoption of HQL assessment. Fortunately, HQL assessment has already been incorporated in a number of federally sponsored studies. The past experiences have encouraged adoption of HQL assessment because they have demonstrated the feasibility and benefits of including HQL assessment in scientific investigations and in evaluations. Also, many of the studies have contributed to improvements in HQL assessment methodology. To date there is no central or agency policy encouraging the use of HQL assessment for health policy analysis, nor are there any universally adopted standards for designing and evaluating research protocols for HQL on federal studies.

The National Center for Health Services Research (NCHSR), now the Agency for Health Care Policy and Research (AHCPR), has sponsored studies since the 1960s that include methodological work and evaluations of health-care programs that have incorporated HQL assessment. The initial studies were investigator initiated. They received support from midlevel program staff at NCHSR, but not from senior agency officials. That has been the pattern of support in other agencies as well.

The Health Insurance Experiment included HQL assessment as a major part of its research protocol. The experiment was initiated in the early 1970s by midlevel program managers in the now-defunct Office of Economic Opportunity in cooperation with the eventual research investigators. When the Office of Economic Opportunity closed, administration of the experiment was moved to the Office of the Assistant Secretary for Planning and Evaluation, U.S. Department of Health and Human Services. The experiment was designed to assess the effect of different insurance policies on the costs and quality of health care received and on changes in the health status of the participants. The findings from the study remain applicable to the present policy debate. A few of the many findings are summarized here. An insurance policy that requires the patient to pay a substantial deductible amount out of pocket, before receiving any insurance benefits, reduces expenditures 31% relative to an insurance policy that requires no payment by the patient (Manning et al., 1988). Furthermore, the analysis of health status indicated that the extra expenditures on the no-charge health insurance plan did not improve the health status of the person with the mean characteristics in the sample. However, "For poor adults (the lowest 20 percent of the income distribution) who began the experiment with high blood pressure (specifically, who were in the upper 20 percent of the diastolic blood pressure distribution) there was a clinically significant reduction in blood pressure in the free fee-for-service plan compared to the plans with cost sharing" (Manning et al., 1988, p. 265).

A recent, limited survey of the NIH invited each institute to provide information on no more than six of their clinical trials or epidemiology studies that included HQL assessment. Eleven institutes provided 52 responses, and collateral data indicated that HQL measures were included in numerous other studies. The Office of the Director, NIH sponsored a workshop on the subject in 1990, and at least five other workshops have been sponsored by individual institutes. Clinical research proposals to certain divisions within the NIH are now routinely required to consider whether HQL endpoints are appropriate for the proposed study. Again, however, there is no central guidance or standards available regarding the decision to include HQL assessment on sponsored studies or on study design and selection of instruments when it is included.

Health-related quality of life assessment may have received a major boost with the establishment of the Agency for Health Care Research and Policy (Raskin & Maklan, 1991). The thrust of the new program is to identify effective and appropriate health-care practices and to develop practice guidelines. Appropriations for the Patient Outcome Research Program were zero in fiscal year (FY) 1987; $1.9 million in FY 1988; $5.9 million in FY 1989; $37.5 million in FY 1990; and $62.7 million in FY 1991 (Reyes, 1991). The total obligations for 5 to 6 years will be around $600 million. The program is a response to the pressures, discussed previously, to control the costs of Medicare and still maintain access to quality care.

Two types of outcome measures are of interest for the research. The first are the traditional or so-called objective consequences of treatment such as morbidity, mortality, complications, and readmissions. The second group of outcomes are "measured in terms of patients' individual expectations, values, and preferences. This includes satisfaction with care and self-assessments of functional capacity, health status, and quality of life" (Raskin & Maklan, 1991, p. 162).

The AHCPR sponsors the Patient Outcomes Research Teams (PORTs), described as the showcase investments of the Medical Treatment Effectiveness Program (MEDTEP), and more generously funded than traditional health services research grants at up to $1 million per year. The PORTs follow an economical research protocol. They begin with activities that provide answers in the shortest period of time and at lowest cost. They begin with a literature review and synthesis. The next step is analysis of variations in practice and patient outcomes using secondary data. This data could come from a number of sources, but the prototype study would use Medicare claims data from administrative files, possibly merged with clinical data abstracted from clinical records. That analysis naturally focuses on the easier to obtain objective measures of output. The third phase involves primary data collection including HQL assessment. The question of how much time and money will be invested in formal HQL assessments remains open. It is significant that, up to the present time, plans for HQL assessment are investigator initiated with no central push for standardization from senior agency officials, and again, the traditional measures of morbidity and mortality remain dominant.

The Health Care Financing Administration (HCFA), which administers the Medicare and Medicaid programs, is a major sponsor of policy research and evaluation studies, and the administrative and reimbursement records generated on its programs are an important source of data for research on health outcomes (Roper, Winkenwerder, Hackbarth, & Krakauer, 1988). The HCFA is exerting considerable effort to improve the accuracy, ease of use, and accessibility of its administrative claims data files and clinical data sets derived to support peer review activities. In one sense, however, those improvements undermine the use of HQL assessment to the extent that they compete for funding and for influence rather than complement HQL measures as they should.

Potentially one of the most exciting developments is the Medicare Beneficiary Health Registry. If implemented, the Registry will include a sample of approximately 2% of new Medicare enrollees each year (about 40,000 people). They will be resurveyed in 5 years and then at decreasing intervals down to every 2 years. Longitudinal data will include risk factors, functional status, sociodemographic variables, medical history, and quality of life. The data will be collected through self-administered questionnaires supplemented by telephone interviews and personal interviews.

The HCFA and the AHCPR are collaborating to conduct four Post-Hospitalization Outcomes Studies (PHOS). Data on functional and health status following hospitalization will be obtained from telephone interviews.

Other data will be extracted from medical records and from Medicare claims data. The studies are intended to identify types and rates of positive outcomes and complications, to investigate the impact of hospitalization and procedures on the progression of illness and on the maintenance of functional status, and to develop indicators of patients who are at high risk for complications following hospitalization. Four conditions were selected: cholecystectomy, pneumonia, total hip replacement, and colon surgery for cancer.

The Health Care Financing Administration is also conducting nursing home reimbursement demonstrations. Considerable data is being collected on variations in costliness or resource use of nursing home residents, on the quality of care provided, and on such HQL measures as functioning and psychological well-being of residents. These studies were mandated by Congress as a result of revelations by the American Nurses Association of inadequate quality of long-term care and lobbying by that organization for remedial action.

The Health Care Financing Administration also sponsors research on capitated reimbursement, which investigates the use of HQL measures to adjust capitated reimbursement of health maintenance organizations for variations in expected risk (use of health care) of enrollees. Managed care, which includes capitated reimbursement for health plans, is an important part of both regulatory and competitive market health-care reform proposals. One of the problems is the appropriate rate of capitated reimbursement. If potential subscribers to a health plan have obviously different risks or needs for care, there is potential for cream-skimming or adverse risk selection.

INFLUENCE OF HQL ON FEDERAL REGULATION

In the most limited sense, the incorporation of comprehensive, sensitive measures of health in research and evaluation should refine the discussion of the issues and raise the level of debate. However, use of HQL assessment could change the results and the nature of the health-care regulatory process in a more fundamental way.

Health-related quality of life assessment can change perceptions of the relative burden of different diseases, and ultimately, priorities for research and treatment. Documenting the impact on functioning, mental health, health perceptions, and pain tends to emphasize the burden of chronic conditions and emotional disorders that today do not register as important as life-threatening diseases on clinical measures or on such traditional measures of burden as mortality, incidence and prevalence of disease, or sick days. Quantification of HQL provides advocates and analysts a way to make explicit comparisons that are impossible to make with nonquantitative descriptions.

Use of HQL assessment in clinical trials and surveys could help improve clinical practice and inform policymakers who are debating what services to include in insurance benefit plans. Furthermore, quantification of the various dimensions of HQL can provide data to confirm the two-way interaction of HQL factors and the biomedical mechanisms involved in the original illness or the continuing chronic condition. That is, HQL is not simply the result of biomedical treatment, but also plays a reverse role and may modulate or continue to influence the basic biomedical mechanisms. Such HQL data could also be used to document and communicate the benefits of biomedical and behavioral research during the annual budgeting process. It could ultimately influence the level and mix of the health research budget.

Health-related quality of life assessment could contribute to the development of regulations and reimbursement incentives to encourage cost-effective health care. It could move a step closer to evaluation and reimbursement of health care on the basis of the patients' health outcomes rather than on process (adherence to practice guidelines) or credentials (degrees, licenses and board certification of personnel, and licenses and certification of facilities). It could also help to develop better standards and guidelines for clinical practice. Traditionally, structural or process measures have been used as indicators of quality of care. For example, occupational licensure, licensing or accreditation of facilities, practice guidelines, and peer review are frequently used as vehicles to assure and to monitor quality of care. The assumed link between credentials and process on one hand and outcomes on the other could be confirmed and strengthened with the use of HQL analysis.

In private markets, consumers' preferences are communicated through the prices they are willing to pay for goods and services. Competition between suppliers assures that consumers get the best value for their money when markets are working efficiently. Attempts to design government health-care policies for the benefit of the general public must proceed without direct knowledge of consumer preferences and willingness to pay as revealed in the markets for private commodities and services. In the absence of market information, advisory committees, task forces, or peer review groups are used to provide information and expert advice. The problem is studied and more research is proposed. Information on citizen preferences is often sought, but the information is filtered in an uncertain manner and may not reflect the citizens' needs. The opinions of representatives of special-interest groups are heard more frequently than are the results of a systematic survey of "informed" citizen preferences.

Health-related quality of life assessment provides a way to empower the patient or layman because it describes the impact of disease and treatment in terms that are understandable and important to them. It provides a way for them to communicate their perceptions and needs to the policy process and a way to perceive the implications of policy decisions. It facilitates systematic surveys of the multiple dimensions of the burdens of diseases and provides a vehicle to elicit consumer preferences or rankings of different health states.

CONCLUSION

To summarize, HQL assessment could contribute to both the formulation and the evaluation of federal health policy. The adversarial nature of the regulatory process and the progress or evolution of health-care delivery contribute to an increasing need for HQL assessment. A number of federally funded studies that incorporated HQL measures demonstrate the feasibility and benefits of more comprehensive assessments of treatment and health-care outcomes.

The HQL measures will likely increase, but the time, resources, and skill required for success will tend to inhibit adoption. The decision to include HQL assessment will be made on a study-by-study basis after consideration of the benefits of the extra information versus the extra time and resources required.

Advocates of HQL assessment might accelerate the adoption process by repeatedly documenting and communicating the benefits and by easing the burden of federal program staff and investigators who decide whether to include HQL measures. A bewildering array of assessment instruments and methods confront the novice who considers incorporating an HQL assessment into a research protocol. Standards for evaluation, validation, and selection of instruments developed by a coalition of HQL assessment experts could ease the burden. Easier identification of professionals with expertise could also help. The use of HQL measures has usually been initiated by investigators rather than by federal program administrators. Implementation of HQL assessment will probably continue to be primarily investigator initiated in the near future. Advocates and experts, therefore, should form coalitions with or offer services to research teams that are proposing or have been awarded a study. But those advocates should also more actively attempt to educate and familiarize policy and regulatory personnel with respect to HQL assessment in order to encourage wider use of the methodology.

REFERENCES

Foley, J. (1992). *Sources of health insurance and characteristics of the uninsured: Analysis of the March 1991 current population survey*. Washington, DC: Employee Benefit Research Institute.

Furberg, C. D., Schuttinga, J. A., Shumaker, S., A. & Wenger, N. K. (Eds.). (1993). *Quality of life assessment: Practice, problems, and promise: Proceedings of a workshop*. Bethesda, MD: The National Institutes of Health.

Manning, W. G., Newhouse, J. P., Duan, N., Keeler, E. B., Leibowitz, A., & Marquis, S. (1988). Health insurance and the demand for medical care: Evidence from a randomized experiment. *American Economic Review, 77*(3), 251-257.

National Institutes of Health. (1992) *NIH data book 1992* (Rep. No. 92-1261). Bethesda, MD.

Phelps, C. E. (1982). *Government and health policy* (Rand Paper No. P-6722). Santa Monica, CA: The Rand Corporation.

Raskin, I. E., & Maklan, C. W. (1991). Medical treatment effectiveness research: A view from inside the agency for health care policy and research. *AHCPR Program Note*. Rockville, MD: Agency for Health Care Policy Research, Public Health Service, U.S. Department of Health and Human Services.

Reyes, B. S. (1991). *Patient outcome research and practice guidelines: A plan for research and policy* (91-50 SPR), Washington DC: Congressional Research Service, The Library of Congress.

Roper, W. L., Winkenwerder, W., Hackbarth, G., & Krakauer, H. (1988). Effectiveness in health care: An initiative to evaluate and improve medical practice. *New England Journal of Medicine, 319*, 1197-1202.

Sonnefeld, S. T., Waldo, D. R., Lemieux, J. A., & McKusick, D. R. (1991). Projections of national health expenditures through the year 2000. *Health Care Financing Review, 13*(1), 1-15.

Ware, J., Jr. (1993). Evaluating measures of general health concepts for use in clinical trials. In C. D. Furberg, J. A. Schuttinga, S. A. Shumaker, & N. K. Wenger (Eds.), *Quality of life assessment: Practice, problems, and promise: Proceedings of a workshop* (pp. 51-63). Bethesda, MD: The National Institutes of Health.

3 Years of Healthy Life: Charting Improvements in the Nation's Health

Pennifer Erickson
Ronald Wilson
Ildy Shannon
National Center for Health Statistics

Increasingly, Americans view living long and healthy lives as what they want from the health system. To realize this goal, people are willing to undergo invasive medical procedures such as liver transplantation for the purpose of surviving to experience the joy of an event such as a child's wedding. People are also beginning to realize that by accepting responsibility for their own health they can increase their healthy life span, thereby enhancing their quality of life. One indication of this new-found accountability is that people are willingly modifying their behaviors by giving up harmful habits, such as cigarette smoking, and by adopting healthy behaviors, such as jogging and other forms of exercise, to extend healthy life.

In formulating health promotion and disease prevention strategies for the next decade, policymakers have captured this desire for long and healthy lives for all Americans in the overall goals set forth in *Healthy People 2000* (DHHS, 1991). Specifically, the first goal calls for increasing the healthy life span as part of a national strategy for improving the health of the nation. In setting this goal, policymakers recognize that the level of health of the nation encompasses more than survival or quantity of life. Quality of life is also recognized as an important component of the nation's health.

The term *quality of life,* however, has different meanings depending on the context in which it is used. In health promotion and disease prevention activities, *quality of life* is generally used synonymously with health status. Although this term can also have many meanings, the most frequently cited definition of *health* is as "a state of complete physical, mental, and social well-being, and not merely the absence of disease or infirmity" (World Health Organization, 1948).

Tracking progress toward increasing the healthy life span requires a measure that combines the survival and health experiences of the population. This chapter describes the conceptual framework that underlies such a measure, namely one that combines morbidity and mortality. The specific measure for tracking progress in increasing the healthy life span in response to *Healthy People 2000* is a measure called years of healthy life. Data sources and methods for calculating years of healthy life are discussed and estimates of years of healthy life for the U.S. population in 1990 are presented and interpreted. The last section outlines areas for future research.

YEARS OF HEALTHY LIFE DEFINED

Years of healthy life, also referred to as *quality-adjusted life years* or *well-life expectancy*, combines health-related quality of life (HQL), which is the value assigned to impairments, functional status, perceptions, and social opportunities, with mortality rates to determine the number of years that a population lives with and without dysfunction. Years of healthy life uses a life expectancy model in which standard life table data are adjusted by the level of HQL of a population. Measures of HQL represent many different concepts and domains of life quality, including symptoms and subjective complaints; mental, physical, and social functioning; general health perceptions, and social opportunities (Patrick & Erickson, 1993).

Many definitions and indicators of health and well-being may be used to measure these different concepts and domains. For example, symptoms usually involve the assessment of physical and psychological sensations, such as pain and feelings of anxiety, that are not directly observable. Social functioning may be measured in terms of an individual's limitation in performing a usual social role, whether this be work, school, or housework; physical functioning may be measured in terms of health-related limitation in mobility such as being confined to a bed, chair, or couch due to health reasons. Health perceptions are assessed in terms of subjective evaluations of health and satisfaction with health. Resilience, an indicator of social opportunity, can be measured in terms of one's capacity for health and ability to cope with stress.

Combining measures of different domains of HQL into a single score requires the adoption of a conceptual model that considers health as a continuum that ranges from perfect health on one end to death on the other. In between these two endpoints lie a number of discrete and mutually exclusive health states that are defined in terms of one or more concepts or domains of HQL. For example, when HQL is defined in terms of perceived health and role limitation, one possible health state is that of being in excellent health and having no role limitations.

To convert this conceptual model into an operational definition of HQL, death is assigned a value of 0, and optimal health is assigned a value of 1. Health states falling between these two endpoints are assigned numbers that represent the values that either society as a whole or single individuals place on being in each health state. When years of healthy life are to be used for national policy, as in *Healthy People 2000*, the values placed on each health state should represent society's values for health and well-being. Various methods from economic and psychometric theory have been used to determine the values for different health states (Torrance, 1986).

These values can be interpreted as representing the proportion of time, on average, that an individual spends in optimal functioning over a given time interval. For example, if the person experiences a health state for 1 year that has a value of .75, we say that the person spent 75% of the year in full function; the remaining 25% of the year was spent in various states of dysfunction due to either chronic or acute conditions or both. For groups of individuals, averaging the values assigned to health states experienced by persons in the group gives the mean HQL for that population for the year.

Years of healthy life for a population over its lifetime can be estimated by adjusting the expected duration of remaining life (i.e., life expectancy) by the average HQL observed in the population. This gives the average number of years that the population is expected to spend in a state of optimal function and the average number of years spent in states of less than optimal health.

MEASURING YEARS OF HEALTHY LIFE FOR *HEALTHY PEOPLE 2000*

Measures of years of healthy life for monitoring population health require HQL and mortality data on representative samples of the population. For *Healthy People 2000,* data on health and well-being that can be used to measure HQL for the general population are collected in the National Health Interview Survey (NHIS). In the NHIS, information is collected in an ongoing, nationwide sample of about 50,000 households that represents the resident civilian noninstitutionalized population of the United States living at the time of the interview. The sample does not include persons residing in nursing homes or institutionalized persons, members of the armed forces, or U.S. nationals living abroad (Adams & Benson, 1992). Information on the size of the institutionalized population is available from the 1990 census and can be used to supplement data from the NHIS.

Life expectancy data, which are presented in a life table are used to reflect the mortality experience of the population. Life tables specify the proportion of people living and dying in each age interval and the average number of years of life remaining at the beginning of each age interval. These data represent the current mortality experience and show the long-range implications of a set of age-specific death rates that prevailed in a given year.

The following section describes how data from the NHIS are used to develop a set of health states and the method used for arriving at a set of values for these states. The following section outlines the procedures for combining these states and associated values with information in the life table to develop estimates of years of healthy life.

Defining Health States

Two types of information in the NHIS, namely, perceived health and role limitation, are used to form an operational definition of HQL. Information about perceived health status is obtained for all respondents using the following question: "Would you say your health in general is excellent, very good, good, fair, or poor?" Role limitation captures a person's limitation in social role that is usually associated with his or her particular age group, for example, working, keeping house, or going to school (Adams & Benson, 1992). For this measure of HQL, each person is classified into one of six categories based on his or her age and ability to perform his or her major activity: not limited; not limited in major activity but limited in other activities; limited in major activity; unable to perform major activity; unable to perform instrumental activities of daily living without the help of other persons; and unable to perform activities of daily living without the help of other persons. The criteria used to classify persons into one of these six categories are shown in Table 3.1.

In classifying persons into one of the six levels of role limitation it has sometimes been necessary to make assumptions about their health status. For example, persons with unknown role limitation were considered to be unlimited in their role function. This assumption makes some persons healthier than they actually might be. Upward bias in role limitation also can occur because of the questionnaire design. For example, information about ability to perform self-care activities was not asked of persons 0 to 4 years of age; unable to perform major activity is the most severe functional limitation to which these persons can be assigned. Thus, children less than 5 years of age can not be assigned to the lowest level of functioning. If the number of respondents is relatively large, then the assumption about unknown role and this feature of the questionnaire can increase the population's level of health. This bias may be offset by a questionnaire feature for persons in the 65 years and older category. The major activity

TABLE 3.1
Definitions of Role Limitation Using National Health Interview Survey Items

Not Limited

- Not limited regardless of age; this category includes unknown role performance regardless of a person's age.

Limited in Other Activities

- Limited in other activities regardless of age, or
- Limitation in activity and 65–69 years of age but able to perform activities of daily living (ADLs) and able to perform instrumental activities of daily living (IADLs).

Limited in Major Activity

- 64 years of age and younger—Limited in amount or kind of major activity, or
- 65 years and older—Major activity is considered to be ADL and IADL activities; therefore these people cannot fall in this category.

Unable to Perform Major Activity

- 64 years of age and younger—Unable to perform major activity, or
- 65 years and older—Major activity is considered to be ADL and IADL activities; therefore these people cannot fall in this category. This treatment may result in making the population less healthy than it actually might be.

Instrumental Activities of Daily Living (IADL)

- 0–17 years of age—Not applicable. Children were not asked the question about handling routine needs such as everyday household chores, doing necessary business, and shopping.
- 18–64 years of age—Unable to perform routine needs without the help of other persons and unable to perform or limited in major activity, or
- 65 years of age and older—Unable to perform routine needs without the help of other persons, or

Activities of Daily Living (ADL)

- 0–4 years of age—Not applicable. Children were not asked the question about needing help with personal care needs; therefore unable to perform their major activity is the most severe functional to which they can be assigned.
- 5–64 years of age—Unable to perform personal care needs without the help of other persons and unable to perform or limited in activity, or
- 65 years of age and older – Unable to perform personal care needs without the help of other persons, or

Note: Persons are placed in only one usual activity category. When a person can be classified in more than one group, he or she is assigned to the group with the lowest score.

for these persons is considered to be activities of daily living and instrumental activities of daily living. Thus, these persons cannot be assigned to either of the two categories that reflect limitation in major activity. This questionnaire design feature may make the population seem less healthy than it actually might be.

The operational definition of HQL based on a matrix of five categories of perceived health and the six categories of role limitation results in 30 possible health states ranging from the optimal level of not limited in role performance and in excellent health to the lowest health state defined as needing help to perform activities of daily living and being in poor health. These health states are shown in Table 3.2 along with the percentage of persons in each health state based on data from the NHIS. In 1990, almost 83% of the noninstitutionalized U.S. population, over 202 million persons, had no role limitation and were perceived to be in excellent, very good, or good health. Approximately 1% of the population was in one of the two lowest perceived health categories and were unable to perform their major activity.

According to the 1990 census, approximately 3.3 million Americans were living in institutions, including correctional facilities, nursing homes, long-term stay hospitals, homes for children, or were serving in the military. The institutionalized populations were assigned a health state based on assumed levels of role limitation and perceived health status. Persons in correctional facilities were considered as limited in major activity and in very good health (Colsher, Wallace, Loeffelholz, & Sales, 1992). The nursing home population is assumed to be limited in activities of daily living and in poor health, whereas persons in long-term stay hospitals are assumed to be limited in instrumental activities of daily living and in good health. Children living in juvenile homes were considered to be limited in other than their major activity and in good health. The military population of 1.7 million persons in 1990 comprises a basically healthy, that is, in very good or excellent health and with no limitations in usual social role, group of individuals; their health status is assumed to be represented by the civilian noninstitutionalized population.

Valuing Health States

Values have been assigned to each of the 30 health states in the matrix defined by perceived health and role limitation using multiattribute utility

TABLE 3.2
Percent of Persons in Health States Based on Role Limitation and Perceived Health Status, NHIS 1990

	Perceived Health Status				
Role Limitation	*Excellent*	*Very Good*	*Good*	*Fair*	*Poor*
Not limited	38.1	26.3	18.2	3.3	0.3
Limited-other	0.6	1.1	1.8	1.3	0.4
Limited-major	0.5	0.7	1.3	0.7	0.2
Unable-major	0.1	0.2	0.5	0.6	0.5
Limited in IADL	0.1	0.2	0.5	0.6	0.6
Limited in ADL	<0.1	0.1	0.2	0.3	0.5

scaling (Keeney & Raiffa, 1976). Scores have been assigned by assuming that the highest level of function for each of the domains in the matrix is 1 and the lowest is 0. Scores for levels within this range have been assigned by examining data from the NHIS. Correspondence analysis was used to help quantify the distance between different levels of each of the two dimensions of health (Greenacre & Hastie, 1987). This analysis led to the following scores for levels within role limitation: 1, 0.75, 0.65, 0.40, 0.20, 0; and for levels within perceived health status: 1, 0.85, 0.70, 0.30, and 0 (Erickson, Wilson, & Shannon, 1994).

The value of the healthiest state, that of having no role limitations and having an excellent perceived health status, is assigned a value of 1; the value of the most dysfunctional health state in this matrix, namely being limited in activities of daily living and in poor health, is assigned a value of 0.1. The Health Utility Index (Drummond, Stoddart, & Torrance, 1987) was used to obtain a score for being in excellent health and limited in activities of daily living, 0.47 in the lower left cell of the matrix. Scores for levels within role limitation and perceived health status plus the values assigned to three of the four corners of the health state matrix, that is, 1, 0.10, and 0.47, have been used to develop values for each cell in the matrix using a model in which the two dimensions are interdependent. A detailed discussion of the procedures for defining the values in the matrix is given in the *Statistical Notes* by Erickson et al. (1994). The values that result from this calculation are shown in Table 3.3.

Although no other set of health states exists that assigns values to both role limitation and perceived health, selected research studies allow some comparison for validation of these values. Role limitation can be compared with the Role Function dimension of the Health Utility Index Mark I (HUI) developed by Torrance (1982). The HUI defines performance of usual social role in terms of being able to eat, dress, bathe, and go to the toilet with or without help and presence or absence of limitations in playing,

TABLE 3.3
Values for the Interim Measure of Years of Healthy Life

	Single Attribute Score	*Perceived Health Status*					
		Excellent 1	*Very Good 0.85*	*Good 0.70*	*Fair 0.30*	*Poor 0*	*Dead*
Not limited	1	1	0.92	0.84	0.63	0.47	
Limited-other	0.75	0.87	0.79	0.72	0.52	0.38	
Limited-major	0.65	0.81	0.74	0.67	0.48	0.34	
Unable-major	0.40	0.68	0.62	0.55	0.38	0.25	
Limited in IADL	0.20	0.57	0.51	0.45	0.29	0.17	
Limited in ADL	0	0.47	0.41	0.36	0.21	0.10	
Dead							0.0

going to school, or working. These functions are similar to those used in the NHIS limitation of activity questions. Scores for the three lowest HUI Role Function levels rescaled from 0 to 1 and those derived for the role limitation dimension are similar, indicating concurrence between these two independent sources of information about values placed on performance of usual social role.

Validity of the single attribute scores assigned to the levels within perceived health, (Table 3.3), is indicated by comparing these scores with results from the Medical Outcomes Study (Stewart, Hays, & Ware, 1988). In this study, Stewart and colleagues showed that perceived health status is a nonlinear scale, with *excellent*, *very good*, and *good health* being closer in scores than are *fair* and *poor health*. This result supports the findings of the correspondence analysis on data from the NHIS, which also indicated that the levels within the perceived health status scale are nonlinear.

YEARS OF HEALTHY LIFE

Following the method for adjusting life expectancy using national health status data that was first implemented by Sullivan (1971), calculation of years of healthy life starts with two data sets, an abridged life table and age-specific estimates of HQL of the U.S. population. The life table for estimating years of healthy life starts with the age intervals of a relevant population, the number of persons alive at the beginning of the age interval (l_x), the number of people in the stationary population in each of the age intervals ($_nL_x$) and a column showing age-specific average estimates of HQL of the population. Procedures used to calculate life tables for the United States are discussed in the annual volumes of vital statistics (National Center for Health Statistics, 1990b). The average quality of life scores are multiplied by the number of person years in each age interval ($_nL_x$), represented in column 3, to obtain the quality-adjusted person years lived in each age interval, which is represented in column 5. These adjusted person years are then summed from the bottom to the top of the table to obtain the number of quality-adjusted person years in each age interval as well as in all subsequent intervals. Dividing the adjusted person years, (T_x') by the number of persons alive at the beginning of the interval (l_x) results in the number of years of healthy life remaining, as shown in Table 3.4.

Table 3.4 shows that for persons 45–50 years of age, the number of adjusted person years in this and subsequent intervals is 2,394,938. Dividing this by the number of persons alive at the beginning of the age interval, 94,179, results in 25.5 years of healthy life remaining. Of the 38 life years remaining for persons in this age group, shown in column 8, approximately two thirds will be spent in a health state defined by excellent perceived health and no role limitations.

TABLE 3.4
Calculation of Years of Healthy Life for the Total U.S. Population, 1990

Age Interval	l_x	${}_nL_x$	*Q*	$Q^*{}_nL_x$	T_x'	*YHL Remaining*	*Life Years Remaining*
0–5	100,000	495,073	.94	465,369	6,403,747	64.0	75.4
5–10	98,890	494,150	.93	459,560	5,938,379	60.1	75.1
10–15	98,780	493,654	.93	459,098	5,478,819	55.5	71.2
15–20	98,653	492,290	.92	452,907	5,019,721	50.9	66.3
20–25	98,223	489,794	.91	445,713	4,566,814	46.5	61.3
25–30	97,684	486,901	.91	443,080	4,121,102	42.2	56.6
30–35	97,077	483,571	.90	435,214	3,678,022	37.9	51.9
35–40	96,334	479,425	.89	426,688	3,242,808	33.7	47.2
40–45	95,382	474,117	.88	417,223	2,816,120	29.5	42.6
45–50	94,179	466,820	.86	401,465	2,398,897	25.5	38.0
50–55	92,420	455,809	.83	378,321	1,997,431	21.6	33.4
55–60	89,735	439,012	.81	355,600	1,619,110	18.0	29.0
60–65	85,634	413,879	.77	318,687	1,263,510	14.8	24.8
65–70	79,590	378,369	.76	287,560	944,823	11.9	20.8
70–75	71,404	330,846	.74	244,826	657,263	9.2	17.2
75–80	60,557	270,129	.70	189,090	412,437	6.8	13.9
80–85	47,168	197,857	.63	124,650	223,347	4.7	10.9
85+	31,892	193,523	.51	98,697	98,697	3.1	8.3

Legend:
Age Interval: Period of life between two exact ages stated in years
l_x : Number living at beginning of age interval
${}_nL_x$: Stationary population in the age interval
Q : Average health-related quality of life of persons in the age interval
$Q^*{}_nL_x$: Quality-adjusted stationary population in the age interval
T_x' : Quality-adjusted stationary population in this and all subsequent age intervals

For the total population, the life expectancy at birth in 1990 was 75.4 years; the corresponding expectancy of years of healthy life was 64. This means that the total population is expected to experience 11.4 years of less than optimal function throughout its lifetime, assuming the same mortality and health situations as experienced in 1990. This dysfunction represents the sum of impacts of chronic conditions and injuries that occur throughout the population's lifetime as measured by role limitation and perceived health. For persons 65 years and over, the average number of life years remaining was 20.8; the corresponding years of healthy life was 11.9. That is, of the 20.8 expected life years remaining, 8.9 years, or approximately 40% of the life years remaining, are expected to be lived with some dysfunction.

Years of healthy life have been calculated for African-American and White persons, as well as for the total population, using these methods. Years of healthy life and life expectancy at birth are compared in Fig. 3.1. In 1990, African Americans had a life expectancy at birth of 69.1 years with 56 of those being years of healthy life. The disparity between life expectancy and years of healthy life for African Americans, 13.1 years, indicates that almost 20% of the average life span for African Americans will be spent in some less than optimal health state. In contrast, Whites have a life expectancy at birth of 76.1 years and a corresponding 65 years of healthy life, which indicates that slightly less than 15% of the life span of Whites is spent in less than the optimal state of excellent health and no role limitation.

Policy goals for improving health should be to raise the years of healthy life for population subgroups to the highest level. Using the data in Fig. 3.1, the life expectancy at birth for Whites of approximately 76 years may be considered the highest level. Within this constraint, improvements in the healthy life span for adults will be accomplished by raising HQL. For the African-American population, on the other hand, the number of healthy life years can be increased by raising both quantity of life and quality of life. Raising life expectancy of the African-American population to that of the White population and assuming no concurrent improvements in HQL raises the number of years of healthy life to 60.8. To further increase the healthy life span for the African-American population improvements will have to be made in HQL.

Another issue of current policy concern, especially since the passage of the Americans with Disability Act, is the health status of persons with disability. For the many disabled persons who feel that they are healthier than their physical limitations suggest, an HQL measure that includes perceived health will be more representative of their overall HQL than a measure that is based on role limitation alone. For example, approximately 300,000 noninstitutionalized civilians are limited in activities of daily living but report themselves in very good or excellent health. If health is measured

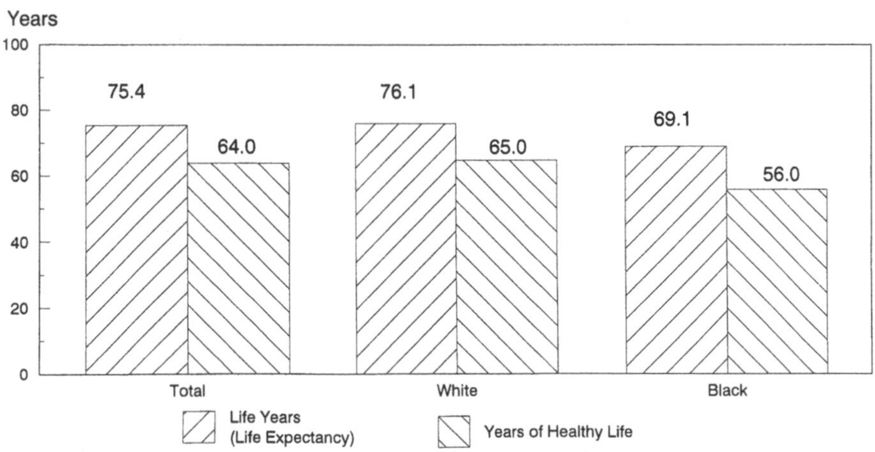

FIG. 3.1. Life years and years of healthy life total population, 1990. (Sources: U.S. Vital Statistics, NHIS Census Bureau).

solely in terms of role limitation, they would be given a score of 0. By also considering perceived health, these persons receive a score of either 0.41 or 0.47. This sensitivity suggests that in addition to being useful for charting the Nation's health for *Healthy People 2000*, this measure can supply useful information for other policy concerns.

FUTURE RESEARCH

The inclusion of years of healthy life in *Healthy People 2000* has stimulated the development of an interim measure of HQL. The best, currently available information for monitoring population health status annually has been included in this measure. A potential problem, however, is the use of two single dimensions, role limitation and perceived health. Current state-of-the-art measures, such as the EuroQol (EuroQol Group, 1990), the Health Utility Index Mark III (Berthelot, Roberge, & Wolfson, 1994), and the Quality of Well-Being Scale (Kaplan & Bush, 1982) include at least four dimensions and use values that are based on data from representative samples of the population. The limited number of dimensions and the assumptions made to develop a set of values may result in a measure that is relatively insensitive to health states that are less than optimal and one that is unable to detect changes in health over time.

In addition to examining these aspects of the interim measure, participants at a workshop sponsored by the National Center for Health Statistics (NCHS) recommended that research and development toward a more comprehensive measure continue with emphasis on identifying concepts to include in an expanded measure, methods for valuing health states, and special population concerns.

Identifying Concepts of HQL

The measure used for charting changes in the nation's health through the 1990s includes three concepts, namely, role limitation, perceived health, and death. Although these concepts have been shown to be important indicators of health, it is unclear whether or not they are sufficiently inclusive to represent all deviations from an optimal function level. For example, the almost 85% of the population in the top three health states, shown in Table 3.2, may experience some other functional limitation, or reduced level of satisfaction that is not reflected in the interim measure. If so, then this measure will not only miss changes in this other dimension (or dimensions) but may also fail to identify areas where change in health policy might bring about improved health or where changes in policy have resulted in a worsening of HQL.

One way of identifying concepts to be included in the expanded measure is through an analysis of the interrelationships between different dimensions of HQL using existing data sets. The first step in such an analysis is to examine the relationship between role limitation and perceived health for different age and racial and ethnic subgroups of the population using data collected in the NHIS. Additional concepts, such as depression, can be analyzed similarly to observe response patterns among the different subgroups. Concepts that are found to be independent of each other are likely candidates for inclusion in an expanded measure.

After a set of concepts has been identified, a classification system analogous to the matrix shown in Table 3.2 needs to be developed. This classification will consist of a number of mutually exclusive levels within each of the concepts. By choosing one level from each of the concepts to be used in the new measure, a comprehensive set of health states can be defined. Classification of concepts based on physical and social function can use existing systems, such as the HUI and the Quality of Well-being Scale, as guides for development, whereas classification of dimensions that include affective components, such as depression, will have fewer models to follow. Thus, any dimensions in an expanded classification system that include mental health will be new and are apt to require extensive research before a set of mutually exclusive levels can be identified. Following the development of a classification system that includes all of the dimensions, a questionnaire needs to be developed and pretested before it can be included in a national survey such as the NHIS.

Valuing Health States:

Although research is proceeding to identify concepts to be included in the expanded measure, existing data and procedures for data collection can be examined from the perspective of estimating values for health states. On the one hand, the values used in the interim measure can be recalculated using different assumptions, for example, about the value assigned to the least functional health state and scores assigned to levels within role limitation and perceived health. Such sensitivity analyses will indicate the robustness of values, those used in the interim measure as well as more generally, to such changes.

On the other hand, methods for collecting data on the values can be studied for their suitability for use within the context of the NCHS. If information on the value that members of the U.S. general population place on health are needed, then the best method for collecting these data will have to be determined. One option is that data on values be collected in the ongoing general population surveys conducted by NCHS. In this case, the methods will have to be compatible with the design of either the NHIS or the National Health and Nutrition Examination Survey. Another option is the use of an ad hoc survey to collect data on the values. A special survey, by removing the constraint of compatibility with existing surveys, would allow greater flexibility in the design and implementation of methods for collecting information on values. With either option, survey design constraints may require the modification of existing methods to ensure that data on values can be collected within a reasonable time from persons with diverse cultural, educational and sociodemographic backgrounds.

Assessing Special Populations:

Concern about the HQL for special populations extends beyond the collection of valid information about the values these people place on health. For example, current information on the institutionalized population is limited to that collected in the decennial census. Although the census indicates the size of the various institutionalized populations, it contains little on the health of these individuals. By the middle of this decade, 1990 estimates on the number of institutionalized persons will be increasingly less accurate. If there is a major shift, for example, toward institutionalizing persons who are mentally ill, this change in policy will not be reflected in estimates of years of healthy life calculations. Thus, more information is needed about the health status of persons in institutions and the flows of persons into and out of institutions over time.

Also, to estimate years of healthy life for various subpopulations, for example, disabled persons, children with developmental disabilities, and persons with chronic disease, specific life tables are needed. Currently, national life tables are routinely available for 12 subpopulations defined in terms of race and gender. Cause-eliminated life tables are of limited value for estimating years of healthy life for persons with chronic disease because they ignore comorbidities and complications (Curtin & Armstrong, 1988). For example, eliminating diabetes as a cause of death overestimates the years of healthy life for persons with diabetes because this life table ignores deaths due to cardiovascular diseases, which are widely known to be complications of diabetes.

Further research in these three areas will lead to a greater understanding of the strengths and weaknesses of years of healthy life for monitoring improvements in population health status. A potential danger in the short run is succumbing to the temptation to use the interim measure for evaluative and allocative purposes. Such applications are beyond the intent of the development of this measure. Persons interested in extending the application of the interim measure are urged instead to join with the NCHS in its commitment to improving the measure of HQL and years of healthy life. Better understanding of the interim measure will indicate how responsive the U.S. health-care system, reflected by its health-care programs, is to giving Americans the longer and healthier lives they desire.

REFERENCES

Adams P., & Benson, V. (1992). Current estimates from the Health Interview Survey, 1991. *Vital and Health Statistics, 10*(184). Hyattsville, MD: National Center for Health Statistics.

Berthelot, J. M., Roberge, R., & Wolfson, M. (1994). The calculation of health-adjusted life expectancy for Ontario using a health status index. In *Proceedings of the 1993 Public Health Conference on Records and Statistics: Toward the year 2000: Refining the measures* (pp. 28–33). Hyattsville, MD: National Center for Health Statistics.

Colsher, P. L., Wallace, R. B., Loeffelholz, P. L., & Sales, M. (1992). Health status of older male prisoners: A comprehensive survey. *American Journal of Public Health, 82*(6), 881–884.

Curtin, L. R., & Armstrong, R. (1988). *Cause-eliminated life tables for the United States.* Hyattsville, MD: National Center for Health Statistics.

Department of Health and Human Services. (1991). *Healthy people 2000: National health promotion and disease prevention objectives* (DHHS Pub. No. PHS 91–50212). Washington, DC: U.S. Government Printing Office.

Drummond, M. F., & Stoddart, G. L., Torrance, G. W. (1987). *Methods for the economic evaluation of health care programmes.* New York: Oxford University Press.

Erickson, P., Wilson, R. W., & Shannon I. (1994). *Years of healthy life. Statistical notes, 6*(pp. 1–8). Hyattsville, MD: National Center for Health Statistics.

EuroQol Group. (1990). EuroQol—A new facility for the measurement of health-related quality of life. *Health Policy, 16,* 199–208.

Greenacre, M. & Hastie, T. (1987).The geometric interpretation of correspondence analysis. *Journal of the American Statistical Association, 82*(398), 437–447.

Kaplan, R. M., & Bush, J. W. (1982). Health-related quality of life measurement for evaluation research and policy analysis. *Health Psychology, 1,* 61–80.

Keeney, R. L., & Raiffa, H. *Decisions with multiple objectives: Preferences and value tradeoffs.* New York: Wiley.

National Center for Health Statistics (NCHS). (1990a). National health and nutrition examination survey III: Data collection forms. Hyattsville, MD: Public Health Service.

National Center for Health Statistics (NCHS). (1990b). *Vital statistics of the United States. Volume II. mortality, Part B.* Washington, DC: U.S. Government Printing Office.

National Center for Health Statistics (NCHS). (1992). *Health United States 1991 and prevention profile.* Hyattsville, MD: Public Health Service.

Patrick, D. L., & Erickson, P. (1993). *Health status and health policy: Quality of life in health care evaluation and resource allocation.* New York: Oxford University Press.

Stewart, A. L , Hays, R. D., & Ware, J. E. Jr. (1988). The MOS short-form general health survey: Reliability and validity in a patient population. *Med Care, 26*(7), 724–735.

Sullivan, D. F. (1971). A single index of morbidity and mortality. *HSMHA Health Reports, 86*(4), 347–355.

Torrance, G. W. (1982). Multiattribute utility theory as a method of measuring social preferences for health states in long-term care. R. L. Kane & R. A. Kane, (Eds.), *Values and long-term care* (pp. 127–156). Lexington, MA: Lexington, Books.

Torrance, G. W. (1986). Measurement of health state utilities for economic appraisal. *Journal of Health Economics, 5(1), 1–30.*

World Health Organization. (1948). *Constitution of the World Health Organization basic document.* Geneva, Switzerland: World Health Organization.

4 Quality of Life Assessment: A Pharmaceutical Industry Perspective

Robert S. Epstein
Eva Lydick
Merck Research Laboratories

It is generally agreed that in order to preserve a good quality of life, one needs to assure a healthy "state of complete physical, mental, and social well-being, and not merely the absence of disease or infirmity," as was stated in the constitution of the World Health Organization (WHO, 1946). Some investigators collect health-related quality of life (HQL) data by determining how well individuals perform on tests of physiologic activities of daily living, mental health functioning, and emotional functioning. Others feel that HQL is intrinsically a perceptual issue that requires assessment by a clinical investigator, caregiver, or participant using questionnaires. The increase in attention to HQL within the pharmaceutical industry has predominantly focused on the latter approach, resulting in the rapid proliferation and application of HQL questionnaires to drug development.

As one would expect, industry's approach to this field reflects the divergent philosophical views of what is meant by HQL and what its potential role should be in appreciating the benefit or consequence of pharmacologic intervention. The purpose of this chapter is to highlight some of the issues and tensions within the corporate environment that affect industry-sponsored studies and to speculate on how today's concerns will likely affect the future direction of HQL research.

OVERVIEW OF CURRENT DIRECTIONS WITHIN HQL RESEARCH

That rapid growth of health-related quality of life assessment can be appreciated through a review of the recent medical literature (see Fig. 4.1).

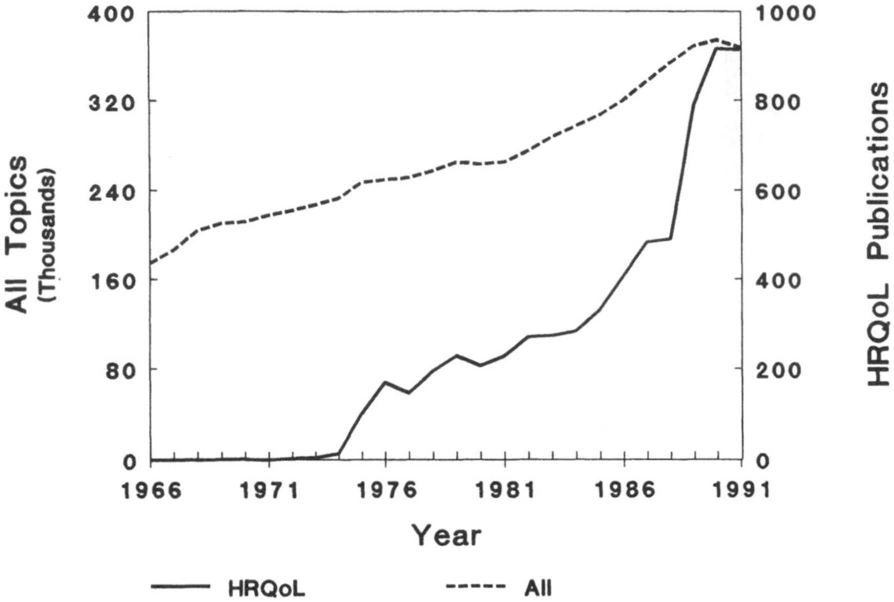

FIG. 4.1. Publications: "All" topics vs "HQL", Medline 1966–1991.

Since the early 1970s, the total number of published studies has grown, from none to nearly 1,000 per year, proportionally a far greater increase than has been seen in the general medical literature. A similar growth has occurred within the subset of industry-sponsored HQL studies. In recent years, there have been numerous educational programs and textbooks geared specifically toward HQL in pharmaceutical development (Drug Information Association, 1993a, 1993b; International Society for Pharmacoepidemiology, 1992; *On-Line Guide to Quality of Life Assessment*, 1992; Spilker, 1990; Spilker, Molinek, Johnston, Simpson, & Tilson, 1990).

The motivation for this increased interest within the pharmaceutical industry stems from a mixture of corporate objectives. Generally, companies are responding to clinician- and patient-driven interest in quantifying the effect of interventions on a person's sense of well-being. It is this shift from concentrating on specific physiologic or anatomic outcomes to patient-perceived outcomes that is driving the increase in HQL research, within both the pharmaceutical industry and clinical medicine as a whole.

Most industry-sponsored studies address one or more of the following objectives:

1. To demonstrate that an intervention improves HQL.
2. To demonstrate that an intervention does not adversely affect HQL.

3. To demonstrate that an intervention halts or slows the decline in HQL associated with a given disease.
4. To demonstrate the trade-off between increased cost and benefit, in economic terms.
5. To describe the level of HQL of study participants.
6. To compare the participants' HQL to another population.

Clearly few studies can fulfill all of those objectives (and may not need to). The first step in designing clinical trials to collect HQL data, as in other clinical trials, is to clearly establish the objective(s). The degree to which this is well-executed depends on whether the trials are *de novo* or add-on protocols to other already-designed studies. Anecdotal discussions with members of other companies reveal that few industry-sponsored studies currently ongoing were designed solely to obtain HQL data. The implications of collecting HQL data from add-on protocols relate to the imposed study design, which can lead to limited power to detect a true difference between treatment groups and potentially uninterpretable findings,

When designing an HQL study to examine a specific objective, an understanding of the natural history of the disease under study is necessary. Disease processes are, of course, highly variable. Some conditions are self-limited, others chronic and intermittent, and other still are chronic and progressive. Additionally, some conditions can be present, but cause no apparent symptomatology or functional impairment. Typically, pharmaceutical research tailors the study design to the specific objective, bearing in mind the epidemiology of the disease.

For example, if a decline in health status due to a disease can be improved with a given therapy (e.g., asthma), then a likely objective of the study may be to demonstrate an improvement in HQL (Objective 1). For diseases that are chronic, perhaps asymptomatic, but require therapy (e.g., hypertension), it may be important to demonstrate no adverse effect due to a given therapy (Objective 2). For diseases that are chronic, progressive, and, in some cases, fatal, and for which therapies are palliative, it may be unrealistic to expect improvement of HQL. It is instead more likely that the intervention will keep the HQL at baseline, which without treatment would slip downward (Objective 3). Finally, there are those who are interested in incorporating HQL into economic assessment. In this instance, the question is how much quality-adjusted life per unit cost is gained compared to another intervention or standard therapy (Objective 4)?

By incorporating HQL assessment into the baseline evaluation of a clinical trial, one can obtain an understanding of the impact of disease on the participants (Objective 5), and potentially compare this to another population (Objective 6): a general population, another study's population with the same disease process, or another population with some other disease. This objective of comparing the HQL requires that both populations under study have used precisely the same questionnaire administered under very similar conditions, because, for example, it has been shown that interviewer-administered and self-administered assessments do not always provide the same answers (Cook et al., 1993). Because most clinical trials enroll participants with highly selected patient characteristics (e.g., the healthy volunteer phenomenon), inferences about the impact of the disease on the overall HQL using these baseline data from a clinical trial will undoubtedly underestimate how participants in the real world with real disease feel.

Whatever objective is chosen ultimately depends in large measure on an understanding of the natural history of the disease. These epidemiologic data may be obtained either prospectively or, more commonly, retrospectively using data from well-published sources of longitudinal HQL data (Costa et al., 1987; Stewart et al., 1989). The ultimate choice of study objective guides the ensuing selection of the patient population, questionnaire to assess HQL, and the development of the study methodology (sample size, time frame, data analytic strategy, etc.).

The questionnaire selected may be a disease-specific or a generic measure (i.e., designed to be used across many disease conditions). Often, particularly in the case of generic questionnaires, the instrument chosen will be a standard, such as the Nottingham Health Profile (NHP; Hunt et al., 1980), or the SF-36 (Ware & Sherbourne, 1992). With disease-specific questionnaires, there may be no standard or pre-existing questionnaire. Then the measure must be a new one, developed for that specific trial, or one previously used in a different disease or therpeutic area. In any event, validity of the instruments must be demonstrated in the disease condition under study. Demonstration of validity requires evidence that the questionnaire is appropriate, reproducible, responsive to change when the disease in question progresses or regresses, and meets some criteria of construct or content validity (Kirschner & Guyatt, 1985).

The further distinction between generic health profiles, such as the NHP or SF-36, and generic utility measures (often referred to as indexes), such as the Quality of Well-being Scale, is important when contemplating the application of the study findings to a health economic objective. To date, there have not been published methodologies to translate the generic health profiles into utilities, although ongoing research is promising (Fryback et al., 1993). Currently, if there is a need to have an economic argument, then the trial typically includes a generic utility measure alongside the other HQL questionnaires (Bombardier et al., 1986).

HQL instruments have also been traditionally characterized as being either evaluative, discriminative, or predictive (Kirschner & Guyatt, 1985).

Evaluative questionnaires measure the change in the level of HQL in a population or subpopulation over time; discriminative ones attempt to separate groups on a cross-sectional basis, for example, those with a disease from those without a disease. Finally, predictive instruments are designed to predict the occurrence of a specific outcome in a group of individuals (Guyatt, Kirschner, & Jaeschke, 1992). As most researchers within the pharmaceutical industry are interested in developing assessments that can be incorporated into clinical trials, the incentive is to develop and validate measures that are evaluative.

CURRENT TENSIONS WITHIN INDUSTRY

Within companies, levels of enthusiasm and expectation may differ between company divisions. Medical affairs divisions typically undertake specific studies in order to gain drug approval. Marketing divisions, although sharing this interest, are charged with obtaining additional data that may be useful in the competitive environments of pricing and sales. Such information may require studies that, for example, differentiate one product from the next, meet the interests of a specialty physician, or provide information on special subpopulations of patients.

Regulatory divisions must assure compliance with all requests and guidelines from regulatory authorities. Often, the regulatory background for HQL studies differs within divisions of a single national regulatory agency as well as between countries. The philosophy of a particular division within the regulatory agency may or may not be expressed as formal guidelines for the submission of new drug applications for pharmaceutical agents. HQL studies may be encouraged in submissions to the oncology division of the Food and Drug Administration (FDA; Shoemaker, Burke, Dorr, Temple, & Friedman, 1990), but may not be viewed as important to another division. In addition, corporate regulatory divisions often fear that HQL changes may require reporting as adverse events, thus increasing their workload considerably and possibly endangering or delaying a potential product license.

Even if all agree on the need to conduct a HQL study, the anticipated favorable result may not be defined in the same manner by each division. For example, the regulatory division may be satisfied with demonstrating that a new product does not impair HQL (a safety outcome), whereas marketing may want to show net improvement (an efficacy outcome). Others still may only be interested in HQL if an economic argument is attached (as in cost-utility assessment).

CURRENT INTERACTIONS BETWEEN INDUSTRY AND NONINDUSTRY

The majority of HQL instruments used by the industry have been developed by academics, either alone or in consultation with representatives from pharmaceutical companies. In spite of this history of collaboration, there remains the potential for tension between the two regarding the selection, development, validation, and implementation of HQL measures. Applications of HQL data collection within industry-sponsored clinical trials involve usage of questionnaires across multiple study centers and sometimes multiple countries and languages. Because of the vast amount of data required to be collected on each individual, study participants face a substantial respondent burden before even encountering the HQL assessment. There is often little time for the training of investigators in these new measures. Specific common complaints about HQL questionnaires center around the length of questionnaires, the mode of administration (interviewer vs. self), and the meaningfulness of changes. All of these issues are apparent to industry researchers, but not always understood by their academic or consulting colleagues.

Outside industry, however, public health and academic researchers often have interests in characterizing populations on a cross-sectional basis (Costa et al., 1987; Stewart et al., 1989). Those who are interested in using HQL as a covariate for baseline status or who wish to assess the likelihood of an outcome favor the development of predictive instruments. Clearly, industry objectives of an evaluative instrument may be discordant with those of HQL researchers outside of industry.

In addition, the academic community may view industry efforts with skepticism. It is sometimes felt that instruments may be tailored to demonstrate the superiority of one aspect of a product over another and not cover the broader range of health parameters that impact on a patient's health-related quality of life. Admittedly, this tailoring of questionnaires has occurred in the past; however, this practice is discouraged by regulatory agencies (*F-D-C Reports,* 1991). Nevertheless, researchers outside industry often feel that instruments developed by themselves are apt to be less biased and more relevant to the disease under study. Finally, there is potential for conflict about the proprietary nature of the questionnaires, in that at times the outside researcher, the company, or both expect to hold copyright to the instrument.

Goverment agencies, beyond research arms such as AHCPR, the National Institutes of Health (NIH), and NCHS, are primarily reviewers of HQL data and they are unlikely to take an active role in the development or utilization of HQL measures. In the case of drug licensing or drug regulating bodies, agencies may encourage, discourage, or circumscribe the use of HQL results. In 1991, one country and one province of another responded to growing interest in the impact of drugs on the overall quality of life of patients and issued draft guidelines requiring future applications for new drug approvals to be accompanied by HQL results (Commonwealth of Australia, 1990; Minister of Health, Ontario, Canada, 1991). It remains to be seen how many other countries will follow this example and how soon this will occur, but current perception within the industry is that these two cases may not remain isolated examples.

Frequently, companies wish to use HQL results as a marketing advantage, to distinguish their product from a crowded field of similar products (Morris, 1990). Quality of life, as a catch phrase, has in the past been used very broadly, implying anything from frequency of reporting a single symptom to increased ability to function and survival (Schumacher, Olschewski, & Schulgen, 1991). Currently, under U.S. FDA guidelines, advertising that discusses improvement in quality of life requires the same rigorous demonstration as for other claims. Briefly, such claims must be based on randomized blinded controlled studies designed to support quality of life claims and marketers may not present data for only those claims for which their product proved superior to a competitor or placebo (*F-D-C Reports*, 1991).

When governments bear responsibility for either dispensing or reimbursing for pharmaceutical products, the price of prescription drugs is also likely to be established with a government agency. Here HQL results may be one way to justify a premium price. In fact, intricate health economic models that sometimes incorporate HQL are created to persuade governments that a new entity will provide savings in monetary terms or in terms of human suffering and thus warrant a price that will compensate the pharmaceutical company for the development costs (Revicki, Rothman, & Luce, 1992). Because new entities often treat diseases for which no treatment existed before, actual cost saving is rarely expected. Thus HQL is used to express the intangible improvement in pain and disability due to the disease. Ironically, quality of life measures have been used so often in these economic models that HQL is often thought of within the industry and some governmental agencies as an economic tool and not ostensibly a clinical measure of outcome.

FUTURE DIRECTIONS

If the current interest in this field continues to increase, HQL assessment will likely shift from being primarily a marketing tool to a clinical measure routinely collected for licensure. This would potentially result in several consequences, both within industry and within health practice in general.

Within industry, planning for drug development studies in humans begins during the preclinical phase, and continues up through and past the time when products are approved for licensure. As HQL outcomes become important to regulatory agencies, their assessment will increasingly become a routine part of a company's clinical trial planning. Companies will therefore need to assess the potential for including HQL studies early on in the planning time period. The earlier planning would require information on the expected rate of change in HQL among untreated persons with the disease, in order to compute the sample size needed for the potential study. Hence, more HQL clinical trials may likewise increase the number of industry-sponsored cohort studies that incorporate HQL.

Information would also be needed on the clinically meaningful difference expected between treated and untreated groups. One of the most common questions regarding the interpretation of HQL studies is "Does a difference of 0.3 (for example) on this quality of life scale really mean something to the patient?" A few methods have been proposed for relating HQL units to actual patient experiences (Jaeschke, Singer, & Guyatt, 1989; Lydick & Epstein, in press; Testa, 1987). It can be expected that as HQL measures are increasingly incorporated into intervention trials as efficacy or safety endpoints, questions regarding the meaning of the reported difference will increase. And with the increase in questions, additional answers will hopefully be developed.

The issue of interpreting HQL outcome data is complicated further when the data arise from multiple countries or cultures. Most researchers believe that cross-cultural use of questionnaires requires more than simple translation into another language. Questions that mean one thing in one culture can mean quite another in another culture. This problem will likely receive even more attention in this era of cross-national clinical trials. If the data from multiple cultures are to be combined, it is imperative that there be some cross-cultural validation of questionnaires. This question, which has been the source of much attention lately, will undoubtedly continue to receive much attention over the next few years.

By incorporating HQL into clinical studies, it is conceivable that providers will obtain a better sense for how the participant is feeling, and the participant may feel more investment in the study and provider. Often, participants complain about their care and feel that providers emphasize their health as measured by biochemical tests and expensive imaging equipment, but do not address how they actually feel. Thus, increased use of HQL assessment in clinical trials may build stronger relationships between a provider and participant.

Given that this field is expanding rapidly, we expect that the current proliferation of HQL questionnaires will eventually taper off for the more common diseases. Already there are numerous questionnaires that have been developed for heart diseases (25 questionnaires), asthma (17 questionnaires), and arthritis (19 measures; *OLGA*, 1992). Comparability across studies that employ different questionnaires is thus not possible, and so we believe that consensus will eventually emerge on the one or two acceptable questionnaires per disease. Consensus building has been attempted in the past for the generic HQL questionnaires (The Portugal Conference, 1987), but to date, there are no industry or agency standards for either generic or disease-specific questionnaires.

The advantages of having fewer questionnaires that become identified as industry standards are readily apparent. Firstly, the planning of future clinical trials would become more efficient, with the development and validation of new instruments rarely required. Also, fewer questionnaires would result in more published data on the psychometric properties of any given questionnaire and its application to various populations. With the use of a standard set of questionnaires, agency reviewers and practitioners may feel less concerned about the potential for selecting a questionnaire that is somehow tailored to highlight the superiority of one product over another. Finally, a consensus on a common generic quality of life measure would better summarize the totality of adverse reactions experienced by patients in clinical trials, rather than the current method of tabulating individual adverse reactions.

However, there are also reasons that fewer questionnaires may not be better. A single questionnaire cannot be expected to address all levels of severity of a given disease (Bindman, Keane, & Lurie, 1990). For example, a questionnaire developed for moderately affected persons may capture improvement among severely affected persons, but may not capture further decline because of a floor effect (where baseline scores are so low that follow-up scores cannot detect further decline) in the design of the questionnaire. Standardization could stifle innovation in an evolving field and halt the search for a better questionnaire.

Although there are obvious advantages for companies to encourage the adoption of standard instruments and to include these questionnaires in their trials, there are also some disadvantages with standardization. Companies that develop and validate their own questionnaires have the ability to make certain that the questionnaires reflect the company needs. That is, the format (interviewer vs. self-administered), length of questionnaire, cross-cultural translations, and even the focus can be selected by those who develop the questionnaire. Also, companies that take the initiative to develop a questionnaire can receive a competitive advantage in that they have had the benefit of time and experience with the questionnaire prior to its usage.

Finally, we see HQL measures being used by the pharmaceutical industry in areas other than intervention trials. Describing the overall burden of disease on society when justifying a treatment will more often include tangibles using HQL measures, as distinguished from the current emphasis on physician visits, hospitalization, drug utilization, and mortality. In addition, HQL instruments may be included in the estimation of the effectiveness (Brook & Lohr, 1985) of a treatment in a population. Just as therapeutic interventions are examined today for their ability to make an impact, in the future, effectiveness may include measures of HQL in addition to conventional measures of morbidity and mortality.

In conclusion, the concept of totality of health and the interest in an individual's health status as perceived by him are relatively new, both in clinical medicine and within drug development. However, the growth and acceptance of HQL measures over the past decade have been impressive. There is no indication that HQL is a passing fancy and all indicators point toward the continuous growth in understanding and use of these measures within the pharmaceutical industry as well as within clinical medicine as a whole. The subjective nature of the HQL indices used in drug development is both their greatest strength and their greatest weakness. Interpretation of the results is difficult for clinicians, regulators, and consumers; however, the desirability of collecting information on the perception of health status by the patients themselves is rarely disputed. Future research will likely answer many of today's questions about the appropriateness and significance of HQL measures.

REFERENCES

Bindman, A. B., Keane, D., & Lurie, N. (1990). Measuring health changes among severely ill patients: The floor phenomenon. *Medical Care, 28,* 1142–1152.

Bombardier, C., Ware, J., Russell, I. J., Larson, M., Chalmers, A., & Read, J. L. (1986). Auranofin therapy and quality of life in patients with rheumatoid arthritis: Results of a multicenter trial. *American Journal of Medicine, 81*, 565–578.

Brook, R. H., & Lohr, K. N. (1985). Efficacy, effectiveness, variations, and quality: Boundary-crossing research. *Medical Care, 23*, 710–722.

Commonwealth of Australia. (1990). *Guidelines for the pharmaceutical industry on preparation of submissions to the Pharmaceutical Benefits Advisory Committee: Including submissions involving economic analysis.* Canberra, Australia: Author.

Cook, D. J., Guyatt, G. H., Juniper, E., Griffith, L., McIllroy, W., Willan, A., Jaeschke, R., & Epstein, R. S. (1993). Interviewer versus self-administered questionnaires in developing a disease-specific health-related quality of life instrument for asthma. *Journal of Clinical Epidemiology, 46,* 529–534.

Costa, P. T., Jr., Zonderman, A. B., McCrae, R. R., Coroni-Huntley, J., Locke, B. Z., & Barbano, H. E. (1987). Longitudinal analyses of psychological well-being in a national sample: Stability of mean levels. *Journal of Gerontology, 42,* 550–555.

Drug Information Association. (1993a, April). *Quality of life evaluation: The 1st Annual Symposium of Contributed Papers on Quality of Life,* Charleston, SC.

Drug Information Association. (1993b, February). *Quality of Life Workshop,* Nice, France.

F-D-C Reports. (1991, January 21). Quality of life ad claims should not be based on open-label "seeding" studies; FDA has continuing "concerns" about quality of life claims in general, pp. 15–16.

Fryback, D. F., Dasbach, E. J., Klein, B. E. K., Dorn, N., & Peterson, K. (1993). The Beaver Dam Health Outcomes Study—Initial catalog of health-state quality factors. *Medical Decision Making, 13,* 89–102.

Guyatt, G. H., Kirschner, B., & Jaeschke, R. (1992). Measuring health status: What are the necessary measurement properties? *Journal of Clinical Epidemiology, 45,* 1341–1345.

Hunt, S. M., McKenna, S. P., McEwen, J., Backett, E. M., Williams, J., & Papp, E. (1980). A quantitative approach to perceived health status: A validation study. *Journal of Epidemiology and Community Health, 34,* 281–286.

International Society for Pharmacoepidemiology. (1992, February). *Quality of life methods: Evaluation pharmaceutical agents,* Sarasota, FL.

Jaeschke, R., Singer, J., & Guyatt, G. H. (1989). Measurement of health status: Ascertaining the minimal clinically important difference. *Controlled Clinical Trials, 10,* 407–415.

Kirschner, B., & Guyatt, G. (1985). A methodological framework for assessing health indices. *Journal of Chronic Diseases, 38,* 27–36.

Lydick, E., & Epstein, R. S. (in press). Interpretation of quality of life changes. *Quality of Life Research, 2.*

Ministry of Health, Drug Programs Branch, Ontario, Canada. (1991). *Guidelines for preparation of economic analysis* (to be included in submission to Drug Programs Branch for listing in the Ontario Drug Benefit Formulatory Comparative Drug Index). Toronto, Canada: Author.

Morris, L. A. (1990). A marketing perspective. In B. Spilker (Ed.), *Quality of life assessments in clinical trials* (pp. 171–182). New York: Raven Press.

The on-line guide to quality-of-life assessment. (1992). Kensington, MD:

The Portugal Conference. (1987). Measuring quality of life and functional status in clinical and epidemiological research [Special issue]. *Journal of Chronic Diseases, 40,* 459–460.

Revicki, D. A., Rothman, M., & Luce, B. (1992). Health-related quality of life assessment and the pharmaceutical industry. *PharmacoEconomics, 1,* 394–408.

Schumacher, M., Olschewski, M., & Schulgen, G. (1991). Assessment of quality of life in clinical trials. *Statistics in Medicine, 10,* 1915–1930.

Shoemaker, D., Burke, G., Dorr, A., Temple, R., & Friedman, M. A. (1990). A regulatory perspective. In B. Spilker (Ed.), *Quality of life assessments in clinical trials* (pp. 193–201). New York: Raven Press.

Spilker, B. (Ed.). (1990). *Quality of life assessments in clinical trials.* New York: Raven Press.

Spilker, B., Molinek, F. R., Jr., Johnston, K. A., Simpson, R. L., Jr., & Tilson, H. H. (1990). Quality of life bibliography and indexes. *Medical Care, 28*(Suppl. 12).

Stewart, A. L., Greenfield, S., Hays, R. D., Wells, K., Rogers, W. H., Berry, S. D., McGlynn, E. A., & Ware, J. E., Jr. (1989). Functional status and well-being of patients with chronic conditions: Results from the Medical Outcomes Study. *Journal of the American Medical Association, 262,* 907–913.

Testa, M. A. (1987). Interpreting quality-of-life clinical trial data for use in the clinical practice of antihypertensive therapy. *Journal of Hypertension, 5*(Suppl), S9-S13.

Ware, J. E., Jr., & Sherbourne, C. D. (1992). The MOS 36-item Short Form Health Survey (SF-36): I. Conceptual framework and item selection. *Medical Care, 30*, 473–483.

World Health Organization. (1946). *Constitution of the World Health Organization.* Geneva, Switzerland: Author.

5 A Commentary on the Pharmaceutical Industry's Sponsorship of Health-Related Quality of Life Research

Robert A. Freeman
*Sterling Winthrop, Inc., New York**

Research arrangements between pharmaceutical manufacturers and universities are commonplace, and a long history of mutual cooperation and understanding exists with regard to issues such as intellectual property rights, scientific independence and integrity, contractual issues, and academic freedom. In recent years, pharmaceutical manufacturers have expressed an interest in developing and validating health-related quality of life (HQL) instruments either in the randomized clinical trial (RCT) setting or in independent studies parallel to a RCT. This chapter discusses the reasons underlying a pharmaceutical manufacturer's interest in funding HQL research within the context of medical, regulatory, and marketing uses of the research. The chapter also reviews some of the ethical issues surrounding industry-sponsored research. The issue of ethical conduct of industry-sponsored pharmacoeconomic research was raised by Hillman et al. (1991) and is addressed within the context of this discussion.

THE SPONSOR'S MOTIVES

The pharmaceutical manufacturer's decision to become involved with the sponsorship of HQL research is influenced by a number of factors, some of which are primarily commercial in nature (e.g., increase a product's sales), whereas others are predominantly medical or scientific (e.g., demonstrating

*The opinions expressed herein are those of the author and do not necessarily reflect those of his current employer.

clinical efficacy through documented improvements in patients' HQL outcomes). In most instances, the pharmaceutical manufacturers have initiated HQL research programs in reaction to changes in the marketplace, which now demands comparative economic analyses of quality of life assessments of new drug therapies. This observation is especially relevant as we move through an area of increasing price sensitivity and concern about the value of medical technology in relation to its cost.

Regardless of the underlying and often complex motives, the utility of the HQL assessments to the sponsoring company ultimately relies on the production and dissemination of information that influences positively the prescription drug's use in medical practice. Ultimately, the manufacturer's investment in HQL research has to be justified by linking research outcomes to the achievement of a corporate goal: increased sales, regulatory approval, or obtaining favorable pricing, reimbursement, or coverage by a third-party payer.

GENERAL USES OF HQL RESEARCH

One of the driving factors behind the pharmaceutical industry's investment in HQL research is the recognition that the field is evolving and that significant resources are required to develop, validate, and replicate both general and disease-specific instruments for HQL. It is also recognized that federal funding for basic research is lacking, and that the pharmaceutical industry's involvement as a funding source is necessary. Additionally, the need to develop instruments to be used in cross-national clinical studies and RCTs is recognized and financed. Finally, it is also commonly recognized that widespread dissemination and adoption of newly developed instruments are essential to their acceptance by the research community; hence, although much of the research funded by the industry is somewhat proprietary, investigators are encouraged to publish outcomes of HQL research without undue restriction.

In essence, it is often the sponsor's objective to influence the medical and regulatory decision-making environments by promoting the adoption of its instruments as standards for HQL assessment of specific therpeutic agents. In particular, the investment required to undertake HQL developmental research, which requires cross-national translation and validation, is substantial, often involving several years of ongoing support and expending in excess of $1 million. It would seem apparent that the sponsoring company would pursue the adoption of its HQL instrument as the "gold standard" for HQL assessment by public and private decision makers in specific disease areas. In so doing, the sponsoring company can, in effect, influence the evaluation of other future interventions using its approach. In this instance, a pharmaceutical company may view HQL as both a tactical product support strategy and an overall competitive marketing and policy strategy.

Because of the multinational conduct of clinical research, it should come as no surprise that HQL research is typically undertaken in several key geographic markets. Because regulatory bodies responsible for approving new drugs for marketing do not necessarily use the same criteria for considering HQL information, the utility of the research also varies among countries. Freeman (1991) observed several uses of HQL assessments by sponsoring companies (Table 5.1).

As noted in Table 5.1, HQL assessment has a number of related, but somewhat distinct applications. Because prescription drug advertising and promotion is stringently regulated throughout the industrialized world, regulatory approval for specific claims is required before a product can be marketed to physicians. In some instances, HQL information from randomized clinical trials and studies may be submitted as part of the registration dossier or New Drug Application (NDA). At present, certain European regulatory agencies responsible for drug approval appear to be receptive to granting approvals for certain indications based on the submission of HQL information. The U.S. Food and Drug Administration (FDA) is interested in HQL information, but the prevailing sentiment in the pharmaceutical industry is that the FDA will not grant a general HQL claim in approved labeling; rather, the FDA regulates HQL under its authority to regulate pharmaceutical marketing practices to ensure truth in advertising and promotion. Review sections within the U.S. FDA are thought to vary substantially according to their willingness to consider HQL information.

TABLE 5.1
Uses of Health-Related Quality of Life Research

Pharmaceutical Marketing
Product differentiation
Advertising and promotion
Reimbursement and coverage decision
Formulary inclusion
Medical and Regulatory Affairs
Secure new indications
Project exisiting indications
Justify product line extensions/dosing regimens
Justify price/reimbursement coverage
Public Policy
Influence regulatory decisions
Establish the value of drug therapy

Oncology products, for example, have profound effects on patients' HQL, and their registration dossiers (NDA) are routinely supported by comparative HQL assessments. Regardless, HQL information derived from the RCT is routinely submitted as part of the NDAs filed on a worldwide basis.

Health-related quality of life information is also frequently submitted as part of pricing dossiers during the formal negotiations that take place between the company and a governmental pricing authority. (The United States is the only major country that does not set the price of new products following market approval.) There is debate within the pharmaceutical industry as to the ultimate value of HQL information in supporting pricing and reimbursement negotiations in relation to the utility of cost-effectiveness analyses of new products. In general, there is not a consensus that reimbursement agencies actually consider HQL information as a significant criterion in a pricing or reimbursement decision; rather, such agencies emphasize the net fiscal impact of the new therapy. Alternatively, there is a prevailing belief that HQL is more important to the patient, to the primary caregivers in the family, the attending physician, and perhaps, the patient's employer.

ORGANIZATIONAL ISSUES

Because HQL has numerous applications in pharmaceutical marketing and medical affairs, the functional unit within the corporation that sponsors this type of extramural research may vary among companies. Zitter (1993) noted that there is a slight majority of companies who choose to locate HQL functions in the marketing division. The second most common locus is in the medical division. It is also not uncommon to find two units responsible for HQL assessment within the same corporation: one in the marketing division to manage product support studies for current products (Phase III-B, Phase IV clinical research), and one located in the medical division (Phases II through IV) to support future products. We should also note that the functional unit responsible for HQL assessments also carries the responsibility for conducting economic analyses of pharmaceutical products and, frequently, outcomes research. Hence, the units are typically named health economics, pharmacoecomonics, health services research, or outcomes research.

Location, more so than the unit's name, is a controversial issue within the industry with no clear consensus on the optimal choice. The key issues are as follows: Marketing is the end user of HQL information. Outcomes of HQL research must be disseminated to clinicians, pharmacists, and formulary decision makers in a format that is understandable, relevant, and timely. Because HQL is a form of product differentiation, marketing would argue that theirs is the more appropriate location for this function, as they are closer to the customer and are more experienced in communicating directly to the customer via advertising, communications pieces, and other promotional devices. The basic argument for locating the function within the medical division is that the randomized clinical trial setting is the appropriate paradigm under which HQL assessments are conducted. Moreover, the use of multinational clinical sites and the existence of long-term collaborative relationships are fundamental reasons for locating the function in the medical affairs division.

Both points are valid but fail to recognize the shortcomings of each location. First, marketing managers tend to turn over relatively quickly due to promotions and transfers, which is not particularly good for managing complex, long-term investigations. Priorities of product managers also vary among individuals, meaning that the value of HQL will change due to changes in personnel. Finally, and perhaps most significantly, marketing managers for the most part do not have formal training in HQL and do not completely understand the clinical/trial study environment. Having a dedicated health economics unit within a marketing division does mitigate some of these concerns. Regarding location in medical affairs, the most significant limitations include budgets and priorities. Health-related quality of life assessment is not universally accepted as a clinical outcome, and clinical development programs that concentrate on traditional measures of safety and efficacy will always receive priority. There is also a lingering concern that HQL assessment is not universally accepted as a clinical outcome, and clinical development programs that concentrate on traditional measures of safety and efficacy will always receive priority. There is also a lingering concern that HQL assessment will retard the submission (and FDA approval) of an NDA, which is the key measure of productivity for the medical affairs division. Finally, there is somewhat of a tendency in medical affairs to view the publication of a refereed paper or issuance of a technical report as the final product of a clinical trial or study, a perspective that may not result in the most optimal vehicle for disseminating results to the end user.

Regardless of the exact location of the sponsoring unit, it is important to note that the majority of pharmaceutical manufacturers have created professional units comprised of health economists, epidemiologists, psychologists, medical sociologists, and clinicians (physicians, pharmacists, nurses) to undertake the management of this function. As the process becomes more directly linked to the RCT, management of the function is shifting away from the applied health services researcher at the PhD level in favor of those acting at the MD/MBA level.

SPECIFIC DRUG THERAPIES AND HQL ISSUES

As implied, not all drug therapies are equally suited for HQL assessment. Drug therapies that are designed to treat acute, self-limiting diseases generally do not require substantive HQL support, especially if the clinical endpoints are terminal and universally accepted. On the other hand, disease states that are chronic, recurring, and lacking definitive curative therapies are more appropriate for HQL assessments. In these conditions the clinician's therapeutic choices are limited to managing symptoms, preventing or lessening occurrence of complications associated with the disease's progression, and in designing therapeutic regimens that allow the patient to resume activities of daily living related to work, social function, and leisure. In the case of terminal and other life-threatening conditions, the therapeutic intent is often to lift or ease the burden on the patient's primary caregiver.

Smith (1991) provided a useful summary of pharmaceutical outcomes that are especially associated with HQL outcomes assessment. Paraphrasing Smith, most instances where HQL assessments are appropriate involve diseases where traditional clinical endpoints are inadequate or inappropriate indicators of clinical efficacy. In these instances, HQL outcomes serve to complement physiological and terminal endpoint measures as evidence of efficacy. In addition to cancer, diseases such as acquired immune deficiency syndrome (AIDS), Alzheimer's disease, cardiovascular diseases (stroke, hypertension), asthma, emphysema, diabetes, osteoporosis, arthritis, and other chronic diseases are receiving special attention in HQL research. With industry support, the World Health Organization (WHO) is undertaking a major effort to develop, translate, and validate HQL instruments in mental health.

ETHICAL ISSUES

As mentioned, Hillman et al. (1991) raised the issue of avoiding or minimizing bias in industry-sponsored, pharmacoeconomic research. As a relatively new area of industry-sponsored research, there have been occasions where misunderstandings and disagreements have occurred between sponsoring companies and academic researchers. In essence, the same codes of conduct that apply to RCTs and pharmacoepidemiologic research should also apply to economic and HQL research:

1. Disclosure of financial arrangements between sponsor and research group, including disclosure of equity positions held by researchers.

2. Clear understanding of data ownership (including instruments) and use of data following completion of current study.
3. A clear statement of expectation pertaining to publication rights, including prior review (if any) by sponsor.
4. The existence of contractual arrangements describing interim and final outputs, deadlines and milestones, and mutually agreed upon reasons for termination of study.

Although it would seem obvious that these basic elements should be in place, the exploratory nature of some HQL projects has precluded their implementation in all instances. For example, in the development of a novel HQL instrument, it is not always known a priori if the instrument will work in the study or disease group tested. Issues such as item sensitivity, reliability, and validity are basically unknown, and in the presence of inconclusive evidence, the project may take a radically different form than originally conceived.

Indeed, it is often difficult to express these divergences in contractual language and some degree of flexibility in contracting is necessary. However, it is imperative to minimize the appearance of the reality of bias, and both the sponsor and research group should take all steps to ensure scientific integrity of the process. To a large extent, universities' policies and procedures for sponsored research should address these issues of bias.

A further issue related to ethical conducts is the general consensus that a "gold standard" for either general HQL or disease-specific HQL assessments does not exist. There are, however, strong opinions about existing instruments, leading to equally strong preferences, if not biases, for certain instruments. Although advocacy is not in and of itself inappropriate, the appearance of bias in favor of selected instruments to the exclusion of others is problematic. Until a consensus emerges, if ever, as to the utility of specific instruments as meeting the criteria associated with the existence of a "gold standard," the appearance of bias must be addressed.

SUMMARY AND CONCLUSIONS

Health-related quality of life information provides information to clinical and other decision makers that corroborates traditional measures of safety and efficacy. As such, HQL assessments, under proper design and execution, have become accepted information for formulary inclusion, reimbursement, and coverage by public and private payment programs. In selected European countries, HQL information has been used, in part, to grant marketing approval for certain therapeutic indications.

As in the case of RCTs, a partnership has emerged between the pharmaceutical industry and the academic research community to facilitate the development and testing of HQL instruments for both general and disease-specific use. As a relatively new partnership, additional information needs to be exchanged concerning the motives, intended uses, and business practices associated with industry-sponsored research. As a general guide, existing principles for the conduct of good clinical research should be applied to HQL research. Some degree of tension is normally expected between the two constituencies, but this will decrease as long-term research relationships are developed and maintained.

REFERENCES

Freeman, R. A. (1991). Organizational issues in outcomes management research. *Journal of Pharmacoepidemiology, 4*, 59–67.

Hillman, A. L., et al. (1991). Avoiding bias in the conduct and reporting of cost-effectiveness research sponsored by pharmaceutical companies. *New England Journal of Medicine, 324*, 1262–1265.

Smith, M. C. (1991). Medications and quality of life. *Bulletin of the Bureau of Pharmaceutical Service, 27*, 4.

Zitter, M. (1993). *How manufacturers are organizing for outcomes research: A survey by the Center for Outcomes Evaluation.* San Francisco: The Zitter Group.

II QUALITY OF LIFE AND SPECIFIC ILLNESSES

6 Quality of Life Assessment in Cancer Clinical Trials

Carol M. Moinpour
Fred Hutchinson Cancer Research Center, Seattle, WA
Marguerite Savage
Department of Veterans Affairs Medical Center, Baltimore, MD
Katherine A. Hayden
University of Arkansas for Medical Sciences
Julia Sawyers
Vanderbilt University
Christine Upchurch
Fred Hutchinson Cancer Research Center, Seattle, WA

INTRODUCTION

This chapter emphasizes health-related quality of life (HQL) asssessment in cancer clinical trials conducted by cooperative groups. Cooperative groups are organizations comprised of hospitals, Community Clinical Oncology Programs (CCOPs), other special programs such as Urological Clinical Oncology Programs (UCOPS), and hundreds of physicians, oncology nurses, and data managers around the country. These groups design and conduct studies to evaluate treatments for cancer; the trials are funded by the National Cancer Institute (NCI). There are a number of cooperative groups: for example, the Southwest Oncology Group (SWOG), Eastern Oncology Group (ECOG), Cancer and Leukemia Group-B (CALG-B), and the National Surgical Adjuvant Breast and Bowel Project (NSABP). The HQL assessment procedures described in this chapter reflect those followed by SWOG, but the conceptual approach is consistent with HQL assessment in other cooperative groups.

In late 1988, a review of the HQL literature along with considerations of SWOG needs and constraints led to a set of policies to guide inclusion of HQL measurement in SWOG clinical trials. An important point in this process was internal approval obtained from SWOG's Quality of Life Subcommittee and its parent committee, the Cancer Control Research

Committee; approval from SWOG's Board of Governors signified group-wide support for the assessment policies. The clinical meaningfulness and feasibility of the HQL assessment guidelines owe much to the experience of Katherine Hayden, at the time a SWOG oncology nurse and chairperson of the Quality of Life Subcommittee. These policies also profited from review by researchers outside SWOG such as Ivan Barofsky, Alice Kornblith, and Rosemary Yancik. A summary of these policies was published in Moinpour et al. (1989).

RATIONALE FOR COLLECTING HQL DATA

More patients are surviving cancer or are experiencing a period of significantly extended life as a result of advances in early diagnosis and treatment. However, patients are faced with multiple painful diagnostic and therapeutic events, and pain and other symptoms are experienced in the long interval between disease diagnosis and termination of treatment. Ideally, in addition to prolonging survival and disease-free intervals, treatment for cancer should reduce symptoms associated with the disease (e.g., pain associated with a tumor), not cause noxious side effects (e.g., chemotherapy-related nausea and vomiting), and improve a person's ability to return to a more normal lifestyle. This is a tall order generally not achieved (Byrne, 1992) and, more often, both the disease and its treatment degrade the well-being of the cancer patient, particularly in advanced-stage disease.

Clinical Versus HQL Endpoints

The usual endpoints in cancer clinical trials are survival time, disease-free survival time, tumor response rates, response duration, and toxicities associated with the treatment. To integrate HQL endpoints into the clincial trials database, we must decide their importance relative to the objectives of the therapeutic trial. Barofsky and Sugarbaker (1990) suggested that HQL assessment is secondary to new developments in cancer treatment but should be a critical modulating influence. In trials where cure is unlikely and palliation is the objective (e.g., protocols that address advanced or metastatic disease), HQL becomes the real endpoint (i.e., the evaluation of degree of palliation; Byrne, 1992). A comprehensive assessment of HQL addressing multiple aspects of a person's life can also suggest changes in treatment and survivor rehabilitation needs.

In SWOG trials, HQL and therapeutic endpoints are evaluated as separate outcomes. There are potentially useful approaches for combining these endpoints by describing both the quantity and quality of survival. For example, the TWiST approach defines Time Without disease Symptoms and treatment Toxicities (Gelber, Gelman, & Goldhirsch, 1989). Q-TWiST (Quality-adjusted Time Without Symptoms of disease and Toxicity of treatment; Goldhirsch, Gelber, Simes, Glasziou, & Coates, 1989) adjusts survival time by weighting time with treatment toxicities and time after relapse and adding these quantities to TWiST. Quality-adjusted life years (QALYs; Kaplan & Anderson, 1988; Kaplan & Anderson, 1990; Torrance & Feeny, 1989) is another approach. However, although there is certainly an appeal associated with an overall summary of HQL, there are problems to consider. The laboratory of cooperative group clinical trials is a busy clinic. In this setting, the complex and cognitively demanding data-collection procedures required to obtain patient preferences for different health states become less practical. Before existing preference for health state data can be confidently used in new patient groups, more research is needed regarding what factors affect these preferences and to what extent preferences change over time. Data aggregation also results in information loss, contrary to the rationale for measuring multiple HQL dimensions. Finally, attempts to use time-adjusted measures such as QALYs as a basis for clinical and policy-level decision making is controversial (LaPluma & Lawlor, 1990).

MEASUREMENT ISSUES

Definitions of HQL For Cancer Clinical Trials Research

Constraints In cancer clinical trials, we are concerned with those aspects of a patient's life most likely to be: (a) positively affected by the treatment's ameliorative effect on disease-related symptoms (e.g., pain reduction; given the absence of radiation-induced dementia, prevention of cognitive deterioration through prevention of recurrence of brain metastasis; improvement in physical functioning as a result of symptom improvement); and (b) negatively affected by the treatment itself (e.g., chemotherapy-related nausea and vomiting; sexual dysfunction resulting from prostate cancer treatment; radiation-induced dementia). Determining whether certain symptoms such as fatigue are due to the disease or the treatment is extremely difficult, even with detailed profiles of patient experience over time.

Excluded from this clinical trials definition of HQL are broader aspects of the quality of a person's life unlikely to be affected by cancer treatment but historically included by others as indicators of general HQL, such as satisfaction with occupation or housing, etc. (Andrews & Withey, 1976; Campbell, Converse, & Rodgers, 1976). These broader dimensions are excluded because, in general, medical interventions such as cancer treatment are not intended to change these indicators. The pairing of the term "health-related" with quality of life (Kaplan & Anderson, 1988; Patrick & Deyo, 1989; Patrick & Erickson, 1988) reflects the more restrictive scope of assessment appropriate for the type of cancer clinical trials research conducted by SWOG and other cooperative groups. Definitions encompassing more general indicators of HQL may be suitable for research in single institutions or for research with broader policy objectives. Such definitions require an expansion of the assessment methods presented in this chapter.

World Health Organization (WHO) Definition of Health The WHO (1958) definition of health is multidimensional, addressing both the absence of morbidity and three aspects of well-being (physical, mental, and social). Cancer patients experiencing pain identified the same three aspects of HQL as salient (Padilla, Ferrell, Grant, & Rhiner, 1990). A more recent WHO (1980) characterization describes several levels of the impact of disease on individuals: (a) the occurrence of a disease or disorder, (b) an impairment due to experienced symptoms, (c) a disability when ability to carry out activities of daily living is restricted, and (d) a handicap when the consequences affect the social realm of the person's life with potential for social disadvantages and discrimination.

Multidimensional HQL Models The three dimensions of health identified by WHO (1958) guide selection of dimensions in most health status and HQL measures. Shumaker, Anderson, and Czajkowski (1990) suggested that a multidimensional assessment approach is particularly important when we know little about the effects of the disease or treatment of the disease on the individual.

Cella and Tulsky (1990) asserted that a multidimensional HQL measure requires inclusion of at least three of the following HQL dimensions frequently assessed in research with cancer patients: functional ability (activity), occupational functioning, social functioning, emotional well-being, family well-being, spirituality, future orientation (planning, hope), sexuality/intimacy (including body image), and physical concerns (symptoms, pain). Schipper (1990) considered the four dimensions of somatic sensation, psychologic functioning, social functioning, and physical and occupational functioning as key domains of HQL. Ferrans (1990) and Ferrans and Power (1985) measured health and functioning, socioeconomic, psychological-spiritual, and family dimensions.

A multidimensional assessment of HQL informs clinicians and researchers about the following: specific effects of treatments on patients, risk-benefit trade-offs associated with a particular treatment, areas for improving cancer treatments, and survivor rehabilitation needs. The value of HQL data for suggesting change in cancer treatment was documented by the work of Sugarbaker, Barofsky, and colleagues. Quality of life findings for soft-tissue sarcoma patients who received limb-sparing surgical procedures with adjuvant therapy versus findings for those receiving amputation ran counter to expectation. The results led to changes in the surgery, the radiotherapy, and physical therapy (Barofsky & Sugarbaker, 1990; Sugarbaker, Barofsky, Rosenberg, & Gianola, 1982). Quality of life assessments obtained after these treatment revisions showed improved patient functioning (Hicks, Lampert, Gerber, Glatstein, & Danoff, 1985).

Patient Versus Proxy Report of HQL

In the past, the Karnofsky performance status scale (KPS; Karnofsky & Burchenal, 1949) was the accepted measure among physicians of the impact of treatment on the patient's overall functioning; this measure is still routinely used in clinical trials to judge functional capability of cancer patients or to stratify patients into subgroups. Examples of other commonly used physician-rated scales are the shorter version of the KPS endorsed by WHO and known variously as the ECOG, Zubrod, or WHO performance status scale (Cella & Cherin, 1987; Selby & Robertson, 1987; WHO, 1979; Zubrod et al., 1960); physician-rated toxicity scales used in cooperative group trials (Green & Weiss, 1992); and the Spitzer QL-Index, a brief index of five dimensions of HQL that can be completed by physicians, other health professionals, family members, and patients (Spitzer et al., 1981).

The validity of scales like the KPS has been documented (Orr & Aisner, 1986). However, often KPS ratings are not obtained with standardized administration procedures and reliability is affected (Cella & Cherin, 1987; Clark & Fallowfield, 1986; Frank-Stromberg, 1984; Hutchinson et al., 1979; Schag, Heinrich, & Ganz, 1984; Yates, Chalina, & McKegney, 1980). Proxy reports are distinguished from patient reports and can involve family member/significant other as well as health-care professional ratings. However, the literature indicates poor agreement between proxy and patient reports both for physician proxies (Brody, 1980; Fossa, et al., 1989; Martin et al., 1976; Martini & McDowell, 1976; Nelson et al., 1983; Slevin, Plant, Lynch, Drinkwater, & Gregory, 1988; Wartman, Morlock, Malitz, & Palm, 1983) and for family member/spouse proxies (Clarridge & Massagli, 1989; Magaziner, Simonsick, Kashner, & Heber, 1988; Slevin et al., 1988). See Sprangers and Aaronson (1992) for a comprehensive review of the agreement between patient and health-care provider/significant other ratings. For example, in general, health-care providers and significant others report patient HQL as worse than that reported by the patient (although there are studies where proxy ratings overestimate patient HQL). However, health-care providers fail to detect the intensity of pain experienced by patients and underestimate this symptom when compared to the patient's report. Sprangers and Aaronson concluded that significant others and health-care providers appear to be equally inaccurate reporters of patient HQL. For significant others, the more concrete the HQL dimension being rated, the better the agreement; closer physical contact between the significant other rater and the patient also improves agreement, but accuracy is also reduced given greater perceived caregiver burden on the part of the rater.

In SWOG trials, patient measures do not substitute for physician measures but supplement them. With respect to HQL, however, patient report is viewed as more important because we believe that the discrepancy between patient and proxy measures is the result of information that only the patient can provide. Although patient and proxy measures do not demonstrate good concordance, proxy measures can provide useful additional measures with certain patient groups (e.g., patients with brain metastases).

Other Measurement Issues

The following issues face a researcher in selecting measures to assess HQL: generic versus disease-specific measures; core plus module approach; a single instrument versus a battery of measures and, a related issue, total versus HQL dimension (separate scale) scores; and psychometric properties of the HQL scales.

Generic Versus Disease-Specific Measures. Patrick and Deyo (1989) discussed the distinction between generic and disease-specific scales. Generic health status or HQL measures address the effect of the disease and/or treatment on normal, everyday functioning and are not worded to reflect a specific disease or treatment approach. Many of the generic measures were developed to assess the health status of normal populations as well as that of different patient groups. The Medical Outcomes Study Short Form-36 (MOS SF-36) is an example of a generic HQL or health status scale (Stewart et al., 1989; Stewart, Hays, & Ware, 1988; Stewart & Ware, 1992; Ware & Sherbourne, 1992). This instrument has been used with groups of healthy individuals and in the evaluation of treatments for a variety of diseases and medical conditions. Disease-specific items are relevant to the disease (e.g., cancer or arthritis) and/or treatment (e.g., chemotherapy) of interest in the clinical trial.

Core Plus Module Approach. The core plus module approach combines a core set of items (either generic or disease-specific) addressing multiple HQL dimensions with a set of disease-specific and/or treatment-specific items. The core items are always included in the HQL battery while the module varies with the disease and/or treatment under evaluation. The European Organization for Research and Treatment of Cancer (EORTC) quality of life core questionnaire (the QLQ-C30) is an example of the core plus module approach used in cancer clinical trials (Aaronson, Ahmedzai, Bergman, et al., 1993; Aaronson, Ahmedzai, Bullinger, et al., 1991; Aaronson, Bakker, et al., 1987; Aaronson, Bullinger, & Ahmedzai, 1988). The SWOG Quality of Life Questionnaire (Moinpour et al., 1989; Moinpour, Hayden, Thompson, Feigl, & Metch, 1990) discussed in more detail in the following section is also an example of a core plus module HQL assessment strategy.

Total Score Versus Dimension Scores. Examples of single scales providing a total score are the Cancer Evaluation Rehabilitation System (CARES; Ganz, Rofessart, Polinsky, Schag, & Heinrich, 1986; Ganz, Schag, Lee, & Sim, 1992; Heinrich, Schag, & Ganz, 1984; Schag & Heinrich, 1990; Schag, Heinrich, Aadland, & Ganz, 1990), the Functional Living Index-Cancer (FLIC; Morrow, Lindke, & Black, 1992; Schipper, Clinch, McMurray, & Levitt, 1984; Schipper & Levitt, 1985), and the Functional Assessment of Cancer Therapy (FACT) scale (Cella, et al., 1993). It is not always possible to identify one instrument that includes all relevant HQL dimensions. Another approach, then, is to combine several separate instruments into an HQL battery as was done with the SWOG HQL Questionnaire. In this case, each HQL dimension might be measured by a separate scale.

Adequate Psychometric Properties. Evidence of acceptable psychometric properties is a critical criterion for selection of an HQL measure for any type of research. Of particular interest is the ability of an HQL measure to describe change over time given that treatment for cancer occurs over a period of weeks or months. In some trials, a shorter, more intensive treatment, is compared to a standard, less intensive dose that may be delivered over a longer period. There is some debate regarding the classification of sensitivity or responsiveness to change as an additional aspect of validity (Hays & Hadorn, 1992) versus its treatment as a separate psychometric property, distinct from the concepts of reliability and validity (Deyo, Diehr, & Patrick, 1991; Guyatt, Deyo, Charlson, Levine, & Mitchell, 1989; Guyatt, Walter, & Norman, 1987).

Quality of Life Assessment References

A number of HQL scales are available for use in cancer clinical trials. A report of an HQL assessment workshop conducted by NCI describes HQL instruments (Nayfield, Ganz, Moinpour, Cella, & Hailey, 1992) as do several books addressing the topic (Osoba, 1991; Spilker, 1990; Tchekmedyian & Cella, 1991). The reader is also directed to a number of review papers addressing both conceptualization and procedural issues in HQL assessment in cancer clinical trials (Aaronson, 1988, 1990; Barofsky & Sugarbaker, 1990; Cella & Cherin, 1987; Cella & Tulsky, 1990; Clark & Fallowfield, 1986; de Haes & van Knippenberg, 1987, 1988; Donovan, Sanson-Fisher, & Redman, 1989; Fayers & Jones, 1983; Frank-Stromberg, 1984; Gotay, Korn, McCabe, Moore, & Cheson, 1992a, 1992b; Hollandsworth, 1988; Moinpour et al., 1989; Najman & Levine, 1981; Osoba, 1992; Schipper, 1990; Selby & Robertson, 1987).

QUALITY OF LIFE ASSESSMENT IN SWOG CLINICAL TRIALS

SWOG HQL Questionnaire

This section describes components of the SWOG HQL Questionnaire. Table 6.1 indicates the HQL dimensions assessed in SWOG's HQL Questionnaire and the method by which each dimension is assessed. The questionnaire is a combination of generic (MOS SF scales) and symptom scales, including items assessing general symptom status (Symptom Distress Scale) and side effects of treatment (treatment-specific items). The core includes all items except the treatment-specific set, which is revised for each clinical trial depending on the disease site and treatments evaluated in the trial. In SWOG clinical trials, HQL is assessed at least three times: randomization, during treatment, and at the conclusion of the protocol-delivered treatment. The number and timing of assessments is based on the natural course of disease, the treatment schedule, and the disease stage. In three current SWOG trials, HQL assessments are occurring at least four times during the trial; one study involves annual follow-up assessments for 5 years.

Table 6.2 documents the reliability of the questionnaire's component scales and supports the use of generic scales such as the MOS-SF for research with cancer patients. These preliminary estimates of reliability are based on sample sizes available prior to completion of two of the three trials; one protocol (SWOG-9045), an advanced colorectal study, is closed. Internal consistency reliability has not yet been estimated for the treatment-specific items. It may not be possible to report a total score for the treatment-specific items; they may require reporting by item as with physician ratings of toxicities obtained in clinical trials.

TABLE 6.1
Southwest Oncology Group Quality of Life Questionnaire

	Instrument	*Number of Items*
Primary Endpoints		
Disease Treatment specific symptoms	a. Developed for protocol	Varies
	b. Symptom Distress Scale	11*
Physical functioning	MOS SF-36 Physical Functioning scale[2]	10
Emotional functioning	MOS SF-36 Mental Health Index[2]	5
Secondary Endpoints		
General symptoms	Symptom Distress Scale[1]	11*
Role functioning	MOS SF-20 role Functioning scale[2]	2
Social functioning	MOS SF-36 social Functioning scale[2]	2
Global HQL	Uniscale from LASA+[3]	1
Global health-related HQL	MOS SF-36 general health rating item[2]	1
Co-morbidity	Single item	1

*The SWOG HQL Questionnaire uses 11 of the 13 Symptom Distress Scale items.
+LASA = Linear Analogue Scale Assessment

References:
[1]Symptom Distress Scale—Benoliel and McCorkle (1980), McCorkle (1987), McCorkle and Benoliel (1983), McCorkle et al. (1989), McCorkle and Young (1978), Young and Longman (1983).
[2]MOS SF—Stewart Hays and Ware (1988), Stewart et al. (1989), Ware and Sherbourne (1992), Stewart and Ware (1992).
[3]LASA Uniscale—Selby, Chapman, Etazadi-Amoli, Dalley, and Boyd (1984), Selby, Campbell, Chapman, Etazadi-Amoli and Boyd (1984).

SWOG Quality Control Procedures

Missing Data. There are two types of missing data problems: failure to obtain questionnaires at all scheduled assessments, and failure to obtain complete questionnaires when they are submitted (i.e., patients do not answer all items). Quality control procedures are essential in order to obtain questionnaires at all assessment points. Minimizing loss-to-follow-up (to avoid biased samples) presents greater challenges in multicenter trials. In addition, care must be taken to ensure that complete data (i.e., a response to each item in the questionnaire) are obtained for each patient at each assessment period.

Poor submission rates for the HQL questionnaires in an earlier SWOG trial led to implementation of more quality control procedures in subse-

TABLE 6.2
Quality of Life Scales: Coefficient Alpha in Southwest Oncology Group Trials
MOS Short Form Scales/Symptom Distress Scale

Trial	*Physical Functioning*		*Role Functioning*		*Emotional Functioning*		*Social Functioning*		*Symptom Distress Scale*	
	ALPHA	*n*	*ALPHA*	*n*	*ALPHA*	*n*	*ALPHA*	*n*	*ALPHA*	*n*
SWOG-8994 Early Prostate	.90	92	.93	95	.84	94	.76	94	.86	86
SWOG-9039 Advanced Prostate	.94	417	.92	421	.78	426	.72	423	.84	412
SWOG-9045 Advanced Colorectal	.93	264	.93	275	.79	277	.74	276	.82	262

quent trials. The FLIC was administered in SWOG-8313, Multiple Drug Adjuvant Chemotherapy for Patients with ER Negative Stage II Carcinoma of the Breast. The HQL study was added to the ongoing therapeutic trial in December 1986 but was closed January 1989 due to poor compliance with the HQL assessment schedule (i.e., failure to obtain HQL assessments at the scheduled times). For example, of 236 patients eligible for the therapeutic trial, only 181 (77%) had the prerandomization assessment and only 109 (46%) had both a baseline and 4-month assessment. Submitted questionnaires also had missing item data. A report regarding HQL submission rates and within-questionnaire missing data for this trial is available (Hayden et al., 1993). The need to close the HQL portion of the trial led to a substantial revision of SWOG quality control procedures for HQL studies, as described here and elsewhere (Moinpour, Feigl, et al., 1989; Moinpour, Hayden, et al., 1990).

Mandatory HQL Assessments. The Southwest Oncology Group's HQL studies, since the adoption of the HQL assessment policies in 1989, have been companion studies to therapeutic trials; that is, these studies involve separate protocols (but a single consent form) for the therapeutic and HQL studies. If a patient can speak or read English (validated translations of the questionnaire do not exist), he or she cannot be registered to the therapeutic trial unless registered to the HQL protocol. This prevents biased samples for the HQL conclusions regarding study treatments and sends a message regarding the importance of the HQL data. Subsequent HQL studies will be incorporated within therapeutic trials, minimizing the need for a second protocol. However, the principle of mandatory HQL assessments (given ability to complete the questionnaire in English) will still be followed. (We were recently awarded research funds by NCI to translate the SWOG HQL Questionnaire into Spanish and validate the translation.)

Quality of Life Study Coordinator. Whether the HQL study is included within the therapeutic trial or activated as a separate study, we recommend identifying an HQL study coordinator. In SWOG, this person is usually an oncology nurse and is responsible for sending reminders to participating institutions regarding the HQL assessment schedule and being the primary contact person for questions about the HQL component.

Quality of Life Institutional Liaisons. In addition, in SWOG, we have tried to identify an HQL liaison at each major assessment site. This person can be contacted when HQL assessments are missing or when data are incomplete.

Training. The Southwest Oncology Group conducts HQL assessment training at biannual Group meetings. A video training tape recently prepared for SWOG by Burroughs Wellcome Company has greatly enhanced our ability to standardize data collection procedures and helped address the frequent staff turnover problems experienced in large cooperative groups. The Group Newsletter published quarterly is also used to highlight HQL data collection problem areas and to remind institution staff about key features of the HQL studies.

Centralized Monitoring. It has become necessary for SWOG's Statistical Center to initiate centralized monitoring of the HQL data collection schedule with regular inquiries when data are not submitted on time. A cover sheet is required with each submitted HQL questionnaire indicating whether or not the assessment was completed, the reason for nonsubmission if not completed, and report of any assistance the patient required to complete the form. In addition, institutions delinquent in submitting HQL questionnaires are now listed in monthly SWOG reports that previously included only missing clinical data; resolving such missing data has implications for an institution's standing within the cooperative group. When HQL studies were first initiated, HQL data appeared quite different and it was difficult to integrate these data into SWOG's data monitoring system. However, the same level of attention devoted to monitoring medical status data is now being applied to the HQL data.

See Moinpour, Feigl, et al. (1989), Moinpour, Hayden, et al., 1990), and Hayden et al. (1993) for a more detailed discussion of training and quality control procedures employed in SWOG HQL studies.

CONCLUSIONS

We believe that the future is bright for HQL assessment in cancer clinical trials. There is increasing physician interest and support for inclusion of

HQL endpoints in SWOG trials. Interest at the national level is also apparent. The NCI workshop on HQL assessment (Nayfield et al., 1992) allowed the cooperative groups to share experiences and suggest guidelines for assessment, quality control procedures, selection of protocols, and analysis approaches. A recent Request for Proposals released by the Division of Cancer Prevention and Control/NCI invited applications for HQL methodological research for special populations. The Food and Drug Administration (FDA) is increasingly open to consideration of HQL outcome data in the licensing of new oncologic drugs, but its definition of HQL is less multidimensional and emphasizes the amelioration of disease-related symptoms by a new drug (FDA/NCI Working Group, 1990; Johnson & Temple, 1985; Shoemaker, Burke, Dorr, Temple, & Friedman, 1990).

Although some HQL scales have been developed specifically for cancer patients (e.g., the FLIC), others have been used with patients experiencing chronic diseases and with normal populations (e.g., the MOS SF scales). The general approach used by cancer clinical trials groups such as SWOG to conduct multicenter HQL assessment is exportable to other disciplines and research settings.

ACKNOWLEDGMENTS

Dr. Moinpour was supported by grant CA 37429 from the National Cancer Institute, the National Institutes of Health, United States Public Health Service.

REFERENCES

Aaronson, N. K. (1988). Quality of life: What is it? How should it be measured? *Oncology, 2,* 69–74.

Aaronson, N. K. (1990). Quality of life research in cancer clinical trials: A need for common rules and language. *Oncology, 4,* 59–66.

Aaronson, N. K., Ahmedzai, S., Bergman, B., Bullinger, M., Cull, A., Duez, N. J., Filiberti, A., Flechtner, H., Fleishman, S. B., de Haes, J. C. J. M., Kaasa, S., Klee, M., Osoba, D., Razavi, D., Rofe, P. B., Schraub, S., Sneeuw, K., Sullivan, M., & Takeda, F. for the European Organization for Research and Treatment of Cancer Study Group on Quality of Life. (1993). The European Organization for Research and Treatment of Cancer QLQ-C30: A quality of life instrument for use in international clinical trials in oncology. *Journal of the National Cancer Institute, 85,* 365–376.

Aaronson, N. K., Ahmedzai, S., Bullinger, M., Crabeels, D., Estape, J, Filiberti, A., Flechtner H., Frick, U., Hurny, C., Kaasa, S., Klee, M., Mastilica, M., Osoba, D., Pfausler, B., Razavi, D., Rofe, P. B. C., Schraub, S., Sullivan, M., & Takeda, F. for the EORTC Study Group on Quality of Life. (1991). The EORTC Core Quality-of-Life Questionnaire: Interim results of an international field study. In D. Osoba (Ed.), *Effect of cancer on quality of life* (pp. 293–305). Boca Raton, FL: CRC Press, Inc.

Aaronson, N. K., Bakker, W., Stewart, A. L., van Dam, F. S. A. M., van Zandwijk, N., Yarnold, J. R., & Kirkpatrick, A. (1987). Multidimensional approach to the measurement of quality of life in lung cancer clinical trials. In N. K. Aaronson & J. H. Beckmann (Eds.), *Monograph series of the European Organization for Research and Treatment of Cancer,* (Vol 17, pp. 63–82). New York: Raven Press.

Aaronson, N. K., Bullinger, M., & Ahmedzai, S. (1988). A modular approach to quality-of-life assessment in cancer clinical trials. *Recent Results in Cancer Research, 111,* 231–249.

Andrews, F. M., & Withey, S. B. (Eds.). (1976). *Social indicators of well-being.* New York: Plenum.

Barofsky, I., & Sugarbaker, P. H. (1990). Cancer. In B. Spilker (Ed.), *Quality of life assessment in clinical trials* (pp. 419–439). New York: Raven Press.

Benoliel, J. Q., McCorkle, R. M., & Young, K. (1980). Development of a social dependency scale. *Research in Nursing and Health, 3,* 3–10.

Brody, D. S. (1980). Physician recognition of behavioral, psychosocial, and social aspects of medical care. *Archives of Internal Medicine, 140,* 1286–1289.

Byrne, M. (1992). Cancer chemotherapy and quality of life. Cancer trials should include measures of patients' wellbeing. *British Medical Journal, 304,* 1523–1524.

Campbell, A., Converse, P. E., & Rodgers, W. L. (Eds.). (1976). *The quality of American life.* Beverly Hills, CA: Sage.

Cella, D. F., & Cherin, E. A. (1987). Measuring quality of life in patients with cancer. In *Proceedings of the Fifth National Conference on Human Values and Cancer* (pp 23–31). New York: American Cancer Society.

Cella, D. F., & Tulsky, D. S. (1990). Measuring quality of life today: Methodological aspects. *Oncology, 4,* 29–38.

Cella, D. F., Tulsky, D. S., Gray, G., Sarafian, B., Linn, E., Bonomi, A., Silberman M., Yellen, S. B., Winicour, P., Brannon, J., Eckberg, K., Lloyd, S., Purl, S., Blendowski, C., Goodman, M., Barnicle, M., Stewart, I., McHale, M., Bonomi, P., Kaplan, E., Taylor, S., IV, Thomas, C. R., Jr., Harris, J. (1993). The Functional Assessment of Cancer Therapy Scale: Development and validation of the general measure. *Journal of Clinical Oncology, 11,* 570–579.

Clark, A., & Fallowfield, L. J. (1986). Quality of life measurements in patients with malignant disease. *Journal of the Royal Society of Medicine, 79,* 165–169.

Clarridge, B. R., & Massagli, M. P. (1989). The use of female spouse proxies in common symptom reporting. *Medical Care, 27,* 352–366.

de Haes, J. C. J. M., & van Knippenberg, F. C. E. (1987). Quality of life of cancer patients. Review of the literature. In N. K. Aaronson & J. H. Beckmann (Eds.), *The quality of life of cancer patients* (pp. 167–182). New York: Raven Press.

de Haes, J. C. J. M. & van Knippenberg, F. C. E. (1988). Measuring the quality of life of cancer patients: Psychometric properties of instruments. *Journal of Clinical Epidemiology, 42, 1043–1053.*

Deyo, R. A., Diehr, P., & Patrick, D. L. (1991). Reproducibility and responsiveness of health status measures: Statistics and strategies for evaluation. *Controlled Clinical Trials, 12*(Supp), 142S-158S.

Donovan, K., Sanson-Fisher, R. W., & Redman, S. (1989). Measuring quality of life in cancer patients. *Journal of Clinical Oncology, 7,* 959–968.

Fayers, P. M., & Jones, D. R. (1983). Measuring and analyzing quality of life in cancer clinical trials: A review. *Statistics in Medicine, 2,* 429–446.

FDA/NCI Working Group on clinical trials endpoints agrees on broader approval criteria: Survival, response rates, time to failure, life quality. (1990). *The Clinical Cancer Letter, 13,* 1–7.

Ferrans, C. E. (1990). Development of a quality of life index for patients with cancer. *Oncology Nursing Forum, 17,* 15–19.

Ferrans, C. E., & Power, M. J. (1985). Quality of life index: Development and psychometric properties. *Advances in Nursing Science, 8,* 15–24.

Fossa, S. D., Aaronson, N., Calais da Silva, F., Denis, L., Newling, D., & Hosbach, G. (1989). Quality of life in patients with muscle-infiltrating bladder cancer and hormone-resistant prostatic cancer. *European Urology, 16,* 335–339.

Frank-Stromborg, M. (1984). Selecting an instrument to measure quality of life. *Oncology Nursing Forum, 11,* 88–91.

Ganz, P. A., Rofessart, J., Polinsky, M. L., Schag, C. C., & Heinrich, R. L. (1986). A comprehensive approach to the assessment of cancer patients' rehabilitation needs: The Cancer Inventory of Problem Situations and a companion interview. *Journal of Psychosocial Oncology, 4,* 27–42.

Ganz, P. A., Schag, C. A. C., Lee, J. J., Sim, M-S. (1992). The CARES: A generic measure of health-related quality of life for patients with cancer. *Quality of Life Research, 1,* 19–29.

Gelber, R. D., Gelman, R. S., & Goldhirsch, A. (1989). A quality-of-life-oriented endpoint for comparing therapies. *Biometrics, 45,* 781–795.

Goldhirsch, A., Gelber, R. D., Simes, R. J., Glasziou, P., & Coates, A. S. (1989). Costs and benefits of adjuvant therapy in breast cancer: A quality-adjusted survival analysis. *Journal of Clinical Oncology, 7,* 36–44.

Gotay C. C., Korn, E. L., McCabe, M. S., Moore, T. D., & Cheson, B. D. (1992a). Building quality of life assessment into cancer treatment studies. *Oncology, 6,* 25–28.

Gotay, C. C., Korn, E. L., McCabe, M. S., Moore, T. D., & Cheson, B. D. (1992b). Quality of life assessment in cancer treatment protocols: Research issues in protocol development. *Journal of the National Cancer Institute, 84,* 575–579.

Green, S., & Weiss, J. R. (1992). Southwest Oncology Group standard response criteria, endpoint definitions and toxicity criteria. *Investigational New Drugs, 10,* 239–253.

Guyatt, G. H., Deyo, R. A., Charlson, M., Levine, M. N., & Mitchell, A. (1989). Responsiveness and validity in health status measurement: A clarification. *Journal of Clinical Epidemiology, 42,* 403–408.

Guyatt, G., Walter, S., & Norman, G. (1987). Measuring change over time: assessing the usefulness of evaluative instruments. *Journal of Chronic Diseases, 40,* 171–178.

Hayden, K. A., Moinpour, C. M., Metch, B., & Feigl, P., O'Bryan, R. M., Green, S., & Osborne, C. K. (1993). Pitfalls in quality of life assessment: Lessons from a Southwest Oncology Group breast cancer clinical trial. *Oncology Nursing Forum, 20,* 1415–1419.

Hays, R. D., & Hadorn, D. (1992). Responsiveness to change: An aspect of validity, not a separate dimension. *Quality of Life Research, 1,* 73–75.

Heinrich, R. L., Schag, C. C., & Ganz, P. A. (1984). Living with cancer: The Cancer Inventory of Problem Situations. *Journal of Clinical Psychology, 40,* 972–980.

Hicks, J. E., Lampert, M. H., Gerber, L. H., Glatstein, E., & Danoff, J. (1985). Functional outcome update in patients with soft tissue sarcoma undergoing wide local excision and radiation. *Archives of Physical Medicine and Rehabilitation, 66,* 542–543.

Hollandsworth, J. G., Jr. (1988). Evaluating the impact of medical treatment on quality of life: A 5-year update. *Social Science and Medicine, 26,* 425–434.

Hutchinson, T. A., Boyd, N. F., Feinstein, A. R., Gonda, A., Hollomby, D., & Rowat, B. (1979). Scientific problems in clinical scales, as demonstrated in the Karnofsky index of performance status. *Journal of Chronic Diseases, 32,* 661–666.

Johnson, J. R., & Temple, R. (1985). Food and Drug Administration requirements for approval of new anticancer drugs. *Cancer Treatment Reports, 69,* 1155–1157.

Kaplan, R. M., & Anderson, J. P. (1988). A general health policy model: Update and applications. *Health Services Research, 23,* 203–235.

Kaplan, R. M., & Anderson, J. P. (1990). The general health policy model: An integrated approach. In B. Spilker (Ed.), *Quality of life assessments in clinical trials* (pp. 131–149). New York: Raven Press.

Karnofsky D. A., & Burchenal J. H. (1949). The clinical evaluation of chemotherapeutic agents in cancer. In C. M. MacLeod (Ed.), *Evaluation of chemotherapeutic agents* (pp. 191–205). New York: Columbia University Press, New York.

LaPluma, J., & Lawlor, E. F. (1990). Quality-adjusted life-years. Ethical implications for physicians and policymakers. *Journal of the American Medical Association, 263,* 2917-2921.

Magaziner, J., Simonsick, E. M., Kashner, T. M., & Hebel, J. R. (1988). Patient-proxy response comparability on measures of patient health and functional status. *Journal of Clinical Epidemiology, 41,* 1065–1074.

Martin, D. P., Gilson, B. S., Bergner, M., Bobbitt, R. A., Pollard, W. E., Conn, J. R., & Cole, W. A. (1976). The Sickness Impact Profile: Potential use of a health status instrument for physician training. *Journal of Medical Education, 51,* 942–944.

Martini, C. J., & McDowell, I. (1976). Health status: Patient and physician judgments. *Health Services Research, 11,* 508–515.

McCorkle, R. (1987). The measurement of symptom distress. *Seminars in Oncology Nursing, 3,* 248–256.

McCorkle, R., & Benoliel, J. Q. (1983). Symptom distress, current concerns and mood disturbance after diagnosis of life-threatening disease. *Social Science and Medicine, 17,* 431-438.

McCorkle, R., Benoliel, J. Q., Donaldson, G., Georgiadou, F., Moinpour, C. M., & Goodell, B. (1989). A randomized clinical trial of home nursing care for lung cancer patients. *Cancer, 64,* 1375–1382.

McCorkle, R., & Young, K. (1978). Development of a symptom distress scale. *Cancer Nursing, 1,* 373–378.

Moinpour, C. M., Feigl, P., Metch, B., Hayden, K. A., Meyskens, F. L., & Crowley, J. (1989). Quality of life end points in cancer clinical trials: Review and recommendations. *Journal of the National Cancer Institute, 81,* 485–495.

Moinpour, C. M., Hayden, K. A., Thompson, I. M., Feigl, P., & Metch, B. (1990). Quality of life assessment in Southwest Oncology Group trials. *Oncology, 4,* 79–89.

Morrow, G. R., Lindke, J., & Black, P. (1992). Measurement of quality of life in patients: Psychometric analyses of the Functional Living Index-Cancer (FLIC). *Quality of Life Research, 1,* 287–296.

Najman, J. M., & Levine, S. (1981). Evaluating the impact of medical care and technologies on the quality of life: A review and critique. *Social Science and Medicine, 15,* 107–115.

Nayfield, S. G., Ganz, P. A., Moinpour, C. M., Cella, D. F., & Hailey, B. J. (1992). Report from a National Cancer Institute (USA) workshop on quality of life assessment in cancer clinical trials. *Quality of Life Research, 1,* 203–210.

Nelson, E., Conger, B., Douglass, R., Gephart, D., Kirk, J., Page, R., Clark, A., Johnson, K., Stone, K., Wasson, J., & Zubkoff, M. (1983). Functional health status levels of primary care patients. *Journal of the American Medical Association, 249,* 3331-3338.

Orr, S. T., & Ainser, J. (1986). Performance status assessment among oncology patients: A review. *Cancer Treatment Reports, 70,* 1423-1429.

Osoba, D. (Ed.). (1991). Effect of cancer on quality of life. Boca Raton, FL: CRC Press.

Osoba, D. (1992). The Quality of Life Committee of the Clinical Trials Group of the National Cancer Institute of Canada: Organization and functions. *Quality of Life Research, 1,* 211-218.

Padilla, G. V., Ferrell, B., Grant, M. M., & Rhiner, M. (1990). Defining the content domain of quality of life for cancer patients with pain. *Cancer Nursing, 13,* 108–115.

Patrick, D. L.,& Deyo, R. A. (1989). Generic and disease-specific measures in assessing health status and quality of life. *Medical Care, 27,* S217-S232.

Patrick, D. L., & Erickson, P. (1988). What constitutes quality of life? Concepts and dimensions. *Clinical Nutrition, 7,* 53–63.

Schag, C. C., & Heinrich, R. L. (1990). Development of a comprehensive quality of life measurement tool: CARES. *Oncology, 4,* 135–138.
Schag, C. C., Heinrich, R. L., Aadland, R. L., & Ganz, P. A. (1990). Assessing problems of cancer patients: Psychometric properties of the Cancer Inventory of Problem Situations. *Health Psychology, 9,* 83–102.
Schipper, H. (1990). Guidelines and caveats for quality of life measurement in clinical practice and research. *Oncology, 4,* 51–57.
Schipper, H., Clinch, J., McMurray, A., & Levitt, M. (1984). Measuring the quality of life of cancer patients: The Functional Living Index - Cancer: Development and validation. *Journal of Clinical Oncology, 2,* 472–483.
Schipper, H., & Levitt, M. (1985). Measuring quality of life: Risks and benefits. *Cancer Treatment Reports, 69,* 1115–1123.
Selby, P. J., Campbell, J. E., Chapman, J. A., Etazadi-Amoli, J., & Boyd, N. F. (1984). Measurement of the quality of life in patients with breast cancer. *Reviews on Endocrine-Related Cancer, 14*(Suppl), 235–247.
Selby, P. J., Chapman, J. A. W., Etazadi-Amoli, J., Dalley, D., & Boyd, N. F. (1984). The development of a method for assessing the quality of life of cancer patients. *British Journal of Cancer, 50,* 13–22.
Selby, P., & Robertson, B. (1987). Measurement of quality of life in patients with cancer. *Cancer Surveys, 6,* 521–543.
Shoemaker, D., Burke, G., Dorr, A., Temple, R., & Friedman, M. A. (1990). A regulatory perspective. In B. Spilker (Ed.), *Quality of life assessment in clinical trials* (pp. 193–201). New York: Raven Press.
Shumaker, S. A., Anderson, R. T., & Czajkowski, S. M. (1990). Psychological tests and scales. In B. Spilker (Ed.), *Quality of life assessment in clinical trials* (pp. 95–113). New York: Raven Press.
Slevin, M. L., Plant, H., Lynch, D., Drinkwater, J., & Gregory, W. M. (1988). Who should measure quality of life, the doctor or the patient? *British Journal of Cancer, 57,* 109–112.
Spilker, B. (Ed.). (1990). *Quality of life assessments in clinical trials.* New York: Raven Press.
Spitzer, W. O., Dobson, A.J., Hall, J., Chesterman, E., Levi, J., Shepherd, R., Battista, R. N., & Catchlove, B. R. (1981). Measuring the quality of life of cancer patients. A concise QL-Index for use by physicians. *Journal of Chronic Diseases, 34,* 585–597.
Sprangers, M. A. G., & Aaronson, N. K. (1992). The role of health care providers and significant others in evaluating the quality of life of patients with chronic disease: A review. *Journal of Clinical Epidemiology, 45,* 743–760.
Stewart, A. L., Greenfield, S., Hays, R. D., Wells, K., Rogers, W. H., Berry, D. S., McGlynn, E. A., & Ware, J. E., Jr. (1989). Functional status and well-being of patients with chronic conditions. Results from The Medical Outcomes Study. *Journal of the American Medical Association, 262,* 907–913.
Stewart, A. L., Hays, R. D., & Ware, J. E., Jr. (1988). The MDS Short-form General Health Survey. Reliability and validity in a patient population. *Medical Care, 26,* 724–735.
Stewart, A. L., & Ware, J. E., Jr. (Eds.). (1992). *Measuring functioning and well-being. The Medical Outcomes Study approach.* Durham, NC and London: Duke University Press.
Sugarbaker, P. H., Barofsky, I., Rosenberg, S. A., & Gianola, F. J. (1978). Quality of life assessment of patients in extremity sarcoma clinical trials. *Surgery, 91,* 17–23.
Tchekmedyian, N. S., & Cella, D. F. (Eds.). (1991). *Quality of life in oncology practice and research.* Williston Park, NJ: Dominus.
Torrance, G. W., & Feeny, D. (1989). Utilities and quality-adjusted life years. International *Journal of Technology Assessment in Health Care, 5,* 559–575.
Ware, J. E., Jr., & Sherbourne, C. D. (1992). The MOS 36-item Short-Form Health Survey (SF-36). I. Conceptual framework and item selection. *Medical Care, 30,* 473–483.

Wartman, S. A., Morlock, L. L., Malitz, F. E., & Palm, E. (1983). Impact of divergent evaluations by physicians and patients of patient's complaints. *Public Health Reports, 98,* 141–145.

World Health Organization. (1958). *The first ten years of the World Health Organization.* Geneva, Switzerland: Author.

World Health Organization. (1979). *WHO handbook for reporting results of cancer treatment* (Offset Pub. No. 48). Geneva, Switzerland: Author.

World Health Organization. (1980). *International classification of impairments, disabilities and handicaps.* Geneva, Switzerland: Author.

Yates, J. W., Chalina, B., & McKegney, F. P. (1980). Evaluation of patients with advanced cancer using the Karnofsky performance status. *Cancer, 45,* 2220–2224.

Young, K. J., & Longman, A. J. (1983). Quality of life and persons with melanoma: A pilot study. *Cancer Nursing, 6,* 219–225.

Zubrod, C. G., Schneiderman, M., Frei, E., Brindley, C., Gold, G. L., Shnider, B., Orieto, C., Gorman, J., Jones, R., Jonsson, V., Colsky, J., Chalmers, T., Ferguson, B., Dederick, M., Holland, J., Selawry, O., Regelson, W., Lasagna, L., & Owens, A. H. (1960). Appraisal methods for the study of chemotherapy of cancer in man: Comparative therapeutic trial of nitrogen mustard and triethylene thiophosphoramide. *Journal of Chronic Diseases, 11,* 7–33.

7 Quality of Life After Breast Cancer: A Decade of Research

Patricia A. Ganz
Anne Coscarelli
University of California, Los Angeles

BACKGROUND

When we began our research with breast cancer patients in the early 1980s, psychosocial oncology was a relatively new discipline (Cohen, Cullen, & Martin, 1982). At that time, much of the research in psychosocial oncology was focused on the patient's coping response to the diagnosis of cancer and its psychosocial consequences (Holland & Jacobs, 1986; Lewis & Bloom, 1978–1979; Meyerowitz, 1980). Pioneering work in cancer rehabilitation had begun in the middle to late 1970s, spurred by the funding of several demonstration projects by the National Cancer Institute (Habeck, Blandford, Sacks, & Malec, 1981; Lehmann et al., 1978; Mellette, 1977) after the passage of the National Cancer Act and Program in 1971. These investigators identified a wide range of physical, psychosocial, and vocational/economic needs in their patients, which were often neglected by health-care providers as part of routine care (Habeck et al., 1981).

Taking insight from both of these areas of research, Schag and Heinrich (Heinrich, Schag, & Ganz, 1984; Schag, Heinrich, & Ganz, 1983) began the development of a problem-focused inventory of situations that cancer patients experienced or faced on a day-to-day basis. This instrument was called the Cancer Inventory of Problem Situations (CIPS),[1] and was developed for use as a component of a competency-based model of coping

[1]The most recent version of this early instrument is called the CAncer Rehabilitation Evaluation System and is available through CARES Consultants, 2118 Wilshire Blvd., Suite 359, Santa Monica, CA 90403.

with cancer (Meyerowitz, Heinrich, & Schag, 1983). In this conceptual model, *coping* is defined as competent responses to problematic situations. The model has three components: problem specification, response enumeration, and response evaluation. The first component identifies the domain of problems with which an individual must cope and provides a normative database. The CIPS was a first effort to describe systematically the problem situations faced by cancer patients on a day-to-day basis.

There were parallel events occuring in the field of health status assessment that substantiated the reliability and validity of various approaches to examining health-related quality of life (HQL; Patrick & Deyo, 1989). Early in the 1980s, researchers in oncology began to develop new tools to assess the multiple dimensions of HQL in cancer patients (de Haes & Welvaart, 1985; Padilla & Grant, 1985; Schipper, Clinch, McMurray, & Levitt, 1984; Spitzer et al., 1981). These instruments were developed specifically for cancer patients who were often more seriously ill than other medical populations, and had specific problems related to the unique toxicities of cancer therapy. Although the CIPS was developed from a coping response and rehabilitation model, by the middle of the 1980s, we recognized that the CIPS also represented a multidimensional instrument that measured quality of life in addition to providing a detailed description of rehabilitation problems (Ganz, Schag, & Cheng, 1990; Schag & Heinrich, 1990; Schag, Heinrich, Aadland, & Ganz, 1990). Thus, much of our subsequent work was presented within the quality of life framework.

Finally, we should note that during this same decade a dramatic change took place in the treatment of breast cancer. Breast conservation treatment was performed rarely in 1980, and the medical establishment had considerable doubt about the survival equivalency of treatment with mastectomy versus breast conservation surgery followed by radiation therapy. The landmark paper published by Fisher and colleagues (1985) in the *New England Journal of Medicine* established the effectiveness of breast conservation treatment. Despite this information, there has been great variability in the adoption of breast-sparing treatment (Farrow, Hunt, & Samet, 1992; Lazovich, White, Thomas, & Moe, 1991; Nattinger, Gottlieb, Veum, Yahnke, & Goodwin, 1992). We should also note that as breast conservation became possible there was a belief held by many, and not documented by prospective research, that women would experience considerably less distress as a result of this new treatment.

In addition, breast cancer was increasingly viewed as a systemic disease at diagnosis, with greater emphasis on early adjuvant therapy with chemotherapy or endocrine therapy, even in women whose tumors were small and had not spread to the axillary lymph nodes. Thus, the intensity of treatment for primary breast cancer increased during the 1980s. Almost all women now receive some form of treatment in addition to surgery (radiotherapy, chemotherapy, tamoxifen), and these treatments can extend primary treatment for 6 months or more after surgery. We were fortunate that our quality of life studies took place during this time, and that we chose to obtain medical and quality of life data in all of our studies.

THE UCLA CANCER REHABILITATION PROJECT

In 1983, we were funded by the National Cancer Institute to develop and evaluate a case management intervention program for breast cancer patients that included rehabilitation needs assessment and referral of patients to community-based rehabilitation resources. The intervention team was staffed by a social worker (and physician consultant) whose role was to perform a comprehensive needs assessment, provide verbal and written information and reassurance, and to make referrals for services as needed. Subsequently, the social worker regularly monitored the status of the patient by telephone (at 4- to 6-week intervals), and documented the content of all intervention activities and referrals. Our case management approach is described in greater detail in our publications (Ganz, 1988; Polinsky, Fred, & Ganz, 1991).

The study design called for examining the impact of the intervention during a 12-month follow-up period after the women received their primary surgical treatment for breast cancer. This design required selection of patients who were likely to have a stable medical status during that follow-up interval, and thus we limited the study eligibiity to newly diagnosed patients with Stage I or II breast cancer. We randomly assigned all patients to the experimental case management intervention or to a minimal intervention control group. The minimal intervention consisted of a full consultation note to the patient's physician describing the results of the initial needs assessment interview. This consultation note was sent to the physicians of all participating patients (control and intervention). To evaluate the effects of the intervention, all subjects were interviewed by an independent evaluator 3, 6, and 12 months after the initial assessment. The evaluator was uninformed about the study design, intervention goals, or randomization procedure, and she conducted an interview that focused on resolution of problems that were identified initially, as well as the type and number of rehabilitation referrals received. In addition, all patients completed a battery of self-administered instruments (CIPS, Profile of Mood States, Functional Living Index-Cancer), which are described in detail in our various publications (Ganz, Schag, & Cheng, 1990; Ganz, Schag, Lee, Polinsky, & Tan, 1992).

Several developmental tasks were required to prepare for the intervention component of the study: the formulation of a comprehensive needs assessment strategy (Ganz, Rofessart, Polinsky, Schag, & Heinrich, 1986) and the creation of a referral resource network (Polinsky, Ganz, Rofessart-O'Berry, Heinrich, & Schag, 1987). For our needs assessment we found that the combination of the results from a self-administered questionnaire (the CIPS) and a clinical interview gave us the most complete picture of the patient's rehabilitation needs and psychosocial status (Ganz et al., 1986). The CIPS also provided a framework for coding the needs assessment interviews. The interview problem list allowed detailed description of rehabilitation problems identified during the interview (Ganz, Schag, Polinsky, Heinrich, & Flack, 1987). Documentation procedures were also developed for the social worker's case management intervention so that we could evaluate the efficiency of the intervention (Polinsky, Fred, & Ganz, 1991). She used the same coded problem list from the interview to track the specific problems she addressed as part of her intervention activities with each patient.

By the time the full study was initiated, it was apparent that community-wide recruitment would be necessary to achieve our accrual goals. Subjects for the randomized trial were identified from the practices of surgeons at University of California, Los Angeles (UCLA), from the clinical faculty in private practice, and from two large hospitals serving a health maintenance organization (HMO) population. This led to considerable patient diversity, with the exception that almost all patients had some form of health insurance.

EARLY RESULTS: DESCRIPTION OF THE REHABILITATION PROBLEMS OF NEWLY DIAGNOSED BREAST CANCER PATIENTS

Between 1983 and 1986, pilot work was performed prior to initiation of the definitive randomized trial in 1987. In the pilot study, patient recruitment had occurred primarily at UCLA Medical Center with some outreach into the community. The pilot study provided valuable prospective data on the rehabilitation problems of newly diagnosed breast cancer patients. Prior to that time, most studies had been cross-sectional and retrospective, and had been conducted in the era prior to breast-conserving surgery. Our work also focused on the wide range of rehabilitation needs (physical, treatment-related, psychosocial, and vocational/economic problems) that had only minimally been described in the past. Our primary source of data for this early work came from the coded problem list that was recorded at the end of the initial needs assessment interview that was conducted 1 month after breast cancer surgery. We also referred to data from the standardized measures (Global Adjustment to Illness Scale, Karnofsky Performance

Status), as well as to a simplified assessment of quality of life using a global rating and a single visual analog scale.

In 1988, we reported on our baseline needs assessment results in the first 50 women who were enrolled in the pilot study. We compared the rehabilitation problems of women receiving modified radical mastectomy with those receiving segmental mastectomy and radiation therapy (Ganz et al., 1987). We found few differences between the two surgical groups. There were no physical or psychosocial differences; however, the mastectomy group reported more difficulty with clothing and body image, whereas the breast conservation group had more disruption of recreation and social activities, probably as a result of the extended treatment period associated with radiation therapy. There were no differences on the independent measures of physical function (Karnofsky Performance Status) and psychological adjustment to illness (Profile of Mood States, Global Adjustment to Illness Scale). Marital adjustment as measured by the Dyadic Adjustment Scale was within the normal range for both groups of patients (Ganz et al., 1987).

In our randomized intervention trial, we added a number of additional independent measures to characterize the psychosocial status and quality of life of the breast cancer patients in our studies. The addition of the Functional Living Index—Cancer (FLIC) provided us with a validated measure of quality life to use as a reference measure. The FLIC also could be used to examine quality of life as an outcome measure because it provided a single score that was continuous. The Profile of Mood States (POMS) is a tool that had been widely used with other samples of cancer patients (Cella et al., 1989; Cassileth, Lusk, Brown, & Cross, 1985; Wolberg, Romsaas, Tanner, & Malec, 1989) and this enabled us to compare the mood and distress of our breast cancer patients with other breast cancer samples.

In 1989, we reported the baseline results from the first 50 patients enrolled in the randomized controlled trial and examined the differences between women receiving adjuvant therapy and those who did not (Ganz, Polinsky, Schag, & Heinrich, 1989). Of this sample, 40% were receiving either chemotherapy or tamoxifen as adjuvant therapy. We found no difference in physical or constitutional problems between the two groups; however, patients on adjuvant therapy reported more frequent psychological problems, including worry about recurrence, anxiety, and depression. They also experienced more treatment-related problems and more difficulty interacting within the health-care setting. Both groups of patients were concerned about their job performance, but patients receiving adjuvant therapy more often lacked information about their health insurance benefits and were concerned about the financial impact of the cancer diagnosis. Although the sample size was too small for statistical comparisons, the adjuvant therapy group had POMS and FLIC scores that were poorer than the no treatment group. These preliminary findings suggested that adjuvant therapy had a negative impact on quality of life as early as 1 month after primary surgery.

Intermediate Studies: Quality of Life and Breast Cancer

In 1990 we published an important methodologic paper that examined the relationship of medical and demographic factors to patient-rated quality of life (Ganz et al., 1990). This paper used data from 109 newly diagnosed breast cancer patients evaluated 1 month after breast cancer surgery in the randomized trial study. Using the FLIC score as the criterion measure of quality of life, we used regression analysis to determine if it would be possible to predict the patient's quality of life. By this time, we had performed further psychometric evaluation of the CIPS (Schag, Heinrich, Aadland, & Ganz, 1990), and the instrument was refined further and renamed the CAncer Rehabilitation Evaluation System (CARES; Schag & Heinrich, 1990). In this paper we demonstrated that the CARES global score had a strong, negative correlation with the FLIC Score ($r = -0.74$, $p < .001$). The correlation was negative because the CARES measures cancer-related problems, and therefore a higher score represents more problems and a poorer quality of life. This study along with others (Schag et al., 1990) led us to conclude that the CARES was a measure of quality of life, and that its five summary scales described five specific dimensions of HQL (physical, psychosocial, medical interaction, marital interaction, and sexual functioning).

We next asked whether certain medical or demographic variables could be used to predict quality of life. That is, if one knows the age, type of surgery, and type of treatment (e.g., adjuvant therapy), can the clinician predict the breast cancer patient's quality of life? Contrary to our a priori predictions, there was no relationship between nodal status or adjuvant chemotherapy and the patient-rated FLIC score, nor was there any relationship to the type of surgery. Furthermore, none of the demographic variables (age, education, marital status, socioeconomic status) were predictive of quality of life. These findings suggested that medical and demographic variables should not be used by the clinician to estimate the patient's quality of life.

Finally, in that report (Ganz et al., 1990), we used the detailed data from the CARES Physical and Psychosocial Summary Scales to describe the frequency of problems experienced by patients with low, medium, and high quality of life scores. Patients with the poorest quality of life had the greatest number of problems on the CARES (see Table 7.1). For example,

TABLE 7.1
Mean Number of CARES Problems in Relation to Quality of Life (QL)

	Low QL	*Mid QL*	*High QL*
Global CARES	54	36	20
Physical[a]	14	9	5
Psychosocial[b]	23	16	10
Med Interact[c]	4	2	1
Marital[d]	7	4	2
Sexual[e]	3	2	1

[a]*Physical* is the Physical summary scale from the CARES and represents those items that relate to the physical changes and disruption of daily activity caused by the disease or its treatment.

[b]*Psychosocial* is the Psychosocial summary scale from the CARES and represents psychosocial items such as psychological issues, body image difficulties, communication, and relationship (other than partner) problems.

[c]*Med Interact* is the Medical Interaction summary scale of the CARES and represents medical interaction and communication with the medical team.

[d]*Marital* is the Marital summary scale of the CARES and represents problems associated with a significant marital-type relationship; only 71 subjects were evaluated using this score.

[e]*Sexual* is the Sexual summary scale of the CARES and represents problems related to interest and performance of sexual activity.

patients with low quality of life scores endorsed an average of 23 psychosocial problems versus 10 problems on average by patients with high quality of life scores. For the subscales of the Psychosocial Summary Scale of the CARES, patients in the high quality of life group had less frequent difficulty in a range of areas (Table 7.2). For example, 88.6% of women with low quality of life scores reported difficulty with body image versus 59.3% of women with high quality of life scores. Thus, in addition to providing a summary evaluation of quality of life (the CARES Global Score), the CARES has the ability to provide detailed information about a

TABLE 7.2
Frequency of Reported Problems in the Psychosocial Subcales of the CARES in Relation to Quality of Life (QL)

Subscale	*Low QL*	*Mid QL*	*High QL*
Pt diff commun with friends/rel[a]	85.7%	65.8%	52.8%
Friends/rel diff commun with pt[b]	74.3%	47.4%	25%
Anxiety in medical situations	97.1%	94.7%	86.1%
Psychological distress	97.1%	97.4%	69.4%
Worry	97.1%	86.8%	52.8%
Cognitive difficulty	80%	57.9%	30.6%
Body image	88.6%	68.4%	59.3%

[a]Patient has difficulty communicating with friends and relatives about the cancer.

[b]Patient thinks friends and relatives have difficulty communicating with the patient about the cancer.

wide range of rehabilitation needs and problems that have an important effect on the patient's reported quality of life.

In a second methodologic paper (Ganz, Lee, Sim, Polinsky, & Schag, 1992), we explored the relationship between age, psychosocial status, and quality of life from the baseline data from the full study sample (N = 229) of newly diagnosed breast cancer patients. We introduced a casement display methodology to examine the influence of demographic and medical variables on the outcome variables of interest (psychosocial status and quality of life) and their relationship to age. The casement display method allows the two variables of interest to be plotted on the ordinate and abscissa in multiple scatterplots, with possible confounding variables shown in subsample windows. This permits visual inspection of each of the subsamples and exploratory evaluation of the influence of each variable on the entire sample and within each subgroup (see Fig. 7.1). This exploratory data analysis approach was advocated by Tukey more than a decade ago (Tukey, 1977). Since then, a number of articles and books (Chambers, Cleveland, Kleiner, & Tukey, 1983; Cleveland & McGill, 1988; Morrow, Black, & Dudgeon, 1991) have demonstrated the value of graphical data presentation techniques in analyzing complicated data sets. This paper (Ganz, Lee, et al., 1992) reflects newer trends in data analysis being used in the social and behavioral sciences (Morrow et al., 1991).

Based on the literature, we predicted a positive relationship between age and psychosocial status, but we were uncertain about the relationship between age and quality of life. For the whole sample, we found a weakly positive relationship between age and measures of psychosocial status and quality of life. However, in the exploratory studies using the casement plots, the positive relationship between age and quality of life was most strong and significant in married women and in women who had received breast conservation surgery (see Fig. 7.1). Among subgroups examined according to marital status and type of surgery, a positive relationship between age, psychosocial status, and quality of life was observed only in married women who received breast conservation surgery. Additional preliminary observations were made about the relationship of household income and age to the outcome variables that were studied. Although statistical inferences could not be made from these exploratory analyses, the evaluation of this data set suggests the important influence of a number of other variables (such as marital status) that must be considered in future studies of quality of life with breast cancer patients.

As the longitudinal data on our patient sample accumulated, we were able to examine the long-term effects of the type of surgical treatment on quality of life and rehabilitation needs. In an analysis of the first 109 patients to complete 1 year of evaluation (Ganz, Schag, et al., 1992), we found no difference in quality of life between women choosing mastectomy or breast

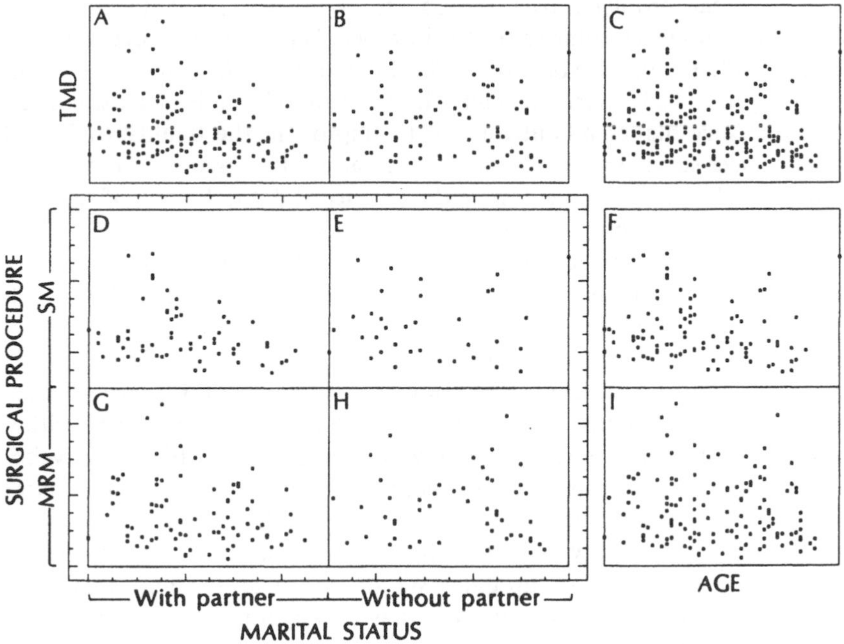

FIG. 7.1. The casement plot for age (abscissa) versus profiles of mood states total mood disturbance (TMD) (ordinate) with additional variables: type of surgery (SM = segmental mastectomy; MRM = modified radical mastectomy) and marital status. The Pearson correlation coefficients and their 95% confidence intervals (C.I.) for age versus TMD in each window are as follows: A, $r = -0.22$, C.I. = (−.37, −.06)**; B, $r = -0.02$, C.I. = (−.23, .19); C, $r = -0.12$, C.I. = (−.24, .01); D, $r = -0.27$, C.I. = (−.49, −.02)*; E, $r = 0.06$, C.I. = (−.28, .39); F, $r = -0.11$, C.I. = (−.31, .09); G, $r = -0.19$, C.I. = (−.39, .03); H, $r = -0.05$, C.I. = (−.31, .23); I, $r = -0.11$, C.I. = (−.28, .06) (* $p < .05$; ** $p < .01$) Reprinted by permission from Ganz et al. (1992).

conservation treatment. This was evidenced by no significant differences in the scores on the all of the independent and self-report outcome measures used for the study (FLIC, the CARES, the POMS, the Karnofksy Performance status score, or the Global Adjustment to Illness Scale). In addition, we found no differences in the dimensions of quality of life (physical, psychosocial, marital, sexual, medical interaction). We observed significant recovery for both surgical treatment groups during the year of follow-up in all of the dimensions of quality of life, with the exception of sexual functioning. However, to evaluate the validity of our assessment, we examined whether the CARES could detect predicted differences in the body image and clothing between the two treatment groups. As expected, we found significant differences between the two surgical groups with the breast conservation patients reporting fewer problems in each of these areas. Nevertheless, both groups of patients showed a significant recovery in body image problems over the course of the year, but no change in difficulties finding clothing to fit, for instance. Our study and several others (Fallowfield, Baum, & Maguire, 1986; Levy et al., 1992; Wolberg et al., 1989) began to tackle systematically the question of whether breast conservation surgery makes a contribution to improving the quality of life of breast cancer survivors. As we mentioned earlier, this assumption has been widely held by many people despite the paucity of data. A body of research on this topic is growing (Kiebert, de Haes, & Van de Velde, 1991).

We have recently begun to analyze the longitudinal data on our final sample of 227 patients. We have now examined all of the 31 CARES subscales. These analyses show that the body image and clothing subscales remain significantly different for the two surgical treatments; however, the remaining subscales of the CARES showed no important differences (Ganz, unpublished data). Thus, we must conclude that women who receive either mastectomy or breast conservation have similar quality of life and psychosocial adjustment after surgical treatment, and that the expected differences in body image occur, but they do not significantly affect the woman's estimation of her quality of life. However, we must note that this is the result of the analysis of group data. We do not mean to imply that for a given individual breast conservation or mastectomy might be preferable and thus affect quality of life.

In some additional studies funded by the American Cancer Society, California Division, we have been able to follow our sample of breast cancer patients in the subsequent years after their primary treatment. Approximately 150 women completed a mailed survey booklet either 2 or 3 years after their primary surgical treatment. The survey included questionnaires that were completed during the first year of the study, as well as the addition of the Medical Outcomes Study Short Form-36 (Ware & Sherbourne, 1992). We also included a number of questions that were specific to breast cancer, such as local problems from surgery, health insurance access problems, and employment problems. A subsample of these breast cancer survivors were also interviewed in person to obtain more qualitative information about their survival experience. Although our final analyses of the survivor sample are not complete, it appears that many of these women had persistent physical symptoms related to the surgical treatment (e.g., numbness and tightness of the axilla or upper arm, increased skin sensitivity), and that they frequently expressed concern about the possibility of recurrence. Nevertheless, the majority of these breast cancer survivors described positive personal outcomes as a result of the cancer experience (Ganz, 1993).

FINALE: PSYCHOSOCIAL RISK ASSESSMENT

Our extensive experience with breast cancer patients has consistently indicated that there are wide variations in the responses and experiences of women with breast cancer. Some patients appear to move through the experience with initial distress but navigate their crises well. Other women have a much more difficult time managing cancer, its treatments, and the attendant discomforts and disruptions. Our extensive prospective database on the psychosocial concerns and quality of life of newly diagnosed breast cancer patients provided us with an opportunity to examine the feasiblity of identifying predictors of psychosocial risk. Although a detailed interview performed by a professional is the current clinical standard for psychosocial assessment, such interviews are usually time consuming and expensive, and thus are rarely performed for screening purposes. In our first analysis (Ganz et al., 1993) we decided to develop a strategy for the rapid identification of newly diagnosed breast cancer patients at high risk for psychosocial morbidity. This was accomplished by having the clinical social worker (who had interviewed all 227 women at baseline) classify each woman for her baseline risk of psychosocial distress in the subsequent year. Specific detailed criteria were developed for the classification procedure, and although the social worker had ongoing contact with half of the patients, the results of the clinical classification had no significant relationship to the intervention or control status of the patient. The social worker's classification was independently validated by ratings of the Global Adjustment to Illness Scale. A logistic regression procedure was used to examine a wide range of variables (age, type of treatment, performance status, CARES scores, FLIC, POMS, etc.) for their ability to classify correctly the risk of psychosocial distress in this sample. The final model included the CARES Psychosocial Summary Scale, the Karnofsky Performance Status score, and age as the best predictors of psychosocial risk (see Table 7.3). Subsequently, these three variables were used to construct a clinically usable risk prediction model.

Although our psychosocial risk prediction model must be validated in a new sample of breast cancer patients, use of the model for screening has the potential to be substituted for the time-consuming clinical interview (1 hour or more) that we used for determining psychosocial risk. The final model selected three predictor variables (CARES Psychosocial score, KPS, age), each of which can be obtained at exceedingly low cost and

TABLE 7.3
Logistic Regression Model Joint Predictors of Patients At Risk for Psychosocial Distress

Variable	*p value*	*Odds Ratio*	*95% CI*
Age	<.001	0.3361	(.1778,.6357)
CARES Psychosocial	<.001	7.039	(3.660,13.55)
Karnofsky score	.005	0.3944	(.2070,.7516)
Constant term	.218	1.497	

Goodness-of-fit: Likelihood ratio statistic on 3 $DF = 84.21$, $p < .001$

professional effort. By using only a single predictor variable (the CARES Psychosocial Score), most of the "at-risk" women will be identified; however, a small number of women with low CARES psychosocial scores are still at risk, and the KPS and age data—both of which are readily available to a clinician without extra cost or effort—will help to identify these additional women. There is considerable simplicity and clinical relevance to this predictive model.

The model has potential value for clinical screening and for directing and guiding preventive and therapeutic psychosocial interventions. Because the CARES provides detailed clinical information on the rehabilitation needs of the patient, in addition to providing a predictive score, the CARES results can be used to tailor the specific psychosocial intervention. It can be the first step in needs identification and will allow the follow-up interviews and planning to be focused and potentially less time consuming.

Knowledge of risk status might also be useful for the primary physician who could be alerted to the woman's needs. This information might alter the physician's management of these women, for example, by providing more support and information, and might also prompt the physician to make referrals for counseling or other resources before difficulties worsen. Further, physicians and their staffs could make certain that these patients receive self-help resources that are available in their community, including existing written materials and support groups. Thus, the old adage, "an ounce of prevention is worth a pound of cure" may realistically be applied in the care of newly diagnosed breast cancer patients.

In a later article (Schag et al., 1993) we detailed the psychosocial needs of the clinically classified "low risk" and "at-risk" women using descriptive data from the CARES and our clinical interview problem list. This report clearly identifies areas in which targeted interventions are needed for newly diagnosed breast cancer patients. Furthermore, it provides validity for the social worker's judgment because patients identified at risk 1 month after diagnosis, continued to have more numerous and more severe problems in all areas (physical, psychosocial medical interaction, sexual function, and marital function) 1 year later (Schag et al., 1993).

Finally, the identification of at-risk patients is important in research settings as well. It will aid the development of new psychosocial interventions and allow testing of these interventions in the most needy population. Targeting interventions in higher risk women in research studies may help facilitate clearer outcomes. As breast cancer is a very common disease, it will be important for this predictive model to be validated in future samples of women with this disease. We are planning such studies, and attention to cost effectiveness will be important to document, especially given the importance of this issue in current medical care.

CODA: WHITHER THE EFFICACY OF THE CASE MANAGEMENT INTERVENTION?

In the final year of funding of our randomized trial, we began the task of examining the data for the major hypothesized outcome of the intervention study. Would a social worker's provision of information, reassurance, and referrals prove to have a significant impact on rehabilitation needs, referrals, and quality of life of newly diagnosed breast cancer patients? Although we have not completed our final manuscript, we have examined our data set in enough detail to know that we are not able to measure an intervention effect. We have examined the effect of the intervention on quality of life, psychosocial function, the number of rehabilitation problems at the end of one year, and the number of referrals received during the course of the year by intervention and control subjects. There was no evidence of an intervention effect for any variable. Our colleague with statistical expertise suggests that by chance, at least one variable should be significant, and the lack of such a finding implies that there may have been a systematic factor in the study design that affected our ability to detect a difference between the two study groups. Although it is possible that our intervention had no measurable effect on the outcome for the women in the intervention group, we discuss next some of our thoughts about problems in the study design and how we might do things differently in future studies.

First, it is important to recall that this was a community-based study with patients identified in the practices of surgeons who were willing to allow their patients to participate in this type of research. (A fair number of surgeons approached about the study flatly refused to participate, and others only referred occasional patients.) By and large, these surgeons were among the most psychosocially enlightened in the community, and most had excellent relationships with their patients. In our design, it should be recalled, we sent a formal consultation note to all of the referring surgeons after our initial needs assessment interview. This comprehensive note described the physical, psychosocial, and vocational/economic concerns of the patient as reported during the interview. We used this procedure because we felt it was the most ethical approach to the performance of the study; however, in retrospect, it is likely that this information was used by some of the surgeons in their subsequent interactions with their patients and that this may have limited our ability to see a significantly different outcome in the control group.

Second, our study included all women, independent of their psychosocial risk, and thus about 44% of these women were at low risk as retrospectively classified by the social worker and were likely to do well without much intervention. The number of referrals reportedly received and utilized was actually somewhat greater in the control group, and this may reflect the excellent coping skills of the low-risk women as well as the wide array of community resources that exist for breast cancer patients. Although we have not yet recalculated the sample size that would have been required to detect a meaningful difference, we believe the measurement of the intervention effect would have been more likely had we targeted the study at a higher risk group of subjects. Another important problem in our evaluation of the randomized trial outcome was that the social worker provided a considerable amount of informal support that eliminated the need for a formal referral. We observed that among the very distressed patients in either control or intervention, mental health referrals were received with the same frequency; however, among the less distressed women, the control group subjects received referrals more frequently than the intervention group subjects, lending some support to our impression that the social worker's contact provided the necessary assistance for these women.

Finally, we are not at all certain that the instruments that we chose, or others that might be available, are sensitive enough to measure the kind of differences in perceived benefit that women in the intervention group experienced. We believe the case management intervention is quite cost effective (Polinsky et al., 1991), in that it makes use of brief telephone counseling and utilizes the available community resources (Polinsky et al., 1987). We know that the women in the intervention group identified the social worker as the first person they would call to help them with a medical concern (from hot flashes to the latest newspaper article on breast cancer), or a wide array of psychosocial and economic problems. However, we are uncertain how this important form of social support can be quantified, and furthermore, how it may impact on quality of life and adjustment. Although we are disappointed about these findings, we hope to share them with others in a final paper that will discuss some of these methodological problems.

In conclusion, this decade of research has moved from the clinical assessment of the rehabilitation needs of breast cancer patients to a predictive model for the identification of women at risk for psychosocial distress in the year after breast cancer (see Table 7.4). During this time we have accumulated extensive descriptive information about the recovery of women after a diagnosis of breast cancer, and have contributed to the understanding of the dimensions of quality of life affected by breast cancer and its treatment. We have been able to share this information with our colleagues in the clinical and behavioral sciences. This body of research provides useful information for clinical intervention with patients and is an important starting point for future research studies with breast cancer survivors.

TABLE 7.4
Summary of Research with Breast Cancer Patients

Comprehensive Approach to Needs Assessment (Ganz et al., 1986)
Short Term Effects of Breast Surgery (Ganz et al., 1987)
Short Term Effects of Adjuvant Therapy (Ganz et al., 1989)
Predictors of Quality of Life in Breast Cancer Patients (Ganz et al., 1990)
Relationship of Age to Quality of Life and Psychosocial Status in Breast Cancer Patients (Ganz et al., 1992)
Longitudinal Follow-up of Breast Cancer Survivors: Does Breast Conservation Make a Difference? (Ganz et al., 1992)
Clinical Description of Women at Risk for Psychosocial Distress after Breast Cancer (Schag et al., 1993)
Development of a Psychosocial Risk Prediction Model for Patients with Breast Cancer (Ganz et al., 1993)

REFERENCES

Cassileth, B. R., Lusk, E. J., Brown, L. L., & Cross, P. (1985). Psychosocial status of cancer patients and next of kin: Normative data from the Profile of Mood States. *Journal of Psychosocial Oncology, 3*, 99–105.

Cella, D. F., Tross, S., Orav, E. J., Holland, J. C., Silberfarb, P. M., & Ralfa, S. (1989). Mood states of patients after the diagnosis of cancer. *Journal of Psychosocial Oncology, 7*, 45–54.

Chambers, J. M., Cleveland, W. S., Kleiner, B., & Tukey, P. A. (1983). *Graphical methods for data analysis*. Belmont, CA: Wadsworth.

Cleveland, W. S., & McGill, M. E. (Eds.). (1988). *Dynamic graphics for statistics*. Belmont, CA: Wadsworth.

Cohen, J., Cullen, J. W., & Martin, L. R. (Eds.). (1982). *Psychosocial aspects of cancer*. New York: Raven Press.

de Haes, J. C. J. M., & Welvaart, K. (1985). Quality of life after breast cancer surgery. *Journal of Surgical Oncology, 28*, 123–125.

Fallowfield, L. J., Baum, M., & Maguire, G. P. (1986). Effects of breast conservation on psychological morbidity associated with diagnosis and treatment of early breast cancer. *British Medical Journal, 293*, 1331–1334.

Farrow, D. C., Hunt, W. C., & Samet, J. M. (1992). Geographic variation in the treatment of localized breast cancer. *New England Journal of Medicine, 326*, 1097–1101.

Fisher, B., Bauer, M., Margolese, R., Poisson, R., Pilch, Y., Redmond, C., Fisher E., Wolmark, N., Deutsch, M., & Montague, E. (1985). Five-year results of a randomized clinical trial comparing total mastectomy and segmental mastectomy with or without radiation in the treatment of early breast cancer. *New England Journal of Medicine, 312*, 665–673.

Ganz, P. A. (1988). Patient education as a moderator of psychological distress. *Journal of Psychosocial Oncology, 6*(1–2), 181–197.

Ganz, P. A. (1993, August 2). Breast cancer survivors: Psychosocial concerns and quality of life (Final Report, Contract PR3–9). American Cancer Society, California Division.

Ganz, P. A., Hirji, K., Sim, M.-S., Schag, C. A. C., Fred, C., & Polinsky, M. L. (1993). Predicting psychosocial risk in patients with breast cancer. *Medical Care, 31*(5), 419–431.

Ganz, P. A., Lee, J. J., Sim, M.-S., Polinsky, M. L., & Schag, C. A. C. (1992). Exploring the influence of multiple variables on the relationship of age to quality of life in women with breast cancer. *Journal of Clinical Epidemiology*, *45*, 473–486.

Ganz, P. A., Polinsky, M. L., Schag, C. A. C., & Heinrich, R. L. (1989). Rehabilitation of patients with primary breast cancer: Assessing the impact of adjuvant therapy. *Recent Results in Cancer Research*, *115*, 244–254.

Ganz, P. A., Rofessart, J., Polinsky, M. L., Schag, C. C., & Heinrich, R. L. (1986). A comprehensive approach to the assessment of cancer patients' rehabilitation needs: The Cancer Inventory of Problem Situations and a companion interview. *Journal of Psychosocial Oncology*, *4*, 27–42.

Ganz, P. A., Schag, C. C., & Cheng, H. (1990). Assessing the quality of life—A study in newly diagnosed breast cancer patients. *Journal of Clinical Epidemiology*, *43*, 75–86.

Ganz, P. A., Schag, C. A. C., Lee, J. J., Polinsky, M. L., & Tan, S.-J. (1992). Breast conservation *versus* mastectomy: Is there a difference in psychological adjustment or quality of life in the year after surgery? *Cancer*, *69*(7), 1729–1738.

Ganz, P. A., Schag, C. C., Polinsky, M. L., Heinrich, R. L., & Flack, V. F. (1987). Rehabilitation needs and breast cancer: The first month after primary therapy. *Breast Cancer Research and Treatment*, *10*(3), 243–253.

Habeck, R. V., Blandford, K. K., Sacks, R., & Malec, J. (1981). *WCCC Cancer Rehabilitation and Continuing Care Needs Assessment Study Report*. (Grant No. NCI-CA-16405). Madison, WI: Wisconsin Clinical Cancer Center, Cancer Control Program.

Heinrich, R. L., Schag, C. C., & Ganz, P. A. (1984). Living with cancer: The cancer inventory of problem situations. *Journal of Clinical Psychology*, *40*, 972–980.

Holland, J. C., & Jacobs, E. (1986). Psychiatric sequelae following surgical treatment of breast cancer. *Advances in Psychosomatic Medicine*, *15*, 109–123.

Kiebert, G. M., de Haes, J. C. J. M., & Van de Velde, C. J. H. (1991). The impact of breast-conserving treatment and mastectomy on the quality of life of early-stage breast cancer patients: A review. *Journal of Clinical Oncology*, *9*, 1059–1070.

Lazovich, D., White, E., Thomas, D. B., & Moe, R. E. (1991). Underutilization of breast-conserving surgery and radiation therapy among women with stage I or II breast cancer. *Journal of the American Medical Association*, *266*, 3433–3438.

Lehmann, J., DeLisa, J., Warren, G., de Lateur, B., Sand-Bryant, P., & Nicholson, C. (1978). Cancer rehabilitation: Assessment of need, development and evaluation of a model of care. *Archives of Physical Medicine and Rehabilitation*, *59*, 410–419.

Lewis, F. M., & Bloom, J. R. (1978–1979). Psychosocial adjustment to breast cancer: A review of selected literature. *International Journal of Psychology in Medicine*, *9*, 1–17.

Levy, S. M., Haynes, L. T., Herberman, R. B., Lee, J., McFeeley, S., & Kirkwood, J. (1992). Mastectomy versus breast conservation surgery: Mental health effects at long-term follow-up. *Health Psychology*, *11*, 349–354.

Mellette, S. J. (1977). *Development and utilization of rehabilitation and continuing care resources and services for cancer patients* (Final report NCI Contract N01—CN—65287). Richmond, VA: Medical College of Virginia/Virginia Commonwealth University Cancer Center.

Meyerowitz, B. E. (1980). Psychosocial correlates of breast cancer and its treatment. *Psychological Bulletin*, *8*, 108–131.

Meyerowitz, B. E., Heinrich, R. L., & Schag, C. C. (1983). A competency-based approach to coping with cancer. In T. G. Burish & L. Bradley (Eds.), *Coping with chronic illness: Research and applications* (pp. 137–158). New York: Academic Press.

Morrow, G. R., Black, P. M., & Dudgeon, D. J. (1991). Advances in data assessment. Application to the etiology of nausea reported during chemotherapy, concerns about significance testing, and opportunities in clinical trials. *Cancer*, *67*, 780–787.

Nattinger, A. B., Gottlieb, M. D., Veum, J., Yahnke, D., & Goodwin, J. S. (1992).

Geographic variation in the use of breast-conserving treatment for breast cancer. *New England Journal of Medicine, 326,* 1102–1107.
Padilla, G., & Grant, M. (1985). Quality of life as a cancer nursing variable. *Advances in Nursing Science, 10,* 45–60.
Patrick, D. L., & Deyo, R. A. (1989). Generic and disease-specific measures in assessing health status and quality of life. *Medical Care, 27,* S217–S232.
Polinsky, M. L., Fred, C., & Ganz, P. A. (1991). Quantitative and qualitative assessment of a case management program for cancer patients. *Health and Social Work, 16,* 176–183.
Polinsky, M. L., Ganz, P. A., Rofessart-O'Berry, J., Heinrich, R. L., & Schag, C. C. (1987). Developing a comprehensive network of rehabilitation resources for referral of cancer patients. *Journal of Psychosocial Oncology, 5*(2), 1–10.
Schag, C. A. C., Ganz, P. A., Polinsky, M. L., Fred, C., Hirji, K., & Petersen, L. (1993). Characteristics of women at risk for psychosocial distress in the year after breast cancer. *Journal of Clinical Oncology, 11,* 783–793.
Schag, C. A. C., & Heinrich, R. L. (1990). Development of a comprehensive quality of life measurement tool: CARES. *Oncology, 4,* 135–138.
Schag, C. C., Heinrich, R. L., Aadland, R., & Ganz, P. A. (1990). Assessing problems of cancer patients: Psychometric properties of the cancer inventory of problem situations. *Health Psychology, 9,* 83–102.
Schag, C. C., Heinrich, R. L., & Ganz, P. A. (1983). Cancer Inventory of Problem Situations: An instrument for assessing cancer patients' rehabilitation needs. *Journal of Psychosocial Oncology, 1,* 11–24.
Schipper, H., Clinch, J., McMurray, A., & Levitt, M. (1984). Measuring the quality of life of cancer patients: The Functional Living Index–Cancer: Development and validation. *Journal of Clinical Oncology, 2,* 472–483.
Spitzer, W. O., Dobson, A. J., Hall, J., Chesterman, E., Levi, J., Shepherd R., Battista, R. N., & Catchlove, B. R. (1981). Measuring the quality of life of cancer patients: A concise QL-index for use by physicians. *Journal of Chronic Diseases, 34,* 585–597.
Tukey, J. W. (1977). *Exploratory data analysis.* Reading, MA: Addison-Wesley.
Ware, J. E., Jr., & Sherbourne, C. D. (1992). The MOS 36-item Short-Form Health Survey (SF-36). I. Conceptual framework and item selection. *Medical Care, 30,* 473–483.
Wolberg, W. H., Romsaas, E. P., Tanner, M. A., & Malec, J. F. (1989). Psychosexual adaptation to breast cancer surgery. *Cancer, 63,* 1645–1655.

8 Blood Pressure and Behavioral Effects of Antihypertensive Medications: A Preliminary Report

Alvin P. Shapiro
Matthew F. Muldoon
Shari R. Waldstein
J. Richard Jennings
Steven B. Manuck
University of Pittsburgh and Shadyside Hospital

A considerable literature exists on the effects of behavior, stress, and personality types in the development and perpetuation of hypertension. Although many questions persist, it does at least seem clear that the behavioral factor must be considered in the mosaic of the predisposition, precipitation, and perpetuation of this disorder. It is not our intention in this brief chapter to review the current status of these sequences, but rather to examine our more recent efforts to look at the other side of the coin, namely the effects of hypertension and indeed its treatment on behavior.

With this in mind, together with the late Robert Miller, we undertook over a decade ago the examination of a set of perpetual, cognitive, and psychomotor behaviors in a group of relatively young, recently discovered, and untreated mild hypertensives. We examined the hypothesis that behavioral deficiencies, albeit of a mild degree, might nevertheless play a role in certain of the overt personality characteristics of hypertensive individuals that have been described by many investigators in the past. A number of subtle performance deficits were noted by neuropsychological testing in these hypertensives, deficits that were not apparent in their usual day-to-day function. In a follow-up study, after treatment with hydrochlorothiazide and/or beta blocking agents, improvement was noted in some of these deficits (Shapiro, Miller, King, Ginchereau, & Fitzgibbon, 1982; Miller, Shapiro, King, Ginchereau, & Hosutt, 1984).

Driven by the fact that since the 1970s the use of antihypertensive medications has escalated to the point where these agents now constitute the most widely used type of prescription medication, many studies have evolved concerning drug side effects that can significantly influence the lives of hypertensive patients. Antihypertensive agents act on a variety of mechanisms that control blood pressure, including the central (CNS) and the autonomic nervous systems (ANS), and consequently symptoms such as fatigue, drowsiness, and impaired concentration are frequently reported and influence daily functioning as reflected in so-called quality of life (QOL) indices as well as various tests of neuropsychological performance.

The results in the literature, however, are somewhat confusing in terms of displaying any consistency of patterns of change (Muldoon, Manuck, Shapiro, & Waldstein, 1991; Muldoon, Shapiro, Manuck, & Waldstein, 1991). Different drugs have different effects. Studies often are not randomized or lack careful controls. Age, gender, and race play a role in these outcomes. There are differences between the changes noted in subjective, often self-scoring, QOL tests and neuropsychological tests in cognitive and other areas, tests that themselves compromise a large battery of sometimes poorly established methods. Results from QOL indices may vary considerably from those obtained or implied by neuropsychological testing. For instance, beta blockers are often noted by patients to cause slowness and fatigue, and yet in some neuropsychological tests they produce improvement in functioning. Because the untreated hypertensive patient shows some deficits, and because these deficits may improve with reduction of blood pressure, the impact of lowering blood pressure per se is not clearly separated from the direct effects of the drugs themselves.

To elucidate some of these inconsistencies in a controlled fashion, we undertook a study of six antihypertensive drugs employing a randomized, placebo-washout, crossover design with 6-week treatment periods for each drug. As of May 1992, 69 White, hypertensive males were studied. In 26 patients, hydrochlorothiazide, at a dosage of 50 mg a day was compared to methyldopa at a dosage of 500 mg a day; metoprolol at 100 mg a day was compared to atenolol at 50 mg a day in 26 patients; and enalapril at 10 mg a day was compared to verapamil at 240 mg a day in 17 individuals. In addition, hydrochlorothiazide at 50 mg a day was compared to metoprolol at 100 mg a day in 29 hypertensive African-American males. The mean blood pressure fall for all six drugs in the 69 White hypertensive males was 9.1/6.8 mmHg. When the drugs were doubled in dosage for those few patients with diastolics greater than 90 mmHg after the first 3 weeks of the 6-week period, the dose-response decrease in blood pressure was not significant.

The declines in blood pressure over the 6-week period were compared among these six different drugs that act by different mechanisms. Hydrochlorothiazide is a diuretic and lowers the blood pressure probably by sodium depletion. Atenolol and metoprolol are both beta blockers, which are somewhat specific as beta-1 central antagonists, but atenolol is hydrophilic and less apt to enter the CNS than metoprolol. Methyldopa is a CNS acting alpha agonist, which results in peripheral blood pressure lowering, and in

QOL scales has been noted to produce drowsiness; verapamil is a calcium blocking agent reported to have few if any CNS side effects. Nevertheless, there was no significant difference in the degree of blood pressure lowering among the six drugs, despite the fact that they act by such varied mechanisms. Compliance was excellent and identical for all six drugs, and the Bulpitt inventory, a QOL scale often used in studies of antihypertensive agents (Bulpitt & Fletcher, 1985), revealed no notable differences amongst the drugs (Fig. 8.1).

On the other hand, in the 29 African-American males, hydrochlorothiazide lowered blood pressure 17.6/10.6 mmHg in contrast to metoprolol which lowered it only 6.7/2.0 mmHg, a difference significant at the .02 level (Fig. 8.1). Again there were no differences in compliance or in scores on the Bulpitt scale.

All patients completed a battery of neuropsychological tests during each drug and placebo period. The results of these behavioral tests for the six different antihypertensives are at the time of this presentation still undergoing completion of detailed analysis. However, a number of observations can be reported. All the medications were associated with a slight reduction

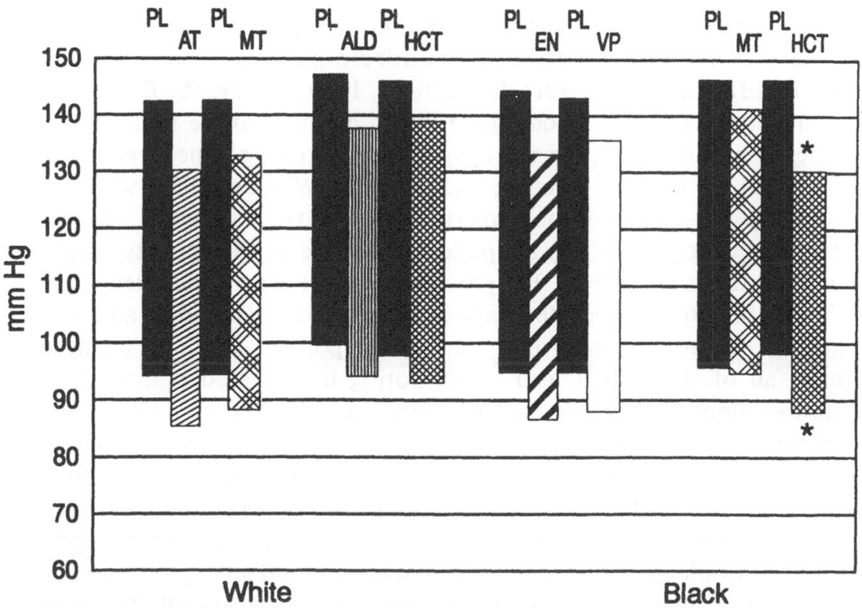

FIG. 8.1. Effects of 6 different antihypertensive drugs on blood pressure in 69 White patients and 29 African-American patients. There is no significant difference between these effects, except for the difference between MT and HCT in African-American males. (PL = placebo; AT = atenolol; MT = metoprolol; ALD = alpha methyldopa; HCT = hydrochorothiazide; EN = enalapril; VP = verapamil).

in mental flexibility as derived from the Trail Making test (Reitan, 1958), perhaps most marked with verapamil. Psychomotor skills and verbal memory were actually improved with beta blockers. Enalapril also improved verbal memory performance, whereas verapamil was associated with diminished memory in both immediate and delayed recall. This preliminary analysis applies only to the White hypertensive group; the data on African-American hypertensives remain to be completed.

DISCUSSION

Although the results from the neurobehavioral testing are preliminary, certain observations can be made at this time. Despite the fact that with these six agents the blood pressure lowering effects were not significantly different, our data suggest that different antihypertensive agents do differentially impact on cognitive and psychomotor performance. There is, however, little evidence to indicate that these neurobehavioral consequences affect normal day-to-day activities, and no particular agent seems to be contraindicated, at least for the period of time represented in these studies, because of its behavioral effects.

What has also been revealing is the inability of QOL scales and other such estimates of behavioral effects garnered from patients' subjective descriptions to differentially measure drug effects. In our study, the Bulpitt scales revealed no differences among the drugs in contrast to the findings, albeit subtle, determined from the neuropsychological testing. One is reminded of the studies of Jachuk, Brierley, Jachuk, and Willcox (1982) who, when examining the effect of antihypertensive agents, had QOL ratings of behavioral changes made by the patients' physicians, the patients' relatives, and the patients themselves. The physicians reported no impairments, about 50% of the patients reported various changes in their mood and affect, whereas the patients' relatives—usually the spouses—reported changes in almost all of them. It is also worth noting in our studies that in some instances improvement in performance seems to occur; this may be particularly true of the beta blockers that have been noted to enhance performance in certain musical and sports activities and have been used by many performers often in an unprescribed fashion (Muldoon, Shapiro et al., 1991; Muldoon, Manuck et al., 1991). On the other hand, verapamil, which we would not have predicted would have effects, produced subtle changes in memory and recall and has been used as a second line agent in manic depression (Eccleston & Cole, 1990). Reasons for effects of calcium channel blockers on CNS function are provided in the literature. These reasons include influences on CNS neurotransmission by affecting receptors and altering properties of membrane mechanisms dependent on calcium channels (Pucilowski, 1992).

We emphasize that our work as well as that by others, although highly suggestive of different neurobehavioral effects of various antihypertensive drugs, remains inconsistent. Carefully controlled studies, done prospectively and with establishment of hypotheses, are necessary to elucidate these areas further and should be part of clinical trials of antihypertensive drugs. Objective neurobehavioral measures, rather than QOL scales alone, should be used. We have now developed the pharmacological skills to control hypertension effectively, but medication for most patients will be long term. Accordingly, behavioral changes will need increased understanding as we fine tune our therapies, which may continue for the lifetime of the patients. Fortunately, for the drugs commonly used at present, the changes noted to date are modest, do not impact greatly on lifestyle, and should not inhibit their use for their beneficial effects on morbidity and mortality in hypertensive and other cardiac disorders.

ACKNOWLEDGMENTS

We appreciate the assistance of Drs. Christopher M. Ryan and Joanna M. Polefrone in these studies. This work was supported by NHLBI Grants HL40962 and HL46328.

REFERENCES

Bulpitt, C. J., & Fletcher, A. E. (1985). Quality of life in hypertensive patients on different antihypertensive treatments: Rationale for methods employed in a multicenter, randomized, controlled trial. *Journal Cardiovascular Pharmacology, 7*(Suppl. 1), S137–S145.

Eccleston, D., & Cole, A. J. (1990). Calcium-channel blockade and depressive illness. *British Journal of Psychology, 15*, 889–891.

Jachuk, S. J., Brierley, H., Jachuk, S., & Willcox, P. M. (1982). The effect of hypotensive drugs on the quality of life. *Journal of the College of General Practitioners, 32,* 103–105.

Miller, R. E., Shapiro, A. P., King, H. E., Ginchereau, E. H., & Hosutt, J. A. (1984). Effect of antihypertensive treatment on the behavioral consequences of elevated blood pressure. *Hypertension, 6,* 202–208.

Muldoon, M. F., Manuck, S. B., Shapiro, A. P., & Waldstein, S. R. (1991). Neurobehavioral effects of antihypertensive medications. *Hypertension, 9,* 549–559.

Muldoon, M. F., Shapiro, A. P., Manuck, S. B., & Waldstein, S. R. (1991). Behavioral sequelae of antihypertensive therapy: A review. In A. P. Shapiro & A. Baum (Eds.), *Perspectives in behavioral medicine: Behavioral aspects of cardiovascular disease* (pp. 287–324). Hillsdale, NJ: Lawrence Erlbaum Associates.

Pucilowski, O. (1992). Psychopharmacological properties of calcium channel inhibitors. *Psychopharmacology, 109,* 12–29.

Reitan, R. M. (1958). Validity of the Trail Making Test as an indicator of brain damage. *Perceptual and Motor Skills, 8,* 271–276.

Shapiro, A. P., Miller, R. E., King, H. E., Ginchereau, E. H., & Fitzgibbon, K. (1982). Behavioral consequences of mild hypertension. *Hypertension, 4,* 355–360.

9 Blood Pressure Affects Cognitive Functioning: The Framingham Studies Revisited

Merrill F. Elias
Penelope K. Elias
The University of Maine

Janet Cobb
Ralph D'Agostino
Boston University

Lon R. White
National Institute on Aging

Philip A. Wolf
Boston University School of Medicine

BLOOD PRESSURE AND COGNITIVE FUNCTIONING

In this chapter we focus on the design features and results of a series of three investigations of relationships between blood pressure and cognitive functioning employing the Framingham Heart Study population (Elias, Wolf, D'Agostino, Cobb, & White, 1993; Farmer et al., 1990; Farmer, White, Abbott, et al. 1987). The results of the Elias et al. (1993) study indicated that blood pressure level and chronicity of hypertension were inversely related to measures of neuropsychological test performance, particularly those measures sensitive to memory processes and learning dependent on memory. This was true even though blood pressure and chronicity of hypertension were assessed 12 to 14 years prior to neuropsychological testing. By reviewing the relevant literature, by comparing the Elias et al. (1993) study with two previous studies of the same population (Farmer et al., 1990; Farmer, White, Kittner, et al., 1987), and by performing additional data analysis for the third, we illustrate design features that may have influenced the outcome of these studies. Such features include using multiple versus single or few measures of blood pressure on one or several occasions, time interval between blood pressure and neuropsychological assessments, medication status of the study participants, and analytic techniques that make use of the full range of test scores (linear regression models) rather than discrete categories (logistic regression models). Finally we discuss the limitations of clinical neuropsychological tests with regard to discriminating among cognitive processes such as attention, memory, and learning, and we discuss several explanatory models relating levels of blood pressure to levels of cognitive functioning.

In recent years many researchers have shown that cognitive performance, especially performance involving memory, attention, learning, and learning-set formation, is lower for hypertensives than for normotensives (Elias & Robbins, 1991; Waldstein, Manuck, Ryan, & Muldoon, 1991). However, carefully treated, essential hypertensives who are free from functionally significant "end organ" change (e.g., left ventricular hypertrophy, eye ground changes, peripheral vascular changes) do not have clinically significant levels of cognitive dysfunction (Elias, Robbins, Schultz, Streeten, & P. K. Elias, 1987). On the other hand, the lower levels of performance among hypertensive cohorts are significant from an epidemiological perspective. Even from an individual perspective, small losses in cognitive functioning can be very important for those persons who must perform at optimum levels. Slight attention, learning, and memory deficits can hinder job performance in areas of rapid technological advance and thus significantly affect the quality of life.

The most common explanation of poor performance by hypertensive cohorts is that such decrements are due to disease-related pathogenic changes in brain, including impaired metabolic function (e.g., Boller, Vrtunski, Mack, & Kim, 1977; Light, 1975; Shapiro, Miller, King, Ginchereau, & Fitzgibbon, 1982; Waldstein, Manuck, et al., 1991; Wilkie & Eisdorfer, 1971). This hypothesis gains indirect support from a recent finding that hypertensive individuals who were not aware of their hypertensive status at the time of neuropsychological testing performed more poorly than normotensive individuals on tests measuring attention, memory, and new learning (Waldstein, Ryan, Manuck, Parkinson, & Bromet, 1991). Using study participants who were unaware of their hypertension was an important control, for it has been argued that knowledge of hypertension could affect emotive or motivational behaviors (e.g., anxiety and depression), which in turn affect cognitive function, especially in testing situations (Robbins, Elias, & Schultz, 1990; Zonderman, Leu, & Costa, 1986).

Aside from asking whether hypertensive cohorts differ from normotensive cohorts, one may also ask if level of cognitive functioning declines with increases in blood pressure. The risk of cardiovascular and cerebrovascular diseases, and related morbidity and mortality, increases directly with increasing blood pressure levels across the full range of human blood pressure values (Dawber, Meadors, & Moore, 1951; Kannel, 1974; Kannel, Dawber, Sorlie, Wolf, & McNamara, 1976; Kannel, Wolf, &Verter, 1970). Thus, it logical to ask whether the same phenomenon is observed for cognitive tests that are sensitive to changes in brain-related vascular pathology.

Are increasing levels of blood pressure associated with decreasing levels of performance across a wide range of blood pressure values? Elias, Robbins, Schultz, and Pierce (1990) argued that findings of inverse associations between blood pressure and cognitive functioning are necessary, although not sufficient, to support the argument that pathophysiological mechanisms are causal with respect to relationships between hypertension and cognitive functioning. Clearly, *failure* to find inverse associations between blood pressure level and cognitive functioning would seriously weaken the pathophysiological-mechanisms hypothesis.

BLOOD PRESSURE-PERFORMANCE RELATIONSHIPS

There is evidence that level of cognitive functioning is related to magnitude of blood pressure. For hypertensive patients, Goldman, Kleinman, Snow, Bidus, and Korol (1974) found a negative correlation between diastolic blood pressure levels and performance on the Halstead-Reitan Categories test, but the sample was extremely small ($N = 12$). With a larger sample of elderly individuals ($N = 96$), Wilkie and Eisdorfer (1971) reported significant negative zero-order correlations between diastolic blood pressure and performance level on subtests of the Weschler Adult Intelligence Scale (WAIS). Light (1975) reported the same phenomenon for individuals who were administered a serial reaction time task ($N = 203$). Using multivariable, linear regression analyses with controls for age, education, and gender, Elias et al. (1990) found inverse relationships between unmedicated systolic and diastolic pressures and cognitive functioning for the Average Impairment Rating, the Categories Test, Tactile Perception Memory Test (TPT-Memory), and Tactile Perception Localization Test (TPT-Localization) from the Halstead-Reitan neuropsychological test battery ($N = 182$). Most important, these relationships were also found for never-treated individuals with blood pressure values ranging from low to borderline ($N = 135$). This finding is indicative of the influence of blood pressure increases across the full range of human blood pressure values.

A positive feature of the studies using correlation/regression analyses of the WAIS and Halstead-Reitan battery is that they were comprehensive and used common clinical measures with either normative scoring systems or cut-scores derived from neurosurgical verification. However, none of them included very large samples as is usually the case when long and comprehensive test batteries are administered.

The need to confirm or refute the finding of a negative relationship between blood pressure and cognitive functioning with a large sample stimulated the first of three investigations using the very large Framingham Heart Study population (Farmer, White, Abbott, et al. 1987). This large-sample analysis of relations between blood pressure levels and cognitive functioning was made possible because a short (25-minute) but comprehensive neuropsychological test battery, the Kaplan–Albert battery (Farmer, White, Kittner, et al., 1987), had been administered to this study population at Examinations 14 and 15.

THE FRAMINGHAM HEART STUDIES

A brief description of the Framingham study helps explain the methodological procedures employed in the research specifically examining relations between blood pressure and cognitive functioning (Studies 1–3). The Framingham Heart study is an extensive longitudinal investigation of cardiovascular disease and its precursors. Blood pressure measurements of the participants have been obtained by a physician at each biennial examination beginning in 1950. There is an ongoing and thorough screening for cardiovascular factors and subsequent events (Belanger, Cupples, & D'Agostino, 1988). Thus it has an ideal database for the study of hypertension-related biological and behavioral processes.

Study 1

The first study of blood pressure–cognitive functioning relationships (Farmer, White, Abbott, et al., 1987) used an impressively large number of subjects ($N = 2{,}023$) and a multivariate, ordinal logistic regression model with statistical control for age, education, cigarette smoking, alcohol consumption, and use of antihypertensive medications. In this cross-sectional study, the investigators expected to find a stronger relationship between blood pressure and cognitive functioning when both phenomena were measured concurrently at the only examination in which each participant received the Kaplan–Albert neuropsychological battery.

Negative Findings. Results of Study 1 failed to confirm the hypothesis of a relationship between blood pressure level and cognitive functioning. However, the negative results may have been related to one or several of the following design features. First, one or the average of two blood pressure measurements was used as the independent variable predicting cognitive functioning. The importance of multiple blood pressure measurements to obtain a more reliable blood pressure profile has been well established (Llabre et al., 1988). When relations between blood pressure and a dependent variable are strong (e.g., cardiovascular or cerebrovascular outcome measures are used), associations between these variables may be seen with few measurements of blood pressure. Otherwise, lack of reliability and consequent validity of measurement may influence study outcome. Second, Farmer, White, Abbott, et al. (1987) used blood pressure values that were measured on the same occasion that neuropsychological tests were administered. It is known that psychological testing is associated with an increase in blood pressure levels and variability (Steptoe, 1981) and differential effects may be observed depending on the initial levels of blood pressure (Sternbach, 1966). Thus, it is important to separate blood pressure measurement from assessment of neuropsychological performance when the goal is to assess the effect of the former on the latter.

In Study 1, Farmer, White, Abbott, et al. (1987) used ordinal regression analyses (Hosmer & Lemeshow, 1989) with trichotomized neuropsychological test measures expressed as good, intermediate, or poor performance categories. Ordinal regression is an excellent method to assess risk. However, this analytic procedure may be insensitive to blood pressure–cognitive performance relationships if, as Elias and his colleagues (Elias & Robbins, 1991; Elias, Robbins, & Schultz, 1987) argued, these relationships are observed primarily within a normal range of cognitive functioning and when study samples do not include individuals with complicated (e.g., cardiovascular and cerebrovascular sequelae) or secondary forms of hypertension.

Study 2

Averaged Blood Pressure Values. The importance of obtaining average blood pressure values based on multiple measurements taken at widely separated occasions was confirmed in a second study using the Framingham Study population (Farmer et al., 1990). Again, cognitive performance was measured with the Kaplan–Albert neuropsychological test battery. Methods employed were similar to those of the first study except that blood pressure profiles were obtained by averaging blood pressure values from 13 biennial examinations. The averaged blood pressure values were used as the independent variables in multiple logistic regression analyses, and an independent measure of duration of hypertension was formed from them (i.e., the chronicity variable). Chronicity was defined as the proportion of examinations in which blood pressure was in the definitely hypertensive range. Averaged blood pressure levels and chronicity of hypertension were inversely related to cognitive functioning on the composite score of the neuropsychological test battery.

Logistic Regression Analyses. Logistic regression analyses using two or three categories of cognitive performance were applied to the data of this second study (Farmer et al., 1990). Therefore, we can conclude that using dichotomous and polychotomous categories of performance as dependent variables did not preclude positive findings. However, it is still possible that use of dichotomous or even polychotomous performance categories results either in (a) increased Type II error (failure to reject the null hypothesis) with respect to tests of blood pressure/cognitive functioning relations or (b) diminished magnitudes of association.

Study 3

To verify and extend the results of the second study we conducted a third study of the same population and used a multiple linear regression analysis (Elias et al., 1993). Scores on the Kaplan–Albert battery were used in their naturally continuously distributed form rather than forced into categories as in ordinal-logistic or logistic regression analyses. In addition, fundamental objectives and design features of the third study distinguished it from the first two (Farmer, White, Abbott, et al., 1987; Farmer et al., 1990) and from others in the literature. Examination of Fig. 9.1 relates these objectives to key design features.

One major objective was to examine relationships between blood pressure and cognitive functioning in three different samples with the following features: (a) relatively few hypertensives in the sample were treated with antihypertensive medications (Parent Sample); (b) all individuals, hypertensive and normotensive, were untreated during a blood pressure measurement window covering multiple examinations (Subsample 1); and (c) no individuals were ever treated with antihypertensive medications (Subsample 2). The second objective was to determine whether blood pressure-cognitive performance relations would be observed for each of these samples when an extensive period of time intervened between blood pressure measurement and assessment of cognitive functioning.

In the earlier years of the Framingham study (1950–1960), there were many fewer types of antihypertensive medications available, and these were given only to those patients with severe hypertension (Kaplan, 1986). For example, alpha-methyldopa was first used only in 1962, and the monoamine oxidase (MAO) inhibitors were first used in 1963. The latter drugs enjoyed popularity until 1970 when propranolol came into use. Thus, we could develop a blood pressure profile for each participant based on measurements at a time when the second generation of medications was largely

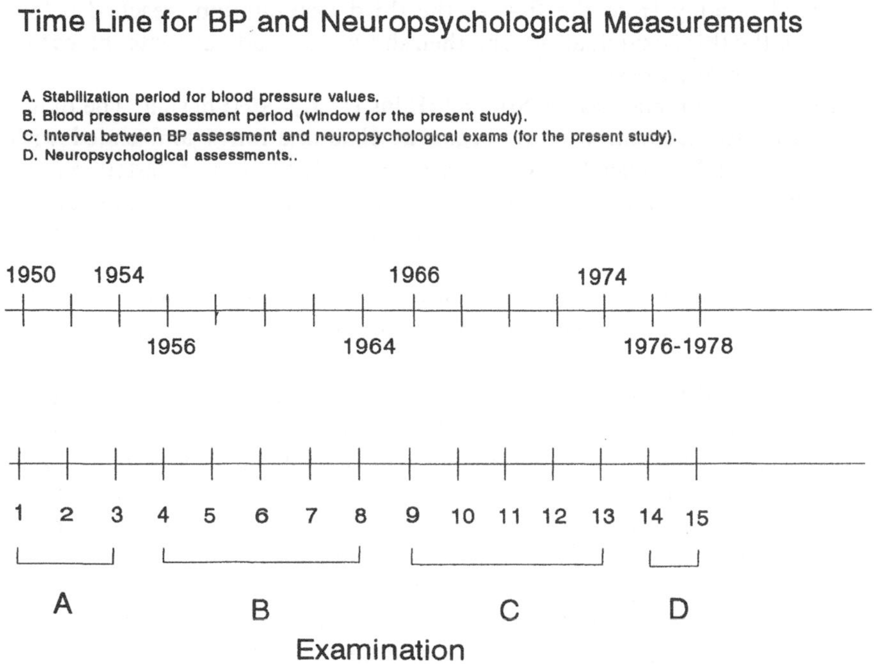

FIG. 9.1. Fundamental design features of the third study (Elias et al., 1993) of blood pressure and cognitive functioning employing the Farmingham Heart Study participants. The same design was used in the subsequent analyses reported in the present chapter.

unavailable, and only severe forms of hypertension were treated aggressively (Examinations 4–8, 1956–1964, see Fig. 9.1).

An equally important feature of our third study was the extended period of time between this "blood pressure measurement window" and administration of the Kaplan–Albert neuropsychological test battery. The battery was not introduced into the study protocol until 1976 (Examination 14). It was given on only one occasion to each subject during a 2-year period spanning Examinations 14 and 15 (1976–1978). The total number of study participants receiving the battery was 2,123.

We made use of this extended time period between the blood pressure measurements and the administration of the Kaplan–Albert battery to test whether the blood pressure profiles obtained over multiple examinations were associated with cognitive functioning measured 12 to 14 years later. The profile was constructed from the average blood pressure values obtained from four or five evaluations, always including Examination 4 values and those from either three or four subsequent evaluations (Examinations 5–8). Exclusion of blood pressure measurements from Examinations 1 to 3 was based on the finding that blood pressure in this cohort declined steadily from the first to the third examination, reached a low point at the third examination, and then showed a steady increase thereafter (Belanger et al., 1988).

Figure 9.1 summarizes the Study 3 (Elias et al., 1993) design. The blood pressure measurement window began at Examination 4 and ended with Examination 8. Depending on whether a participant was tested on the Kaplan-Albert battery at Examination 14 or 15, six to seven examinations intervened between the window and neuropsychological testing. Clearly, blood pressure was not measured concurrently with the measurement of cognitive functioning, and the design provides a very stringent test of the robustness of associations between blood pressure and cognitive performance over time.

After excluding 126 individuals who had experienced stroke at some time during the study period, 1,702 individuals met study criteria and completed all the tests. This stroke-free sample, which included treated (with antihypertensive medication) and untreated participants, was referred to as the Parent sample and was further classified into two subsamples. One group (Subsample 1, $n = 1{,}485$) included only those participants who had not taken antihypertensive medications at any time from Examinations 4 through 8 (i.e., during the blood pressure measurement window). The second (Subsample 2, $n = 1{,}038$) included participants who were untreated throughout the entire study period (Examinations 4–14/15). It is very important to note that no individual in the study reported antihypertensive medication use at the three examinations that preceded the study period (i.e., Examinations 1–3).

Neuropsychological Battery. The 20- to 25-minute Kaplan–Albert battery (Farmer, White, Kittner et al., 1987) was given at Examination 14/15 (1976–1978) and utilized tests described in Table 9.1.

A standardized score (z) was obtained for each of the eight individual test scores (i.e., $z = [\bar{X} - X]/SD$; Downey & Starry, 1977). The composite score was the sum of the z scores for each test divided by 8 (the number of tests). This linear transformation allows scores on psychometric tests of ability (which have no absolute zero point or ratio measurement properties) to be compared and averaged meaningfully.

Blood Pressure Measurement. Near the beginning of each biennial examination, systolic and diastolic blood pressure readings had been taken by the examining physician using a mercury sphygmomanometer on the left arm of seated study participants (Belanger et al., 1988; Dawber et al., 1951). These readings were used as the blood pressure values for each of the examinations included in the blood pressure measurement window.

TABLE 9.1.
A Brief Description of the Tests Making Up the Kaplan-Albert Neuropsychological Test Battery[a]

Logical Memory-Immediate Recall WMS-Form 2, Passage A. A short story is read to the examinee who is subsequently asked to retell the story. Scoring is based on the number of predetermined story elements recalled correctly by the individual. Tests short-term memory, particularly immediate recall for verbal ideas.

Visual Reproductions WMS-Form 2. Cards with designs printed on them are shown to the examinee for 5 seconds. The examinee is then asked to draw the design based on what he or she remembers of it. Scoring is based on the number of correctly drawn whole parts of the figure, accuracy of detail, and relations among figure parts. This test measures visual organization as well as visual reproductions (cf. Lezak, 1983).

Paired-Associates Learning WMS-Form 1. Fourteen word pairs representing easy and difficult word pairs are read to the examinee, and then, in a series of trials, the examinee is given one of the words and asked to give the other. Scoring is based on a weighted sum of correct number of easy and hard associations. The test places heavy demands on learning-dependent memory for new information.

Number of Digits Forward[b] WAIS Subtest. The individual is given sequences of numbers increasing in length on each of a series of trials, and then asked to repeat them correctly. The score is the greatest number of digits forward remembered correctly. The test places heavy demands on attention, or "passive span of apprehension."

Number of Digits Backward WAIS Subtest. Same as preceding, although digits are to be given back in reverse order. The score is the largest number of digits given in correct order. The test places heavy demands on "double tracking," that is, memory and reversing operations must take place at the same time.

Word Fluency[b] Multilingual Aphasia Exam. The individual is asked to say as many words as he or she can think of that begin with a designated letter of the alphabet, excluding the same word with a different suffix, proper nouns, and numbers. The score is the total number of acceptable words produced during three trials of 1 minute duration. The test measures how quickly (and presumably how easily) the examinee can produce words.

Similarities[b] WAIS Subtest. The examinee is asked in what way two words are alike and the abstractness of the similarities increase as the sequence of word pairs continues. Scoring is based on if, or how well, the similarities are described. This test places heavy demands on verbal comprehension and concept formation.

Delayed Recall (Boston Variant) WAIS Form 1, Passage A. About 20 minutes after the logical recall test is given, the individual is asked to recall the first story read. Other tests in the battery are given during the time intervening between administration of the logical memory test and the delayed recall version. Scoring is the same as for the Immediate Recall Test. Presumably this variation of the immediate recall test places more demands on memory for verbal ideas as the material must be recalled after a longer period and with interference from intervening tests and related activity.

[a]The Kaplan-Albert Neuropsychological Test Battery incorporates subtests from the Wechsler Memory Scale (WMS), the Wechsler Adult Intelligence Scale (WAIS), and the Multilingual Aphasia Examination. For descriptions of these tests see, respectively, Wechsler (1945), Wechsler (1958), and Benton and Hamsher (1976). See Lezak (1983, pp. 316–317, 325, 463–466) for evaluations, review papers, further discussion of intellectual domains measured, and for data relevant to clinical implications of significantly lowered levels of performance.

[b]Test showed nonsignificant results in multivariate regression analysis.

The predictor variables, averaged diastolic blood pressure (mmHg), averaged systolic blood pressure (mmHg), and chronicity were entered separately (along with each of the control variables) into a multiple regression analysis. Chronicity was defined as the proportion of examinations (in the blood pressure measurement window) for which blood pressure values were in the hypertensive category as defined by Framingham study criteria (Dawber et al., 1951). A systolic pressure under 140 mmHg and a diastolic pressure under 90 mmHg defined normotensive blood pressures. Either a systolic blood pressure above 160 mmHg or a diastolic pressure above 95 mmHg was defined as a definite hypertensive blood pressure value. The number of examinations for which an individual was defined as definitely hypertensive was divided by the number of examinations for which blood pressure data were available. Thus, possible chronicity values were: .00, .20, .25, .40, .50, .60, .75, .80, and 1.00.

Sample Characteristics. Mean values for averaged levels of diastolic blood pressures were 82, 81, and 80 mmHg for the Parent sample, Subsample 1 and Subsample 2; means for systolic blood pressures were 131, 128, and 123, respectively. The percentages of hypertensives in each sample declined (29%, 18%, and 8%) for the three samples as increasing numbers of individuals with medication histories were eliminated.

Ages ranged from 55 to 88 years for each sample, and mean ages were 67, 67, and 66 years, respectively. Education, in the Framingham study, is reported in nine levels rather than years; occupation is reported in seven levels ranging from unskilled to professional. No differences among the three samples were observed for mean education or occupational level, and all levels were represented in each sample. A smoker was defined as an individual reporting more than zero cigarettes a day at Examinations 14/15 and a drinker as a person reporting 1 or more ounces of alcohol per week at Examinations 14/15. There were no differences in the percentage of drinkers or smokers across the samples.

Analytic Methods. In the statistical analyses, age, education, lifetime occupation, alcohol consumption, and cigarette smoking were included in the regression model as covariates. Each variable was defined by Framingham Study criteria (Dawber et al., 1951) and, except for occupation, which we added, had been included in Studies 1 and 2. Given the importance placed on reporting data in terms of magnitude of association (rather than strength of association) relations between blood pressure and cognitive functioning (and chronicity and cognitive functioning) were expressed as regression coefficients.

Study 3 Results

With statistical control for age, education, occupation, cigarette smoking, alcohol consumption, and gender, blood pressure levels and chronicity of hypertension were inversely associated with the composite score for all tests and measures of attention, memory, and learning. These results were observed for the Parent Sample, for the subsample untreated with antihypertensive medications during the blood pressure measurement window (Subsample 1), and for the subsample untreated throughout the study period (Subsample 2).

The results of this study are elaborated elsewhere (Elias et al., 1993). In the next section of this chapter, we present data based on a very similar set of analyses, and we present the results of additional analyses performed subsequent to Elias et al. (1993).

Reanalysis of Study 3 Results

Specifically, in Study 3 (Elias et al., 1993) we emphasized a composite of all measures as the outcome variable. Therefore individuals who did not finish every test in the battery were excluded from analyses of each separate test. For data presented in this reanalysis every participant who completed a test within the battery (e.g., Logical Memory) is included in the analysis for that test, although they may not have completed all other tests. In addition to these modifications in reporting of the data, several analyses were conducted in order to make more direct comparisons between our study and Studies 1 and 2. Ordinal regression analyses were performed with (a) averaged diastolic blood pressure and (b) a single blood pressure measurement from Examination 4 used as predictors. Performance scores were divided into quartiles, and individuals received a ranking score of 0, 1, 2, or 3 for the dependent variables. Finally, logistic regression analyses were performed with predictors as in the ordinal regressions and dependent variables based on a split of performance scores into (a) upper and lower halves and (b) upper and lower quartiles.

In Table 9.2, associations between averaged diastolic blood pressure and cognitive functioning are expressed as coefficients of regression (slope coefficients), controlled for all the covariates. In subanalyses involving the Parent sample and Subsample 1 (Table 9.2), a "dummy-coded" variable (ever-medicated versus never-medicated after Examination 8, coded 0 and 1, respectively) was added to the covariate set because some subjects in these samples were medicated after the blood pressure measurement window. The medication variable was not associated with cognitive functioning, and its

TABLE 9.2
Results of Multivariate Linear Regression Analyses Describing the Relation Between Averaged Diastolic Blood Pressure (mmHg) and the Individual Neuropsychological Test Scores (z scores) for Stroke-Free Participants of the Framingham Study, 1950–1978[a]

	Parent Sample[b]		*Subsample 1*[b]		*Subsample 2*[b]	
Variable	*Beta*	*N*[c]	*Beta*	*N*	*Beta*	*N*
Logical Memory	−0.107***	1,789	−0.094***	1,561	−0.145***	1,011
Visual Reproductions	−0.087***	1,771	−0.059***	1,550	−0.088*	1,091
Paired Associates	−0.059*	1,753	−0.048	2,530	−0.071*	1,076
Digit Span Backwards	−0.065*	1,800	−0.061*	1,572	−0.112**	1,108
Logical Memory Delayed	−0.075**	1,781	−0.075**	1,554	−0.103**	1,098

[a]Regression coefficients (Beta) for averaged diastolic blood pressure express decrements in performance in standard score *z* units per 10 mmHg increments in blood pressure. Regression coefficients and statistical tests are controlled for Age, Education, Gender, Cigarette Smoking, Occupation, Alcohol Use, and, for the Parent Sample and Sample 1, use versus nonuse of Antihyptertensive Medications between Examinations 9 and 14/15 inclusive.

[b]Parent Sample—relatively few hypertensives were treated with hypertensive medications; Subsample 1—all individuals were untreated during a blood pressure measurement window (Exams 4–8); Subsample 2—no individuals were ever treated with antihypertensive medications.

[c]Differences in *N* (subjects) per test between these data and the published report of Study 3 (Elias et al., in press) are due to the fact that subjects finishing any tests (not just those finishing all tests) were included in the analysis, and the analysis including the antihypertensive medication variable in the model is shown.

*$p < .05$. **$p < .01$. ***$p < .001$.

presence in the regression model had no effect on the pattern of significant findings.

It is clear from Table 9.2, that inverse associations between blood pressure and cognitive functioning were observed for all three samples. Expressing the results in practical terms and using the never-treated sample (Subsample 2) as an example, an increase in 10 mmHg for diastolic blood pressure was associated with a decline of 0.14 *z* score (standard score) units for Logical Memory, 0.09 *z* score units for Visual Reproductions, 0.07 *z* score units for Paired Associates, 0.11 *z* score units for Digit Span Backwards, and 0.10 *z* score units for Logical Memory Delayed.

Clearly these are modest changes, but one must consider that measurement of blood pressure and assessment of cognitive functioning were separated by a period of 12 to 14 years. Moreover, Elias and Robbins (1991) pointed out that relations between blood pressure and cognitive functioning are very modest for individuals who have not suffered functionally significant "end-organ" changes associated with sustained hypertension, for example, severe cardiovascular and cerebrovascular disease or stroke (Elias, Robbins, & Schultz, 1987; Elias et al., 1990).

It is also important to consider these results in relation to the full range of blood pressures in this population. Diastolic blood pressure ranged from 56 to 120 mmHg for the Parent sample (29% hypertensive), 56 to 115 mmHg for Subsample 1 (18% hypertensive), and 56 to 99 mmHg for Subsample 2 (8% hypertensive). For Logical Memory, an increment in blood pressure from 60 to 80 mmHg would result in a decline of 0.28 z score units, or slightly more than a quarter of one standard deviation in Subsample 2.

Results for systolic blood pressure paralleled those for diastolic blood pressure, but (as may be seen in Table 9.3) regression coefficients, expressing magnitude of relationship, were consistently smaller for the former using Logical Memory as an example, $\beta = -0.05$ for systolic blood pressure and -0.11 for diastolic blood pressure. Of course, the clinical implications of 10 mmHg increase in diastolic and systolic blood pressures are different. Typically a fall in 10 mmHg diastolic blood pressure and 20 mmHg systolic blood pressure are viewed as clinically significant. Relationships between systolic and diastolic blood pressure and cognitive performance were similar for Subsamples 1 and 2.

Findings for chronicity of hypertension speak more directly to the issue of effects of hypertension on cognitive functioning. These data are most meaningful for the Parent sample where 29% of the participants were hypertensive on at least one examination. As may be seen in Table 9.4,

TABLE 9.3
Multivariate Linear Regression Coefficients (Beta) Describing Relations Between Systolic or Diastolic Blood Pressure and the Individual Neuropsychological Test Scores (z) for the Full Sample of Stroke-Free Participants of the Framingham Study, 1950–1978[a]

Variable		*Systolic BP*	*Diastolic BP*	*N/Test*
Logical Memory	Beta[b]	−0.051***	−0.107***	1789
	SE[c]	0.015	0.026	
Visual Reproductions	Beta	−0.035*	−0.087***	1771
	SE	0.014	0.027	
Paired Associates	Beta	−0.033*	−0.059*	1753
	SE	0.012	0.028	
Digit Span Backwards	Beta	−0.020	−0.065*	1800
	SE	0.016	0.028	
Logical Memory Delayed	Beta	−0.045**	−0.075*	1761
	SE	0.015	0.028	

[a]Regression coefficients and statistical tests are controlled for Age, Education, Gender, Cigarette Smoking, Occupation, Alcohol Use, and Use of Antihyptertensive Medications between Examinations 9 and 14/15 inclusive.

[b]Regression coefficients (Beta) for averaged systolic and diastolic blood pressure express change in performance in standard score units (z) per 10 mmHg increments in blood pressure.

[c]SE = Standard Error.

*$p < .05$. **$p < .01$. ***$p < .001$.

TABLE 9.4
Results of Multivariate Linear Regression Analysis with Regression Coefficients (Beta) Describing the Relation Between Chronicity of Hypertension and the Individual Neuropsychological Test Scores, Expressed in Standard Score Units (z) for the Parent Sample of Stroke-Free Participants of the Framingham Study, 1950–1978[a]

Variable	*Beta*[b]	*Standard Error*	*N/Test*
Logical Memory	−0.222**	0.084	1789
Visual Reproductions	−0.179*	0.085	1771
Paired Associates	−0.102	0.088	1753
Digit Symbol Backwards	−0.054	0.089	1800
Logical Memory Delayed	−0.183*	0.084	1761

[a]Regression coefficients and statistical tests are controlled for Age, Education, Gender, Cigarette Smoking, Occupation, Alcohol Use, and use or nonuse of Antihyptertensive Medications between Examinations 9 and 14/15 inclusive.

[b]Regression coefficients (Beta) express change in performance in standard score units (z) with increases in proportion of examinations for which participants were hypertensive.

*$p < .05$. **$p < .01$.

chronicity was related to poorer performance for Logical Memory, Visual Reproductions, and Logical Memory Delayed ($p < .05$). It is somewhat difficult to translate slope coefficients for chronicity into a practical example of performance deficit because they are expressed in proportions. However, if we use the regression coefficient for Logical Memory, assume a simple univariate regression equation, and calculate $\hat{Y}_i = \beta X_i +$ intercept, it becomes clear that an individual who was hypertensive on every examination in the blood pressure window would drop −0.22 z score units compared to an individual who was not hypertensive at any examination.

Conclusions: Study 1 Versus Study 3

In Study 3, for persons administered antihypertensive medications after a medication-free blood pressure measurement window (Subsample 1) and individuals who were never treated (Subsample 2), increments in blood pressure were associated with modestly lowered levels of cognitive performance for measures of attention, concentration, and memory. Given the negative findings of Study 1 and the positive findings of Study 3 relating blood pressure to cognitive performance, it is important to consider what features of the designs or analyses could have accounted for such opposite results.

Question 1. Would positive results have been observed if for Study 3, as in Study 1 (Farmer, White, Abbott, et al., 1987), blood pressure assessment had been limited to only one or two blood pressure measurements? It is clear from Table 9.5 that the answer is yes, but with some qualifications. Fewer dependent variables were significantly associated with blood pressure across samples, and the magnitudes of association were less consistent when Examination 4 pressure alone was used as the predictor variable. The discrepancy between findings for average blood pressures (Examinations 4–8) versus Examination 4 blood pressures only was greater when systolic, rather than diastolic, blood pressure was the predictor.

Question 2. Would the positive results of Study 3 be observed if, as in Studies 1 (Farmer, White, Abbott, et al., 1987) and 2 (Farmer, et al., 1990), ordinal or logistic regression analyses were performed with a polychotomous dependent variable? The results of our ordinal regression analyses (performed after Study 3 was submitted for publication) are shown in Table 9.6. The table shows results for all three samples, but with averaged diastolic blood pressure (ADBP) from Examinations 4–8 and Examination 4 blood pressure (DBP4) as the predictor variables. In this analysis, individuals received a performance score based on whether they were in the top quartile of performance (3), the second quartile (2), the third quartile (1), or the bottom quartile (0). In these analyses, poorer performance is associated with a higher positive score, but the signs are reversed so as to agree with the previous tables. The ordinal regression does not use the values of the performance scores, only their ordinality. It is not possible to

TABLE 9.5
Results of Multivariate Linear Regression Analysis Describing the Relation Between the Average of One or Two Blood Pressures Taken at Examination 4 and the Individual Neuropsychological Test (*z*) Scores for Stroke-Free Participants of the Framingham Study, 1950–1978[a]

Variable	*Parent Sample*[b] *Beta*[c]	*Subsample 1*[b] *Beta*[c]	*Subsample 2*[b] *Beta*[c]
Logical Memory	−0.072***	−0.072**	−0.096**
Visual Reproductions	−0.076***	−0.060**	−0.089**
Paired Associates	−0.043*	−0.044	−0.057
Digit Span Backwards	−0.037	−0.041	−0.055
Logical Memory Delayed	−0.056**	−0.048*	−0.073**

[a]Regression coefficients and statistical tests are controlled for Age, Education, Gender, Cigarette Smoking, Occupation, Alcohol Use, and use of Antihyptertensive Medications between Examinations 9 and 14/15 inclusive.

[b]Parent Sample—relatively few hypertensives were treated with hypertensive medications; Subsample 1—all individuals were untreated during a blood pressure measurement window (Exams 4–8); Subsample 2—no individuals were ever treated with antihypertensive medications.

[c]Regression coefficients (Beta) for Examination 4 diastolic blood pressure express change in performance in standard score units (*z*) per 10 mmHg increments in blood pressure.

*$p < .05$. **$p < .01$. ***$p < .001$.

TABLE 9.6
Regression Coefficients (Beta) for Multivariate Ordinal Logistic Regression Analysis Describing the Magnitude of the Relationship (in *z* scores) Between Two Independent Variables (averaged diastolic blood pressure and Examination 4 blood pressure) and Individual Neuropsychological Test Scores for Stroke-Free Participants of the Framingham Study, 1950–1978[a]

Variable	*BP Measure*	*Parent Sample*[b] *Beta*[c]	*Subsample 1*[b] *Beta*[c]	*Subsample 2*[b] *Beta*[c]
Logical Memory	ADBP[d]	−0.016***	−0.018**	−0.031***
	DBP4[e]	−0.011**	−0.012**	−0.019**
Visual Reproductions	ADBP	−0.013**	−0.009	−0.010
	DBP4	−0.011**	−0.008	−0.011
Paired Associates	ADBP	−0.008	−0.005	−0.012
	DBP4	−0.012	−0.006	−0.010
Digit Span Backwards	ADBP	−0.005	−0.005	−0.017*
	DBP4	−0.003	−0.005	−0.008
Logical Memory Delayed	ADBP	−0.014**	−0.013*	−0.021*
	DBP4	−0.008*	−0.008	−0.012

[a]Regression coefficients and statistical tests are controlled for Age, Education, Gender, Cigarette Smoking, Alcohol Use, and Occupation. Adding an Antihyptertensive Medication variable to the set of covariates had no effect on results for the Parent Sample or Subsample 1. No one was treated with antihypertensive medications throughout the study for Subsample 2.

[b]Parent Sample—relatively few hypertensives were treated with hypertensive medications; Subsample 1—all individuals were untreated during a blood pressure measurement window (Exams 4-8); Subsample 2—no individuals were ever treated with antihypertensive medications.

[c]Regression coefficients (Beta) for diastolic blood pressure express change in quartile performance score units per 10 mmHg increments in blood pressure.

[d]Averaged diastolic blood pressure (Examinations 4-8).

[e]Average of one or two pressures taken by the physician at Examination 4.

*$p < .05$. **$p < .01$. ***$p < .001$.

compare magnitude of the ordinal regression coefficients directly with those for the multiple linear regression analyses (Table 9.2) because the scales of measurement for the dependent variables are different. However, we can compare the number of significant associations ($p < .05$) observed for each sample.

For averaged blood pressure values (ADBP), increments in blood pressure level were related to poorer performance across all three samples for Logical Memory. This was also true when Examination 4 blood pressures were employed as the predictor variable in the regression analyses. For Visual Reproductions, the relationship was significant only for the Parent sample. For Digit Span Backwards averaged blood pressures were related to performance, but only for Subsample 2 (never-treated individuals). For Logical Memory Delayed, ADBP was related consistently with performance across samples, but for Examination 4 blood pressures, the relationship held only for the Parent sample.

Similar results were obtained when logistic regression analyses were based on a split between those performing in the upper and lower halves of the distribution of scores for each test, but with somewhat less consistency across subsamples. However, when categorizations were made in terms of the upper 75th percentile (presumably normal performance) versus the lower 25th percentile (presumably deficient performance), no significant blood pressure–cognitive performance relationships were observed at all. Thus, for this stroke-free sample, elevated blood pressure was not associated with clinically abnormal levels of performance, although the associations observed were of epidemiological significance.

In summary, some of the statistically significant associations between blood pressure and cognitive functioning observed in Study 3 became weaker or insignificant when analyses were repeated with methods similar to those used in Studies 1 and 2. The greater number of significant associations obtained in Study 3 may be attributed to two main factors acting in concert: (a) Standard linear regression methods are more sensitive to the full range of cognitive functioning than ordinal- or dichotomous-logistic regression analyses; (b) Blood pressures measured on several occasions, some years before assessment of cognitive functions (the procedure used in Study 3) are more reliable (total lower error variance) and more relevant to the underlying pathogenic mechanisms than one or a few blood pressures measured at or shortly before the assessment of cognitive functioning.

OVERALL CONCLUSIONS AND IMPLICATIONS

Methodological Considerations

Multiple measurements of unmedicated blood pressure and multivariate linear regression analyses using a full range of performance scores are clearly desirable design features in studies of blood pressure and behavior. Ordinal regression analyses do not preclude findings of blood pressure-performance relationships, but they are clearly less sensitive to them. Logistic regression analyses featuring simple dichotomies of performance, "good" and "poor," seem particularly insensitive to blood pressure relations. This comes as no surprise given data indicating that blood pressure-performance relations are observed within a wide range of cognitively normal behavior. (Elias, Robbins &, Schultz, 1987: Elias, Robbins, Schultz, et al., 1987).

One point with respect to relative value of logistic versus linear regression models needs to be emphasized. We are not arguing that the results of logistic regression analyses are to be mistrusted or have no utility. Indeed, they are particularly useful when one wishes to examine the relationship of disease variables to clearly defined diagnostic endpoint variables (e.g., normal cognitive functioning vs. dementia). As such they are sensitive to strong associations that are most likely to be of epidemiological and clinical significance. In this context it is important to point out that although *p* values are impressive for several of the associations revealed by our multivariate linear regression models, the magnitude of the influence of blood pressure on cognitive functioning in the Framingham study population (not necessarily in individuals) is modest when one compares it with the influences of age, education, occupation, stroke, or a dementing illness.

Attention, Learning, Memory, and Blood Pressure

The most exciting trend in the literature has been the emerging evidence that attention and memory, and new learning processes (dependent on memory and attention) are particularly vulnerable to hypertension (e.g., Blumenthal, Madden, Pierce, Siegel, & Appelbaum, 1993; Madden & Blumenthal, 1989; Waldstein, Manuck, et al., 1991; Waldstein, Ryan, et al., 1991; Wilkie & Eisdorfer, 1980). The measures for which blood pressure–performance associations were observed in this study place demands on memory and attention, or involve new learning (i.e., paired associates test), which depends on memory and attention. Our emphasis on memory and attention is important, as the relatively pure measure of attention in this study (i.e., Digit Span Forward) was not associated with blood pressure levels, and *p* values were not even close to statistically significant.

The susceptibility of attention and memory processes to hypertension, or sustained increases in blood pressure level, is hardly a new discovery. Based on a review of the literature in 1979 and earlier, Wilkie and Eisdorfer (1980) argued that tests involving memory and attention were among those that discriminated best between hypertensive and normotensive cohorts. As noted earlier, many studies since then led to the same general conclusion. Framingham Studies 2 (Farmer et al., 1990) and 3 (Elias et al., 1993) provide epidemiological credibility to this work by virtue of positive findings with extremely large samples of individuals. Study 3 and data summarized in this chapter add credibility to the argument that inverse relations between blood pressure and attention, memory, and new learning are not an artifact of concurrent treatment with antihypertensive medication or medication history. The magnitudes of the relationships observed were modest, but nonetheless of epidemiological significance, if one considers the impact of blood pressure on cognition for large populations of individuals.

While emphasizing that attention, memory, and new learning appear particularly vulnerable to increasing levels of blood pressure, it is important to recognize two things. First, most uncomplicated, essential hypertensives do not score below the normal range on tests of learning and memory. As a cohort they score significantly lower than a comparable normotensive cohort, but, taken by itself (i.e., without complicating factors such as detectable white matter lesions), essential hypertension is not associated with severe decline in cognitive functioning.

Second, clinical measures are not pure indices of memory and attention or new learning. Lezak (1983) summarized a literature indicating that Logical Memory, Visual Reproductions, and Logical Memory Delayed are weighted heavily with respect to verbal memory but inadequately measure nonverbal memory processes. The Visual Reproductions Test, although designed to measure memory, may actually place heavier demands on visual organization than visual reproduction from memory. Although Logical Memory Delayed was an adaptation of Logical Memory, the two are highly correlated and the latter measures essentially the same recall abilities as the former. Digit Span Forward appears more a pure measure of attention than Digit Span Backward. The latter appears to measure double-tracking and memory. No significant associations were observed for the former measure, but significant associations were observed for the latter. This leads to interesting hypotheses for further study, but it is unlikely that issues of relative vulnerability of memory or attention can be resolved with clinical measures. One cannot expect to isolate underlying latent variables such as attention and memory with clinical assessments. Not only are they impure measures of specific dimensions of cognitive functioning, but they often confound cognitive dimension(s) with task difficulty (Elias & Elias, 1993).

Experimental paradigms from the psychology laboratory can be used to isolate underlying cognitive abilities affected by increasing levels of blood pressure or hypertension. For example, Madden and Blumenthal (1989), and more recently Blumenthal et al. (1993), performed detailed microanalyses of short-term memory processes and found that rate of search through short-term memory was slower, on the average, for cohorts of mildly hypertensive individuals than for normotensive cohorts, although time taken to encode stimuli did not differ. Moreover, increments in diastolic blood pressure were inversely related to rate of search through short-term memory. Consistent with this study, Digit Span Backwards performance was lower for hypertensive than for normotensive cohorts. Quite a few years earlier, Watson (1976) found that the average amount of time to encode stimuli into memory did not differ for hypertensive and normotensive cohorts. Microanalyses of learning and memory processes are important as we attempt to isolate those factors primarily responsible for cohort effects. Information processing designs are also useful for identifying the aspects of job-related tasks that may be at risk for decline in the hypertensive population. This is a significant first step in determining ways to enhance the performance of hypertensive individuals whose employment opportunities may suffer due to less than optimal performance.

Explanatory Models

Much has been written about mechanisms linking blood pressure to poor cognitive functioning. For reviews and interpretive discussions see Elias and Robbins (1991), Waldstein, Manuck, et al., (1991), Light (1975), Shapiro et al., (1982), and Wilkie and Eisdorfer (1971). Of the mechanisms discussed in these papers, the most popular, and possibly most compelling, model is one in which the pathophysiological correlates of increasing blood pressure or hypertension (e.g., changes in cerebral metabolism, microvascular lesions, etc.) are seen as the causes of poorer cognitive performance. There has been little direct evidence for these biological arguments until recently. Recent magnetic resonance imaging studies (Salerno et al., 1992; van Swieten et al., 1991) indicate that hypertension in elderly persons is associated with white matter lesions and cognitive deficit.

Clearly it is important to continue to consider hypotheses that compete with the notion that pathogenic processes provide a direct link between blood pressure and cognition. It is possible that common cerebrovascular processes lead to increasing levels of blood pressure and cognitive deficit, but that blood pressure and cognitive performance are not directly and causally linked via these processes.

Explanatory psychosocial models have been proposed. For example, investigators have argued that knowledge of one's hypertensive status (Robbins et al., 1990; Zonderman, Leu, & Costa, 1986), hypertension-associated anxiety and depression (Elias, Robbins, & Schultz, 1987), nonadherence to medication (Farmer et al., 1990), education (Farmer et al., 1990), and other psychosocial variables may modify biologically based relationships between blood pressure and cognitive functioning. However, blood pressure–performance level relations have been shown to be significant in studies in which these variables have been controlled statistically or via study design (Elias & Robbins, 1991; Waldstein, Manuck, et al., 1991; Waldstein, Ryan, et al., 1991). Although biological explanations for poorer performance with increasing blood pressures seem to have prevailed (Blumenthal et al., 1993; Elias et al., 1993; Waldstein, Manuck, et al., 1991; Waldstein, Ryan, et al., 1991), future studies with magnetic resonance imaging and cerebral blood flow analyses will be important to test the validity of these models.

Shapiro, A. P., Miller, R. E., King, H. E., Ginchereau, E. H., & Fitzgibbon, K. (1982). Behavioral consequences of mild hypertension. *Hypertension, 4*, 55–60.

Steptoe, A. (1981). *Psychological factors in cardiovascular disorders*. New York: Academic Press.

Sternbach, R. A. (1966). *Principles of psychophysiology*. New York: Academic Press.

van Swieten, J. C., Geyskes, G.G., Derix, M. M. A., Peeck, B.M., Ramos, L. M. P., Van Latam, J. C., & Van Gijn, J. (1991). Hypertension in the elderly is associated with white matter lesions and cognitive decline. *Annals of Neurology, 30*, 825–830.

Waldstein, S. R., Manuck, S. B., Ryan, C. M., & Muldoon, M. F. (1991). Neuropsychological correlates of hypertension: Review and methodological considerations. *Psychological Bulletin, 110*, 451–468.

Waldstein, S. R., Ryan, C. M., Manuck, S. B., Parkinson, D. K., & Bromet, E. J. (1991). Learning and memory function in men with untreated blood pressure elevation. *Journal of Consulting and Clinical Psychology, 59*, 513–517.

Watson, W. E. (1976). *Components of reaction time slowing with aging and with hypertension*. Unpublished master's thesis. Syracuse University, Syracuse, NY.

Weschler, D. (1945). A standardized memory scale for clinical use. *Journal of Psychology, 19*, 87–95.

Weschler, D. (1958). *The measurement and appraisal of adult intelligence*. Baltimore: Williams & Wilkins.

Wilkie, F. L., & Eisdorfer, C. (1971). Intelligence and blood pressure in the aged. *Science, 172*, 959–962.

Wilkie, F. L., & Eisdorfer, C. (1980). Hypertension and tests of memory. In M. F. Elias & D. H. P. Streeten (Eds.), *Hypertension and cognitive processes* (pp. 71–82). Mt. Desert, ME: Beech Hill.

Zonderman, A. B., Leu, V. I., & Costa, P. T., Jr., (1986). Effects of age, hypertensive history, and neuroticism on health perceptions. *Experimental Gerontology, 21*, 449–458.

It is important to emphasize again that the associations between blood pressure and cognitive functioning are modest when blood pressure elevations are not associated with medical complications. However, we are impressed with the consistency with which blood pressure-cognitive functioning relationships are reported in the literature and feel that even these modest relationships may have significant implications for some hypertensives. Thus we suggest that a useful applied direction for future studies would be the examination of relationships between blood pressure and cognitive functioning in occupations critical to public safety.

ACKNOWLEDGMENTS

This research was undertaken when M.F. Elias was Visiting Research Professor of Medicine and Visiting Professor of Public Health (Epidemiology and Biostatistics), School of Medicine, Boston University.

We recognize, with much appreciaiton, the following sources of support for this chapter: Framingham Heart Study Visiting Scholars' Fund; National Institutes of Health Research Grants 5-R37-AG03055-11 (M.F. Elias, National Institute on Aging), 1-R01-AG08122-05 (P.A. Wolf, National Institute on Aging), 2-R01-NS17950-11 (P.A. Wolf, National Institute of Neurological Disorders and Stroke); and contract NIH-N01-HC-38038 (P.A. Wolf, National Heart, Blood, and Lung Institute).

REFERENCES

Belanger, R. A., Cupples, L. A., & D'Agostino, R. B. (1988). Section 36. Means at each examination and inter-examination consistency of specified characteristics: Framingham Heart Study, 30-year followup. In W. B. Kannel, P. A. Wolf, & R. J. Garrison (Eds.), *The Framingham Heart Study: An epidemiological investigation of cardiovascular disease* (NIH publication No. 88-2970). Washington, D.C.: National Institutes of Health, Public Health Service.

Benton, A. L., & Hamsher, K. de S. (Eds.). (1976). *Multilingual aphasia examination*. Iowa City: University of Iowa.

Blumenthal, J. A., Madden, D. J., Pierce, T. W., Siegel, W. C., & Appelbaum, M. (1993). Hypertension afffects neurobiological functioning. *Psychosomatic Medicine, 55*, 44–50.

Boller, F., Vrtunski, P. B., Mack, J. L., & Kim, Y. (1977). Neuropsychological correlates of hypertension. *Archives of Neurology, 34*, 701–705.

Dawber, T. R., Meadors, G. F., & Moore, F. E. (1951). Epidemiological approaches to heart disease: The Framingham Study. *American Journal of Public Health, 41*, 279–286.

Downey, N. M., & Starry, A. R. (1977). *Descriptive and inferential statistics* New York: Harper & Row.

Elias, M. F., & Elias, P. K. (1993). Hypertension affects neurobiological functioning: So what's new? [Editorial Comment]. *Psychosomatic Medicine, 55*, 51–54.

Elias, M. F., & Robbins, M. A. (1991). Effects of cardiovascular disease and hypertension on cognitive function. In A. P. Shapiro & A. Baum (Eds.), *Behavioral aspects of cardiovascular disease* (pp. 249–285). Hillsdale, NJ: Lawrence Erlbaum Associates.

Elias, M. F., Robbins, M. A., & Schultz, N. R. (1987). The influence of essential hypertension on intellectual performance: Causation or speculation? In J. W. Elias & P. H. Marshall (Eds.), *Cardiovascular disease and behavior* (pp. 107–149). Washington, DC: Hemisphere Press.

Elias, M. F., Robbins, M. A., Schultz, N. R., & Pierce, T. W. (1990). Is blood pressure an important variable in research on aging and neuropsychological test performance? *Journal of Gerontology: Psychological Sciences Special Issue, 45*, P128–P135.

Elias, M. F., Robbins, M. A., Schultz, N. R., Streeten, D. H. P., & Elias, P. K. (1987). Clinical significance of cognitive performance by hypertensive patients. *Hypertension, 9*, 192–197.

Elias, M. F., Wolf, P. A., D'Agostino, R. B., Cobb, J., & White, L. R. (1993). Untreated blood pressure is inversely related to cognitive functioning: The Framingham Study. *American Journal of Epidemiology, 138*, 353–364.

Farmer, M. E., Kittner, S. J., Abbott, R. D., Wolz, M., Wolf, P. A., & White, L. R. (1990). Longitudinally measured blood pressure, antihypertensive medication use, and cognitive performance: The Framingham Study. *Journal of Clinical Epidemiology, 43*, 475–480.

Farmer, M. E., White, L. R., Abbott, R. D., Kittner, S. J., Kaplan, E., Wolz, M., Brody, J. A., & Wolf, P. A. (1987). Blood pressure and cognitive performance: The Framingham Study. *American Journal of Epidemiology, 126*, 1103–1114.

Farmer, M. E., White, L. R., Kittner, S. J., Kaplan, E., Mars, E., McNamara, P., Wolz, M. M., Wolf, P. A., & Feinleib, M. (1987). Neuropsychological test performance in Framingham: A descriptive study. *Psychological Reports, 60*, 1023–1040.

Goldman, H., Kleinman, K. M., Snow, M. Y., Bidus, D., & Korol, B. (1974). Correlation of diastolic blood pressure and signs of cognitive dysfunction in essential hypertension. *Diseases of the Nervous System, 35*, 571–572.

Hosmer, D. W., & Lemeshow, S. (1989). *Applied logistic regression*. New York: Wiley.

Kannel, W. B. (1974). Role of blood pressure in cardiovascular morbidity and mortality. *Progress in Cardiovascular Disease, 17*, 5–25.

Kannel, W. B., Dawber, T. R., Sorlie, P., Wolf, P. A., & McNamara, P. M. (1976). Components of blood pressure and risk for atheroembolic brain infarction. The Framingham Study. *Stroke, 7*, 327–333.

Kannel, W. B., Wolf, P. A., & Verter, J. S. (1970). Epidemiologic assessment of the role of blood pressure in stroke. The Framingham Study. *Journal of the American Medical Association, 214*, 301–310.

Kaplan, N. M. (1986). *Clinical hypertension* (4th ed.). Baltimore: William & Wilkins.

Lezak, M. D. (1983). *Neuropsychological assessment*. New York: Oxford.

Light, K. (1975). Slowing of response time in young and middle-aged hypertensive patients. *Experimental Aging Research, 1*, 209–227.

Llabre, M. M., Ironson, G. H., Spitzer, S. B., Gellman, Weidler, & Schneiderman (1988). How many blood pressure measurements are enough? An application of generalizability theory to the study of blood pressure reliability. *Psychophysiology*, 25, 97–105.

Madden, D. J., & Blumenthal, J. A. (1989). Slowing of memory search performance in men with mild hypertension. *Health Psychology, 8*, 131–142.

Robbins, M. A., Elias, M. F., & Schultz, N. R., Jr. (1990). Effects of age, blood pressure, and knowledge of hypertension on anxiety and depression. *Experimental Aging Research, 16*, 199–208.

Salerno, J. A., Murphy, D. G. M., Horowitz, B., DeCarli, C., Haxby, J. V., Rapoport, S. I., & Schapiro, M. B. (1992). Brain atrophy in hypertension. A volumetric magnetic resonance imaging study. *Hypertension, 20*, 825–830.

10 Antihypertensive Therapy and Quality of Life: Effects of Drug and Nondrug Interventions on Sleep, Mood State, and Sexual Functioning

Raymond C. Rosen
John B. Kostis
University of Medicine and Dentistry of New Jersey
Robert Wood Johnson Medical School

> The office of medicine is but to tune this curious harp of man's body and reduce it to harmony.
>
> —Francis Bacon

Hypertension is a highly prevalent condition, currently affecting about 50 million people in the United States alone (The Joint National Committee on Detection, Evaluation, and Treatment of High Blood Pressure [JNC-V], 1993). Given the need for lifelong treatment in most cases, along with the potential costs of antihypertensive therapy for the individual and society, attention has shifted to evaluating risks as well as benefits of treatment. In particular, the potential impact of treatment on patients' functional capacity, health perceptions, and cognitive, emotional, and social well-being have been increasingly emphasized (Croog et al., 1986; Fletcher et al., 1990; Wenger & Furberg, 1990). Measurement of these variables, it has been argued, leads to a more comprehensive and clinically meaningful assessment of treatment outcome. As noted by Oberman (1984), "Quality of life data provide an independent evaluation of the success, or lack thereof, of an intervention and may be the deciding factor in the final selection of therapeutic alternatives" (p. 17).

Despite the rapid growth of quality of life (QOL) research in antihypertensive therapy, a number of key conceptual and methodological problems have been insufficiently addressed (Rosen & Kostis, 1985). Furthermore, major discrepancies are apparent in the results of previous research in the area. Specific methodological weaknesses are as follows: (a) the inclusion of a wide range of treatment agents with differing pharmacological properties and mechanisms of action; (b) lack of randomization or use of standardized assessment procedures; (c) patient selection biases—women and elderly patients are underrepresented in most studies; and (d) lack of placebo or nondrug therapy controls. Nondrug therapy provides an important control for the effects of blood pressure lowering per se, independent of the pharmacological effects of a given drug.

In addressing these issues, we have developed a laboratory-based, psychophysiological approach for assessment of adverse side effects of antihypertensive therapy (Kostis & Rosen, 1987; Kostis, Rosen et al., 1990; Rosen, Kostis & Jekelis, 1988). Three major areas of patient function have been selected for investigation by means of this approach: sleep, sexual function, and mood state. Adverse treatment side effects in each of these areas are highly prevalent and are frequently associated with patient noncompliance or withdrawal from treatment (e.g., Lazar, Eisold, Gadson, & Tesch, 1984; Medical Research Council Working Party on Mild to Moderate Hypertension, 1981). Additionally, there is evidence of a strong bias toward underreporting these effects by both patients and physicians (Jachuck, Brierley, Jachuck & Willcox, 1982). In the latter study, marked discrepancies were noted between subjective ratings of physicians, patients, and close family members. Whereas physicians and patients tended to minimize the occurrence of adverse treatment side effects, about three fourths of the patients' spouses rated their husbands or wives as significantly impaired as a result of treatment. Complaints of loss of sexual interest and depressed or irritable mood were commonly reported by the patients' spouses. Changes in sleep quality have also been associated with adrenergic-inhibiting drugs (Rosen & Kostis, 1985), and may lead to complaints of daytime somnolence or fatigue in many patients (Kostis et al., 1990).

Sleep, sexual function, and mood state are viewed as key components of patient's overall quality of life. The effects of antihypertensive therapy on other components of quality of life, such as functional status, social support, and cognitive performance are addressed in detail by other contributors to this volume and are beyond the scope of the present chapter. In addition to evaluating drug effects on sleep, sexual function, and mood state, we report here results of the first laboratory studies of these effects in patients exposed to a multifaceted, nondrug therapy program for hypertension (Rosen, Kostis, & Brondolo, 1989). It is widely assumed that nondrug therapy has unique advantages for patients' QOL, although there is a paucity of empirical data to support this claim JNC-V, 1993). Accordingly, we have compared specific QOL effects of nondrug therapy with both drug and placebo controls in middle-aged and elderly hypertensive males (Kostis et al., 1992; Rosen, Kostis, & Brondolo, 1989). Current research in our laboratory is evaluating nondrug therapy effects on sleep, mood state, and sexual function in hypertensive females, and we have recently begun to investigate these effects in patients with congestive heart failure (CHF). Findings from these latter studies are reported separately.

SLEEP, MOOD STATE, AND SEXUAL FUNCTION IN NORMAL MALES

In our first study (Kostis & Rosen, 1987), a randomized, crossover design was used to evaluate sleep and sexual function effects of four beta blockers with different ancillary properties. Thirty normal male volunteers were randomly assigned to a double-blind, Latin-square crossover-design study with five drug treatment periods of 1 week each, separated by a 2-week, drug-free washout period between each drug condition. Each subject received, in counterbalanced order, atenolol (100 mg qd), metoprolol (100 mg bid), propranolol (80 mg. bid), pindolol (10 mg bid), and placebo. Atenolol is a hydrophilic, $beta_1$-selective blocker; metoprolol is a lipophilic, $beta_1$-selective blocker; and propranolol is a lipophilic, nonselective beta blocker. Pindolol is a nonselective, lipophilic beta blocker that also possesses intrinsic sympathomimetic activity (ISA).

Baseline assessments were performed prior to and following each treatment phase and included objective and subjective measures of sleep and sexual function, as follows: (a) Daily and weekly questionnaires were used to assess a wide range of subjective variables; (b) polysomnographic sleep studies provided a quantitative assessment of sleep architecture and continuity (Rechtschaffen & Kales, 1968); (c) laboratory measures of nocturnal penile tumescence (NPT) were used as an objective index of sexual function (Karacan, Salis, & Williams, 1978); (d) morning blood samples were drawn for hormonal assays following each overnight study; and (e) multistage exercise stress testing was used to demonstrate equipotency of beta blockade at each of the drug dosages selected.

Results indicated that both subjective and objective measures of sleep continuity were affected by each of the lipophilic beta blockers tested (pindolol, propranolol, metoprolol). In particular, sleep was rated as more restless and disturbed on pindolol, propranolol, and metoprolol, as compared with atenolol and placebo, and more interrupted sleep was reported with metoprolol and propranolol. As shown in Fig. 10.1, polysomnographic data showed a significant increase in the total number of awakenings and total wakefulness after sleep onset when subjects received pindolol, propranolol, or metoprolol, compared to both atenolol and placebo. Similar trends were observed on other measures of sleep continuity, such as total sleep time and sleep efficiency.

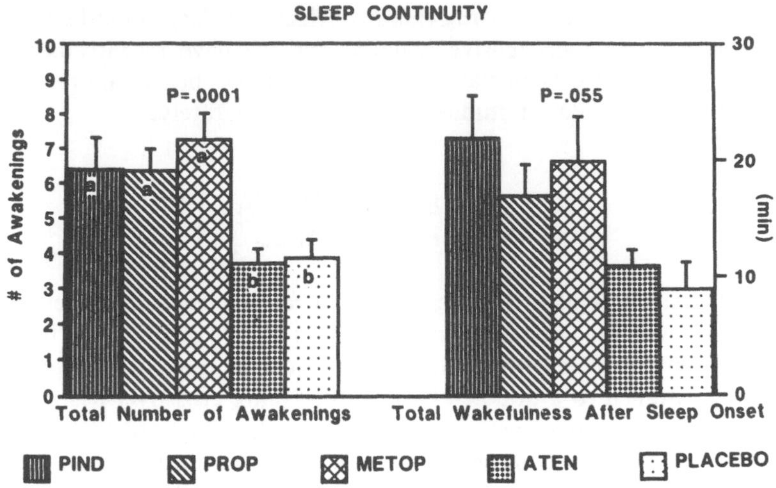

FIG. 10.1. Polysomnographic measures of sleep continuity in normal subjects receiving 1 week of treatment with pindolol (10 mg bid), propranolol (80 mg bid), metoprolol (100 mg bid), atenolol (100 mg qd), and placebo. From Kostis & Rosen (1987). Reprinted by permission from the American Heart Association.

Although all three lipophilic beta blockers (pindolol, propranolol, metoprolol) disturbed sleep continuity, only pindolol altered sleep architecture (i.e., the distribution of sleep stages). Specifically, REM sleep onset was delayed, and total REM time was significantly decreased in the pindolol condition alone. This effect was not observed with the non-ISA beta blockers (atenolol, propranolol, metoprolol). Moreover, none of the study drugs were associated with significant changes in REM activity or REM density, nor were significant changes in dream content or quality reported. This is in contrast to previous reports in the literature of vivid or disturbing dreams in patients receiving propranolol therapy (Rosen & Kostis, 1985). However, it is possible that these latter effects only occur at higher dosages or with chronic drug administration.

Separate analyses were conducted of drug effects on measures of mood state and sexual function (Rosen et al., 1988). A slight, but significant increase in depressed mood was observed in subjects receiving each of the lipophilic beta blockers. Significant drug effects on both total and free testosterone were found with all four beta blockers, although it appeared that the nonselective drugs (propranolol, pindolol) were associated with the greatest reduction in total testosterone (see Fig. 10.2). A similar trend was observed for measures of nocturnal penile tumescence (NPT). Analysis of self-report data indicated that subjects complained more often of sexual difficulties on propranolol, and one subject, in particular, experienced severe erectile difficulties on 4 out of 7 days on the drug. Within each drug

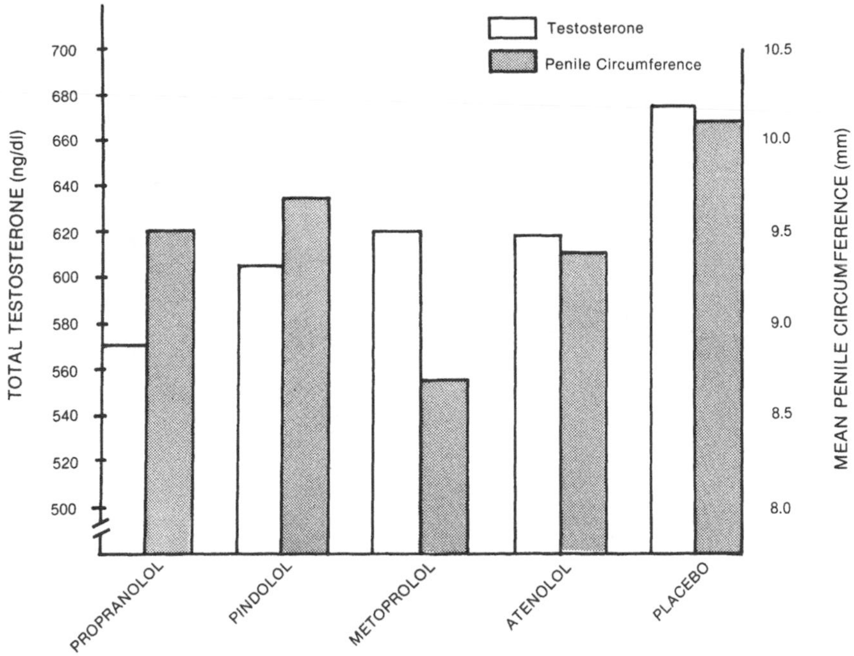

FIG. 10.2. Mean plasma testosterone and NPT responses associated with beta-blocker administration in normal subjects. From Rosen, Kostis, & Jekelis (1988). Reprinted by permission from Plenum Publishers.

condition, testosterone levels were significantly correlated with the frequency of intercourse and the subjective ratings of desire for sex. These findings are consistent with other reports of decreased plasma testosterone levels in patients receiving chronic beta blocker administration (Suzuki, Tominaga, Kumagi, & Sarita, 1988).

Finally, the effects of beta blockade on heart rate (HR) during sleep were evaluated (Rosen, Kostis, Seltzer, Taska, & Holzer, 1991). Electrocardiographic (EKG) signals were converted by a cardiotachometer into HR, which was electronically averaged for each 30-second period during the night. The mean HR for each sleep stage and for each hour of sleep was computed. Each of the beta blockers without ISA (propranolol, metoprolol, atenolol) was associated with a significant reduction in both mean and maximum HR during all sleep stages (see Fig. 10.3). In contrast, pindolol was associated with a significant increase in HR, compared to placebo, in all sleep stages. This effect is consistent with the intrinsic sympathomimetic properties of the drug (Kostis & DeFelice, 1984). A differential effect of pindolol on non-REM/REM sleep analogous to rest–exercise was not observed, however, suggesting that the tachycardia of REM sleep is mediated primarily through nonadrenergic (e.g., vagal) mechanisms. More-

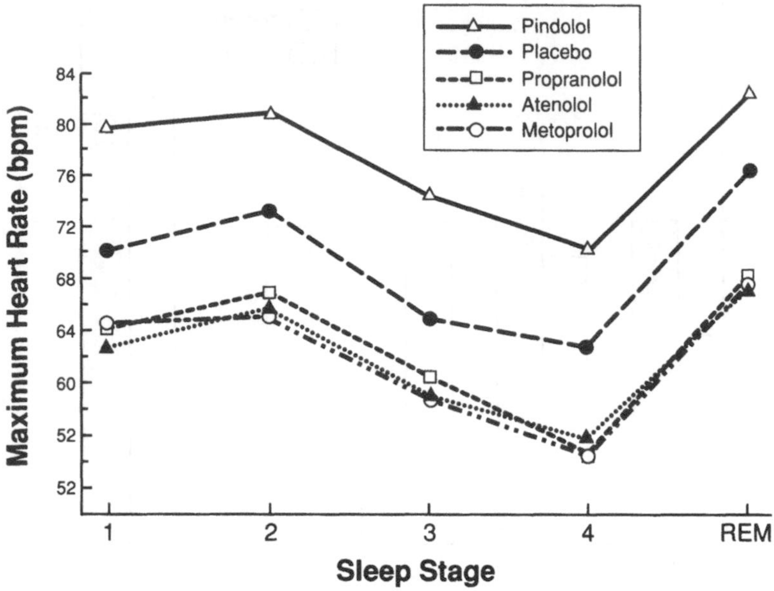

FIG. 10.3. Effects of beta blockers on maximum heart rate at different stages of sleep in normal subjects. From Rosen, Kostis, Seltzer, Taska, & Holzer (1991). Reprinted by permission from the American Sleep Disorders Association.

over, an increase in HR in the early morning hours was not observed, as long as subjects remained asleep.

TREATMENT EFFECTS IN HYPERTENSIVE MALES

Having evaluated QOL effects of beta blockers in healthy, normotensive subjects, a series of prospective studies of treatment side effects in middle-aged and elderly hypertensive patients was conducted. In addition to evaluating side effects of centrally active, antihypertensive drugs (propranolol, clonidine), these studies provided the first controlled comparison of drug and nondrug therapies for hypertension (Kostis et al., 1992; Kostis et al., 1990; Rosen et al., 1989). These studies also served to replicate our earlier results with normal subjects in middle-aged and elderly hypertensive patients. The major findings of this research are briefly as follows.

In our first clinical study (Kostis et al., 1990), 46 middle-aged, mildly hypertensive men were randomly assigned to receive one of two antihypertensive drugs or double-blind placebo in a counterbalanced, crossover-design study. The mean age of the subjects was 54.5 years (age range = 31–78), and the mean baseline blood pressure was 158.2/102.6 mmHg

(SBP/DBP). Treatment drugs for the study were propranolol (20–80 mg bid), clonidine (0.1–0.3 mg bid), and placebo, each of which was administered on the basis of a double-blind, stepped care regimen. Each treatment phase was continued for 3 months and was followed by a 1-month drug-free washout period. Subjects were then assigned to the remaining drug conditions in counterbalanced order with baseline assessments before and after each treatment phase. Treatment compliance was assessed by means of both pill-count and patient self-report after each treatment phase (Kostis et al., 1990).

Polysomnographic studies revealed a significant effect of treatment on four of six primary sleep variables; total sleep time was reduced with both study drugs, as was sleep maintenance, REM latency, and total REM time (see Table 10.1). In particular, clonidine was associated with decreased total sleep time, and a marked increase in REM latency. Propranolol was similarly shown to have disruptive effects on each of the measures of sleep continuity, although these effects were less pronounced than with clonidine. Surprisingly, propranolol was associated with a greater increase in subjective measures of fatigue and daytime sleepiness, compared to both clonidine and placebo. Analysis of NPT data revealed that the duration of penile tumescence was significantly decreased by clonidine, and a similar trend was observed for the effects of propranolol.

Another unexpected finding in this study was that sleep and mood were

TABLE 10.1
Antihypertensive Drug Effects on Sleep Continuity, Sleep Architecture, and Nocturnal Penile Tumescence (NPT)

	Placebo		*Propranolol*		*Clonidine*			
	$\bar{X}$	*SD*	$\bar{X}$	*SD*	$\bar{X}$	*SD*	*F*	*P*
Sleep continuity								
Total sleep time	355.9[a]	48.4	328.4[ab]	49.7	320.1[b]	51.1	3.40	0.04
Sleep latency	25.4	22.5	24.5	27.5	15.2	13.2	2.92	0.06
Sleep maintenance	92.3[a]	5.9	90.7[ab]	7.14	88.2[b]	8.9	3.15	0.05
Total awakenings	7.7	4.7	8.0	4.6	7.3	3.1	0.30	0.74
REM measures								
Percent REM time	18.8[a]	5.6	16.7[ab]	5.7	15.4[b]	7.3	4.84	0.01
REM latency	81.4[a]	37.6	89.9[a]	31.2	116.5[b]	58.4	6.87	0.002
Number of REMPs	3.42[a]	0.95	3.0[ab]	0.8	2.73[b]	0.92	6.12	0.004
REM density (RA/RT)	1.21	0.36	1.22	0.4	1.23	0.44	0.03	0.975
Mean REM heart rate	67.5[a]	7.3	65.9[ab]	8.2	63.7[b]	7.3	4.43	0.019
NPT measures								
Maximum change in mm	34.6	12.6	30.5	15.1	30.1	15.9	2.42	0.105
Duration of maximum tumescence	41.4[a]	34.5	29.4[ab]	28.0	27.0[b]	27.6	4.23	0.026

Note. Means with the same letter are not significantly different at $p < .05$. From Kostis et al. (1990). Reprinted by permission from Springer-Verlag.

less affected in elderly, compared to middle-aged hypertensive males. Only a slight trend toward delayed REM onset was observed with propranolol, whereas other sleep and mood measures showed little or no change with drug therapy (Kostis et al., 1990). In contrast, penile tumescence was significantly decreased (by about 30%) in elderly patients receiving propranolol, compared to those receiving the placebo. Cognitive and psychomotor function were also adversely affected by propranolol in the elderly, compared to middle-aged hypertensive patients. Clonidine was not administered to elderly hypertensives in this study, due primarily to the increased risk of orthostatic hypotension (Wollam & Hall, 1988).

In a second study, we compared the effects of propranolol or placebo with a 12-week, nondrug therapy condition in a randomized trial of 79 mildly hypertensive male patients (Kostis et al., 1992). Dependent variables for this study included a broad range of cardiovascular, metabolic, and QOL measures. Subjects assigned to the nondrug therapy condition ($N = 33$) were required to attend weekly intervention sessions, which were conducted in a group format. Weight loss was strongly emphasized for all patients weighing 115% or more of ideal body weight. Additionally, subjects were required to restrict sodium and alcohol intake and to participate in a graduated program of aerobic exercise. Stress management training was also provided. Propranolol and placebo administration were based on the stepped-care regimen described earlier.

A significant reduction in diastolic blood pressure (DBP) was observed following treatment with both nondrug therapy (-8.0 ± 1.08 mmHg) and propranolol (-9.5 ± 1.46 mmHg), compared to placebo (-0.1 ± 2.01 mmHg). A similar trend was observed for treatment effects on systolic blood pressure (SBP). In addition to lowering blood pressure, nondrug therapy was associated with significant weight loss (-6.5 ± 2.4 kg), lower total and low-density lipoprotein (LDL) levels, lower triglyceride levels, and increased exercise tolerance. In contrast, propranolol therapy was associated with a slight increase in weight and LDL-cholesterol.

Marked changes in sexual function were observed in both treatment conditions. As shown in Fig. 10.4, propranolol was associated with a significant decrease in the number and duration of penile tumescence responses, compared to both placebo and nondrug therapy. A trend toward decreased subjective arousal was also observed in the drug condition. In contrast, patients receiving the 12-week nondrug therapy program reported a significant improvement in self-ratings of sexual arousal and satisfaction following treatment. Specifically, patients receiving nondrug therapy reported increased arousal during sexual activity ($p < .05$), more satisfying ejaculations ($p < .02$), and increased frequency of orgasms ($p < .01$). Similar improvements in subjective ratings of sexual function were reported

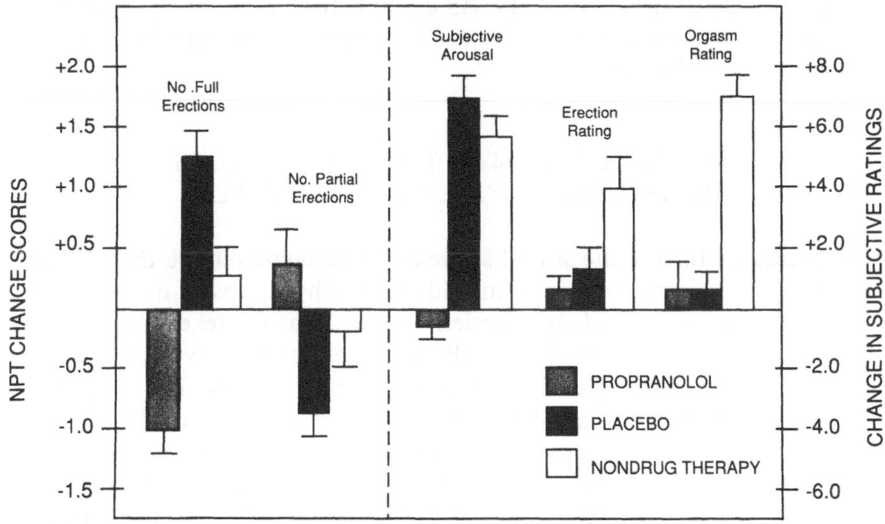

FIG. 10.4. Treatment effects on NPT and subjective measures of sexual function in male hypertensive patients receiving drug (propranolol), nondrug therapy, or placebo. From Kostis et al., (1992). Adapted by permission from Mosby-Year Book, Inc.

in a recent study of dietary changes and vigorous exercise training in sedentary, middle-aged men (White, Case, McWhirter, & Mattison, 1990). Unfortunately, neither study included hormonal measures of sexual function.

Finally, significant effects of treatment were observed on four of the five mood scales recorded. Specifically, patients receiving nondrug therapy rated themselves as significantly more energetic ($p < .02$) following treatment. Both patients receiving nondrug therapy and propranolol rated themselves as more clear-headed ($p < .05$) than those receiving placebo. Patients in the propranolol group also rated themselves as feeling less anxious and unsure than patients in the placebo group. Differences between propranolol and nondrug therapy on these latter measures were not signficant. Positive effects of nondrug therapy on mood state have been reported in the recent multicenter Trial of Antihypertensive Interventions and Management (TAIM), in which patients receiving weight loss and sodium restriction reported less fatigue and depression, compared to patients on atenolol or chlorthalidone therapy (Wassertheil-Smoller, Oberman, Blaufox, Davis, & Langford, 1992).

Current research in our laboratory is evaluating mood and sexual function effects of newer antihypertensive agents (enalapril, atenolol), compared to a similar multifaceted nondrug therapy program. In addition, we are presently evaluating QOL effects of antihypertensive therapy in a sample of elderly female patients. As noted before, none of the studies to date have systematically compared QOL effects of treatment in male and female hypertensive patients.

ANTIHYPERTENSIVE THERAPY EFFECTS IN SEXUALLY DYSFUNCTIONAL MALES

To investigate further the sexual sequelae of antihypertensive therapy, an additional study was conducted in middle-aged hypertensive males with a specific history of sexual dysfunction (Rosen, Kostis, Jekelis, & Taska, 1994). These individuals are potentially at higher risk for adverse treatment side effects, given their past history of sexual dysfunction. The study was also designed to compare physiological, subjective, and hormonal indices of sexual function in a clinically relevant population of hypertensive patients.

Treatment drugs for the study included alpha-methyldopa (500 mg bid), propranolol (80 mg bid), atenolol (100 mg qd), hydrochlorthiazide/triamterene (Dyazide) (50/25 mg bid), and placebo. Each study drug was administered for a 1-month treatment period, followed by a 2-week washout period, according to a counterbalanced, Latin-square crossover design. Twenty-one male patients met the criteria for randomization, and 13 subjects completed all five phases of the study.

As in our previous research, polysomnographic studies indicated that sleep architecture was significantly altered by the centrally active, sympatholytic drugs. In particular, REM latency was increased, and the percentage of REM time relative to total sleep time was decreased by both centrally active drugs, propranolol and methyldopa. A lack of consistent effects on sexual function was observed, however, contrary to the study hypothesis. Specifically, although little change was observed in self-report measures of sexual arousal, free testosterone was significantly reduced with both propranolol and methyldopa. Additionally, a trend toward diminished amplitude and duration of NPT was observed with each of the study drugs. The lack of significant changes in subjective arousal or NPT in the present study may have reflected a "floor effect," in that low baseline levels of arousal were apparent prior to the onset of treatment (Rosen, Kostis, Jekelis, & Taska, 1994).

Significant negative correlations were observed between age and the major sexual function variables in this study. In particular, age was negatively correlated with both total and free testosterone, as well as subjective ratings of erectile function and overall sexual satisfaction. In contrast, no significant correlations were observed between changes in blood pressure and sexual function scores. This latter finding, along with our observations on the effects of nondrug therapy, strongly suggest that it is not the blood pressure lowering effect of the drugs, per se, that is responsible for adverse sexual side effects in these patients. In each of our studies to date, sexual function changes have been related to the type of drug administered (e.g., sympatholytic versus nonsympatholytic agents), rather than reductions in blood pressure, heart rate, or other cardiovascular concomitants of drug administration (Rosen, 1991).

Taken together with the findings of our previous studies, these results do not support the hypothesis that sexually dysfunctional males are at greater risk for adverse sexual side effects when treated with sympatholytic agents or diuretics. In fact, the overall pattern of effects was remarkably similar to that observed with both nondysfunctional, hypertensive males (Kostis et al., 1990), and normotensive controls (Rosen et al., 1988). Furthermore, the correlations observed between age and measures of sexual function are generally consistent with studies of healthy elderly men (e.g., Davidson et al., 1983; Schiavi & Schreiner-Engel, 1988), in which moderately negative correlations were reported between age, testosterone, and NPT. On the other hand, given the relatively brief treatment periods (1 month), and high dropout rate in the present study, these findings need to be cautiously interpreted.

Surprisingly, few studies to date have evaluated the effects of angiotensin converting enzyme (ACE) inhibitors or calcium channel blockers on sexual function. One recent placebo-controlled, crossover study compared the effects of atenolol and nifedipine on self-report measures of sexual function in older men (Morrissette, Skinner, Hoffmann, Levine, & Davidson, 1993). In this study, several patients on nifedipine reported decreased firmness of erections during masturbation. Additionally, Suzuki et al. (1988) reported problems of delayed ejaculation in male patients receiving nifedipine. Current research in our laboratory is comparing the effects of enalapril and atenolol on sexual function in both male and female hypertensive patients.

EFFECTS OF CHOLESTEROL-LOWERING DRUGS ON SLEEP AND SEXUAL FUNCTION

Pravastatin and lovastatin are structurally related hydroxy-methylglutaryl CoA (HMG CoA) reductase inhibitors widely used in the treatment of patients with hypercholesterolemia. Lovastatin is a lipophilic drug that readily crosses the blood–brain barrier, and has been associated with increased nocturnal awakenings and decreased sleep time (Schaefer, 1988; Vgontzas, Kales, Bixler, Manfredi, & Tyson, 1991). Patients complaining of lovastatin-induced insomnia have also been shown to have an increased rate of periodic leg movements (PLMS) during sleep (Corbett & Ehrenberg, 1991). These effects have not been reported in patients taking pravastatin, a hydrophilic HMG-CoA reductase inhibitor. Given the widespread use of these drugs in cardiovascular patients, we extended our previous research by comparing sleep and sexual function effects of lovastatin and pravastatin in a clinical sample of hyperlipidemic male patients. In addition to providing a controlled, polysomnographic assessment of sleep architecture and continuity changes associated with cholesterol-lowering drugs, this study represents the first systematic evaluation of the effects on sexual function of HMG-CoA reductase inhibitors.

Twenty-two hyperlipidemic male patients, ages 35 to 65, were randomly assigned to a double-blind, placebo-controlled, crossover design study. After an initial 3-week placebo lead-in phase, subjects were assigned to three consecutive 6-week treatment periods with pravastatin (40 mg/d.), lovastatin (40 mg/d.), or matching placebo. Treatment periods were separated by a 4-week placebo washout, followed immediately by the next treatment phase. Standardized laboratory measures of sleep and NPT were performed at baseline, at the end of each washout period, and following the second and sixth week of each treatment phase.

Results indicated a significant reduction in both total and LDL-cholesterol with each of the study drugs. Patients showed a 20% to 30% decrease in LDL-cholesterol with both drugs. In contrast, neither drug was associated with significant changes in sleep architecture or continuity. A slight trend was noted toward decreased total sleep time and reduced sleep efficiency with lovastatin, compared to both pravastatin and placebo. No significant differences in subjective measures of sleep were observed.

Analysis of NPT data revealed that both study drugs were associated with a significant increase in the duration of maximum tumescence at 2 weeks of treatment (see Fig. 10.5). A similar trend was observed for measures of maximum tumescence adjusted for total sleep time, peak tumescence, and duration of partial tumescence. On each of these measures, penile tumescence was increased relative to pretreatment baseline levels. Although the trend was maintained, these differences were not significant after 6 weeks of treatment.

The increase in NPT duration at 2 weeks of treatment with both study drugs cannot be explained on the basis of changes in REM sleep or total sleep time alone. Rather, this effect may be due to improved endothelial function and enhanced endothelium-dependent relaxation of corporal smooth muscle in the penis (Azadzoi & Saenz de Tejada, 1991). The effect was not statistically significant at 6 weeks of treatment, however, and may not be clinically significant. In any event, it appears that neither study drug was associated with a worsening of sexual function in these patients. Further studies are needed to determine possible long-term effects of HMG-CoA reductase inhibitors on sexual function in hyperlipidemic patients.

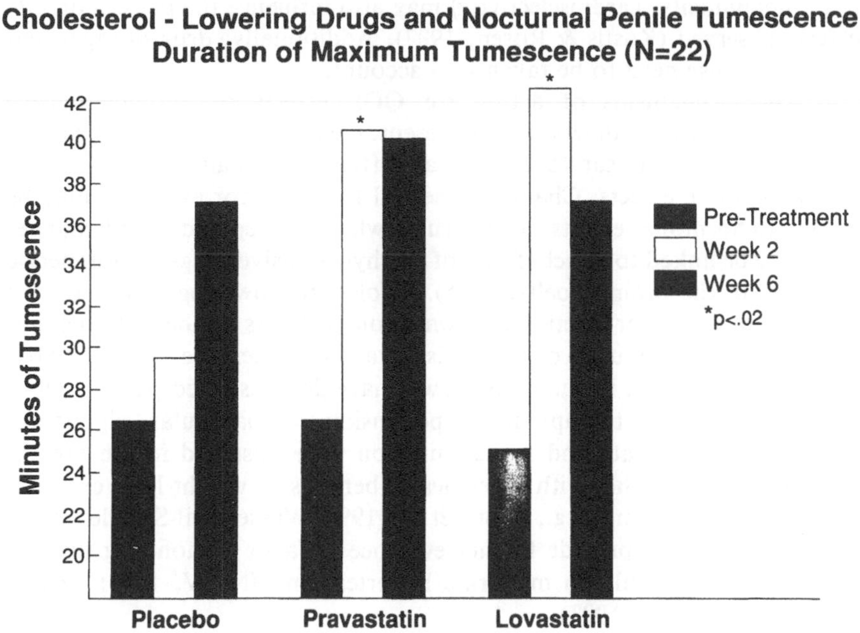

FIG. 10.5. Effects of cholesterol-lowering drugs (pravastatin, lovastatin) on NPT in hyperlipidemic male patients.

Recently there have been several reports of depression associated with clinical use of HMG-CoA reductase inhibitors (Dutts & Bos, 1993; Morgan, Palinkas, Barret-Connor, & Weingard, 1993). In the present study, however, no significant differences were observed in Beck depression scores between either of the two treatment conditions and placebo.

DISCUSSION AND CONCLUSIONS

Given the diversity of treatment options available, and concern with possible adverse side effects of antihypertensive therapy, there is increasing emphasis on evaluating treatment effects on patients' QOL (Wenger & Furberg, 1990). Based on results of these studies, some tentative conclusions can be drawn as follows:

1. Alterations in sleep, mood state, and sexual function are common sequelae of antihypertensive therapy. These effects are more likely to be encountered with beta blockers and other centrally active antihypertensive agents (e.g., clonidine, alpha-methyldopa). Ancillary properties of the drug

(e.g., lipophilicity, cardioselectivity) may also influence the pattern of side effects observed (Kostis & Rosen, 1987). Additionally, drug dosages and duration of use need to be taken into account.

2. The mechanisms of action for QOL effects of antihypertensive therapy are not well understood at present. Considering the overall pattern of results, there appear to be several different mechanisms involved in mediating these effects. Changes in sexual function, for example, may be related to hormonal effects of the drugs, whereas sleep and mood changes appear to be linked to direct effects of antihypertensive drugs on adrenergic receptors in the brain (Koella, 1985). Cholesterol-lowering drugs, on the other hand, may alter erectile function through effects on the endothelium-dependent smooth muscle of the penis (Azadzoi & Saenz de Tejada, 1991).

3. Several studies, including our own, have demonstrated positive QOL effects of nondrug therapy for hypertension. In particular, significant changes in mood state and sexual function were observed in the present studies. Taken together with other health benefits of weight loss, exercise, and relaxation training (e.g., Kostis et al., 1992; Wassertheil-Smoller et al., 1992), these results provide further evidence in favor of nondrug therapy for patients with mild to moderate hypertension (JNC-V, 1993; Rosen, Brondolo, & Kostis, 1993).

4. Male–female differences in QOL effects of antihypertensive therapy have not been sufficiently investigated to date. This is somewhat surprising, given the role of sex differences in patterns of cardiovascular response (Messerli et al., 1987) and the increased susceptibility in women to systemic side effects of antihypertensive drugs (Toner & Ramsay, 1984). Similarly, insufficient research has been conducted on QOL effects of antihypertensive therapy in elderly hypertensives (Rosen et al., 1989). We are currently participating in a multicenter, clinical trial (TONE), in which QOL effects of nondrug therapy in elderly hypertensives are being investigated.

5. Finally, side effects of newer antihypertensive agents, such as the angiotensin converting enzyme inhibitors and calcium channel blockers, are not well understood. Considering the widespread use of these drugs in clinical practice, and the paucity of data available concerning their effects on sleep, mood, and sexual function, further studies are clearly needed. Research on this topic is currently underway in our laboratory.

ACKNOWLEDGMENTS

Research studies were supported by NIH grants #HL33960–04 and #HL48642–02. Additional support for this research was provided by Stuart Pharmaceuticals and Bristol-Meyers Squibb Pharmaceutical Research Institute.

REFERENCES

Azadzoi, K. M., & Saenz de Tejada, I. (1991). Hypercholesterolemia impairs endothelium-dependent relaxation of rabbit corpus cavernosum smooth muscle. *Journal of Urology, 146*, 238–240.

Corbett, K., & Ehrenberg, B. (1991). Excessive periodic limb movements of sleep in hyperlipidemic patients susceptible to lovastatin-induced insomnia. *Sleep Research, 20*, 230.

Croog, S. H., Levine, S., Testa, M. A., Brown, B., Bulpitt, C. J., Jenkins, C. D., Klerman, G. L., & Williams, G. H. (1986). The effects of antihypertensive therapy on the quality of life. *New England Journal of Medicine, 314*, 1657-1664.

Davidson, J. M., Chen, J. J., Crapo, L., Gray, G. D., Greenleaf, W. J., & Catania, J. A. (1983). Hormonal changes and sexual function in aging men. *Journal of Clinical Endocrinology and Metabolism, 57*, 71–77.

Dutts, N., & Bos, F. M. (1993). Depressive symptoms and cholesterol-lowering drugs. *Lancet, 341*, 114.

Fletcher, A. E., Bulpitt, C. J., Hawkins, C. M., Havinga, T. K., Berge, B.S., May, J. F., Schuurman, F. H., van der Veur, E., & Wesseling, H. (1990). Quality of life on antihypertensive therapy: A randomized, double-blind controlled trial of captopril and atenolol. *Journal of Hypertension, 8*, 463-466.

Jachuck, S. J., Brierley, H., Jachuck, S., & Willcox, P. M. (1982). The effects of hypotensive drugs on the quality of life. *Journal of the Royal College of General Practitioners, 32*, 103–105.

Joint National Committee on Detection, Evaluation, and Treatment of High Blood Pressure. (1993). The Fifth Report of the National Committee on Detection, Evaluation, and Treatment of High Blood Presssure (JNC-V). (1993). *Archives of Internal Medicine, 153*, 154–183.

Karacan, I., Salis, P. J., & Williams, R. L. (1978). The role of the sleep laboratory in the diagnosis and treatment of impotence. In R. L. Williams & I. Karacan (Eds.), *Sleep disorders: Diagnosis and treatment* (pp. 248- 263). New York: Wiley.

Koella, W. P. (1985). CNS-related side-effects of beta-blockers with special reference to mechanisms of action. *European Journal of Clinical Pharmacology, 28* (Suppl), 55–63.

Kostis, J. B., & DeFelice, E. A. (1984). *Beta-blockers in the treatment of cardiovascular disease*. New York: Raven Press.

Kostis, J. B., & Rosen, R. C. (1987). Central nervous system effects of beta- adrenergic blocking drugs: The role of ancillary properties. *Circulation, 75*, 204–212.

Kostis, J. B., Rosen, R. C., Brondolo, E., Taska, L., Smith, D. E., & Wilson, A. C. (1992). Superiority of nonpharmacological therapy compared to propranolol and placebo in men with mild hypertension: A randomized prospective trial. *American Heart Journal, 123*, 466–474.

Kostis, J. B., Rosen, R. C., Holzer, B. C., Randolph, C., Taska, L. S., & Miller, M. H. (1990). CNS side effects of centrally-active antihypertensive agents: A prospective, placebo-controlled study of sleep, mood state, and sexual function in hypertensive males. *Psychopharmacology, 102*, 163–170.

Lazar, J., Eisold, J., Gadson, I., & Tesch, D. (1984). Recognition and management of antihypertensive therapy drug side-effects. *Clinical Pharmacology and Therapeutics, 35*, 254.

Medical Research Council Working Party on Mild to Moderate Hypertension. (1981). Adverse reactions to bendrofluazide and propranolol for the treatment of mild hypertension. *Lancet, ii*, 539–543.

Messerli, F. H., Garavaglia, G. E., & Schmieder, R. E., Sundgaard-Riise, K., Nunez, B. D., & Amodeo, C. (1987). Disparate cardiovascular findings in men and women with essential hypertension. *Annals of Internal Medicine, 07*, 158–161.

Morgan, R. E., Palinkas, L. A., Barret-Connor, E. L., & Weingard, D. L. (1993). Plasma cholesterol and depressive symptoms in older men. *Lancet, 341*, 75–79.

Morrissette, D. L., Skinner, M. H., Hoffmann, B. B., Levine, R. E., & Davidson, J. M. (1993). Effects of antihypertensive drugs atenolol and nifedipine on sexual function in older men: A placebo-controlled, crossover study. *Archives of Sexual Behavior, 22*, 99–109.

Oberman, A. (1984). The role of quality of life assessment in clinical trials. In N. K. Wenger, M. E. Mattson, & C. D. Furberg (Eds.), *Assessment of quality of life in clinical trials of cardiovasuclar therapies* (pp. 81- 98). New York: LeJacq.

Rechtschaffen, A., & Kales, A. A. (1968). *Manual for standardized terminology, techniques, and scoring system for sleep stages of human subjects.* Washington, D C: National Institute of Mental Health.

Rosen, R. C. (1991). Alcohol and drug effects on sexual response: Human experimental and clinical studies. *Annual Review of Sex Research, 2*, 119–180.

Rosen, R. C., Brondolo, E., & Kostis, J. B. (1993). Non-pharmacological treatment of essential hypertension: Research and clinical applications. In R. Gatchel & E. Blanchard (Eds.). *Psychophysiological disorders: Research and clinical applications.* (pp. 63–110). Washington, DC: American Psychological Association Press.

Rosen, R. C., & Kostis, J. B. (1985). Biobehavioral sequellae associated with adrenergic-inhibiting antihypertensive agents: A critical review. *Health Psychology, 4*, 579–604.

Rosen, R. C., Kostis, J. B., & Brondolo, E. (1989). Nondrug treatment approaches for hypertension. *Clinics in Geriatric Medicine, 5*, 791-802.

Rosen, R. C., Kostis, J. B., & Jekelis, A. W. (1988). Beta-blocker effects on sexual function in normal males. *Archives of Sexual Behavior*, 17, 241-255.

Rosen, R. C., Kostis, J. B., Jekelis, A., & Taska, L. S. (1994). Sexual sequelae of antihypertensive drugs: Treatment effects on self-report and physiological measures in middle-aged, male hypertensives. *Archives of Sexual Behavior, 23*, 135–152.

Rosen, R. C., Kostis, J. B., Seltzer, L. G., Taska, L. S., & Holzer, B. C. (1991). Beta blocker effects on heart rate during sleep: A placebo- controlled polysomnographic study with normotensive males. *Sleep, 14*, 43–47.

Schaefer, E. J. (1988). Sleep abnormalities in patients on lovastatin. *New England Journal of Medicine, 319*, 1222.

Schiavi, R. C., & Schreiner-Engel, P. (1988). Nocturnal penile tumescence in healthy, aging men. *Journal of Gerontology, 43*, 146–150.

Shumaker, S. A., Anderson, R. T., & Czajkowski, S. M. (1990). Psychological tests and scales. In B. Spilker (Ed.), *Quality of life assessments in clinical trials* (pp. 95–104). New York: Raven Press.

Suzuki, H., Tominaga, T., Kumugai, H., & Sarita, T. (1988). Effects of first-line antihypertensive agents on sexual function and sex hormones. *Journal of Hypertension, 6*(Suppl 4), 5649-5651.

Toner, J. M., & Ramsay, L. E. (1984). Thiazide-induced hypokalemia: Prevalence higher in women. *British Journal of Clinical Pharmacology, 18*, 449–452.

Vgontzas, A. N., Kales, A. A., Bixler, E. O., Manfredi, R. L., & Tyson, K. L. (1991). Effects of lovastatin and pravastatin on sleep efficiency and sleep stages. *Clinical Pharmacology and Therapeutics, 50*, 730–737.

Wassertheil-Smoller, S., Oberman, A., Blaufox, M. D., Davis, B., & Langford, H. (1992). The Trial of Antihypertensive Interventions and Management (TAIM) study: Final results with regard to blood pressure, cardiovascular risk, and quality of life. *American Journal of Hypertension, 5*, 37–44.

Wenger, N. K., & Furberg, C. D. (1990). Cardiovascular disorders. In B. Spilker (Ed.), *Quality of life assessments in clinical trials* (pp. 335–346). New York: Raven Press.

White, J. R., Case, D. A., McWhirter, D., & Mattison, A. M. (1990). Enhanced sexual behavior in exercising men. *Archives of Sexual Behavior, 19*, 193- 209.

Wollam G. L., & Hall, W. D. (1988). *Hypertension management: Clinical practice and therapeutic dilemmas.* Chicago: Year Book Medical.

11 The Effects of Hypertension on Neurobehavioral Functioning

Elizabeth Towner Thyrum
James A. Blumenthal
Duke University Medical Center

Hypertension places as many as 58 million people in the United States at increased risk for a variety of health problems and diseases, including coronary artery disease, peripheral vascular disease, and kidney failure (Joint National Committee, 1988). In addition to the serious medical consequences of chronically sustained blood pressure, this condition has been shown to affect the central nervous system (CNS) on several levels. In the extreme, a variety of clinically overt neurologic complications of advanced hypertension may develop, including convulsions, hypertensive encephalopathy, ischemic stroke, intracerebral hemorrhage, and multi-infarct dementia (Page, 1987). On a more subtle level, hypertensive individuals display less obvious impairments in psychological functioning, which have been observed through poorer performance on perceptual and psychomotor tests, as compared to individuals with normal blood pressure (e.g., Blumenthal, Madden, Pierce, Siegel, & Appelbaum, 1993; Elias, Robbins, & Schultz, 1987; Elias, Robbins, Schultz, & Pierce, 1990; Light, 1978; Madden & Blumenthal, 1989; Oppenheimer & Fishberg, 1928; Waldstein, Manuck, Ryan, & Muldoon, 1991; Wilkie, Eisdorfer, & Nowlin, 1976).

Although numerous studies have shown that hypertension is associated with neuropsychological disturbances, results from empirical investigations have yielded inconsistencies in the types and patterns of deficits observed. These inconsistencies are, in part, due to the relatively few well controlled studies that have compared hypertensives to normotensives. As a result, deficits in specific areas of cognitive functioning (such as verbal memory, figural memory, and attention) and associated mechanisms by which hypertension may influence these changes are not well understood. Furthermore, it is not clear how these alterations in cognitive functioning may impact on quality of life. The relatively few investigations into this relationship have emphasized that the performance differences between hypertensives and normotensives are not associated with compromises in the ability to perform routine activities of daily living, such as occupational or recreational functioning (Elias, Robbins & Schultz, et al., 1987; Friedman & Bennett, 1977).

In general, research studies into the effects of hypertension on psychological functioning have employed two types of assessment approaches. This chapter examines these assessment methods and reviews their respective findings in the area of neurobehavioral functioning associated with hypertension. Future directions for research are also discussed.

RESEARCH USING NEUROPSYCHOLOGICAL TESTING

One approach to the study of neurobehavioral functioning in hypertensive patients consists of a battery of individual, clinical neuropsychological instruments (e.g., Elias, Robbins, Schultz, Streeten, & Elias, 1987; Franceschi, Tancredi, Smirne, Mercinelli, & Canal, 1982; Mazzucchi et al., 1986; Schmidt et al., 1991). Standardized neuropsychological instruments include subtests from the Wechsler Adult Intelligence Scale (WAIS) and the Halstead–Reitan Neuropsychological battery (e.g., Elias et al.. 1990; Elias, Robbins, Schultz, et al., 1987; Elias, Robbins, Schultz, & Streeten, 1986; Elias, Schultz, Robbins, & Elias, 1989; Wilkie et al., 1976). Some of these types of studies compared untreated hypertensives with normotensives and either matched or statistically adjusted for age, education, and other possible confounding factors such as gender, socioeconomic status, and health status (Franceschi et al., 1982; Madden & Blumenthal, 1989; Mazzucchi et al., 1986).

A recent study (Elias et al., 1990) measured neuropsychological functioning in approximately 300 subjects ranging in age from 20 to 75 years. Test measures from the Halstead–Reitan battery, which have been shown to distinguish hypertensives and normotensives, included Digit Symbol Substitution, Categories, Tactile Perception-Total Time, Tactile Perception-memory, Tactile Perception-localization, Finger Tapping, Trails A, and Trails B. The scores on these seven tests also were combined into a single composite performance score, in which hypertensives scored lower than normotensives. Moreover, higher systolic and diastolic blood pressures were associated with poorer neuropsychological performance. In both a continuous analysis of blood pressure and a group comparison of hypertensives and normotensives, subjects with higher blood pressures performed more poorly on Categories, TPT-localization, and TPT-Total, and the single composite score. The remaining tests alone were not significantly different between the two groups. Antihypertensive medication use and medical complications did not help predict neuropsychological performance. It was concluded that hypertension was associated with deficits primarily in tests of memory, but performance of hypertensives and normotensives was mostly within normal limits. Elias et al. (1990) also noted that 2% to 6% of the variance in the single composite score from this study was accounted for by blood pressure, which may be clinically relevant when considering the large population of hypertensive individuals.

This general approach to the measurement of cognitive processes is associated with an interpretive style that classifies global dysfunction into various cognitive domains (e.g., perceptual motor speed, short-term verbal memory, etc.) as a means of identifying cognitive deficits. Dysfunction associated with hypertension generally has been detected through tests believed to measure abstract reasoning, attention, construction, memory, perception, and psychomotor ability (Waldstein et al., 1991). However, the specific instruments that are incorporated into the respective test batteries vary widely among investigators.

In a careful analysis of controlled studies of untreated hypertensives, Waldstein et al. (1991) concluded that abstract reasoning and learning and memory processes are compromised among hypertensives. The various tests of abstract reasoning included Categories, Card Sorting, and Raven Progressive Matrices. Examples of assessment methods of learning and memory included Tactual Performance Test (Localization and Memory tests), Visual Reproductions, Verbal Paired-Associate Learning, Logical Memory, Figural Memory, Rey-Osterreith recall, and Benton Visual Retention Test. According to Waldstein et al. (1991), data on attentional processes, construction, general intelligence, and psychomotor ability are equivocal, and, therefore, their relationship to hypertension is unclear.

These empirical studies examining the relationship between hypertension and neuropsychological functioning have been criticized in several ways, related primarily to the measurement tools. First, global clinical measures employed in neuropsychological batteries do not permit precise analyses of specific functioning (Elias & Elias, 1993). Tests believed to measure memory, learning, or other related functions almost always assess multiple, inseparable components of cognition. As a result, it becomes evident that the classification of tests into neuropsychological function categories is somewhat arbitrary. For example, some investigators classify Digit Span (Backwards) as a test of short-term memory, whereas others consider it to be a test of sustained and directed attention. Second, these test batteries generally are not derived from theoretical paradigms, but are descriptive of brain injury. These limitations of clinical neuropsychological testing have contributed to a portion of the inconsistencies in the research literature.

Despite these problems, it generally is believed that unmedicated hypertensives perform more poorly than normotensives in several areas of neuropsychological functioning. Yet, differences have not been observed on all tests, or in all studies (Waldstein et al., 1991). In addition, studies have concluded that differences between hypertensives and normotensives are not due to antihypertensive medication effects or demographic variables, including age and education.

RESEARCH USING INFORMATION-PROCESSING APPROACHES

Another approach to the assessment of neurobehavioral functioning utilizes methods related to information processing and cognitive theory. Primary measures include reaction time (RT) performance on laboratory-based cognitive tasks (Light, 1978; Madden & Blumenthal, 1989; Spieth, 1964). Information processing procedures are designed to isolate component operations of global cognitive functions and to estimate the duration of the component operations. This approach developed from theoretical characterizations of cognitive functions, whereas neuropsychological testing approaches are more empirically based.

In a previous cross-sectional study (Madden & Blumenthal, 1989) using only an information-processing methodology, it was demonstrated that men with mild hypertension exhibited a slowing of memory search performance relative to normotensive men. Figure 11.1 shows that the estimated rate of search through items held in short-term memory was significantly slower for hypertensives than for normotensives. The rate of search became significantly slower with greater numbers of items.

To date, studies typically have not compared concurrently neuropsychological tests with information-processing assessments in the same sample of subjects. Combining neuropsychological instruments with reaction time tests may provide a more integrated approach to the study of neurobehavioral performance. One study that combined these two test methods (Blumenthal et al., 1993) was conducted to examine the relationship among a relatively broad set of measures of neurobehavioral performance in normotensive and hypertensive men and women. Subjects completed a battery of cognitive tests including both neuropsychological and information processing measures. The study was designed to determine empirically several dimensions of cognitive performance underlying the test measures, to establish the relative contribution of individual measures to these

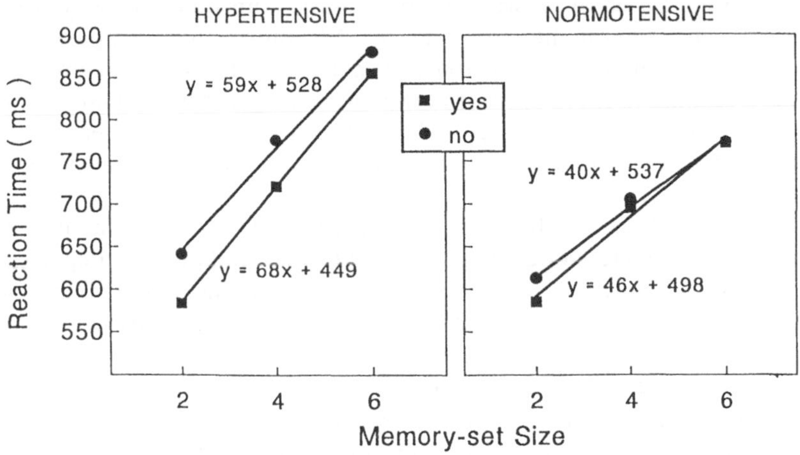

FIG. 11.1. Mean reaction time (msec) across memory-set size for hypertensives and normotensives. Analysis of variance revealed main effects of Memory-set Size (2, 4, or 6) ($p < .0001$) and Response Type (yes or no) ($p < .0129$) as well as interactions of Group (Hypertensive vs. Normotensive) × Memory-set Size ($p < .0004$) and Response Type × Memory-set Size ($p < .0244$). "Yes" represents reaction time when the subjects responded that the digit was a member of the memory set, and "No" represents that the digit was not a member. The least-squares estimate of the best-fitting line is also presented.

performance dimensions, and to examine the relation of individual measures, within performance dimensions, to blood pressure status.

Participating in the study were 68 hypertensives and 32 normotensive individuals. Subjects were screened for other diseases including cardiovascular disease, asthma, and secondary hypertension, and were not taking antihypertensive medications at the time of the study. The neuropsychological component of the test battery included the Russell Revision of the Wechsler Memory Scale (WMS)-immediate and delayed logical and figural memory, Digit Span (Backwards) from the WAIS-R, Trail Making Test (Part B), Stroop Color-Word Test, Paired Associate Learning from WMS, and Vocabulary from the WAIS-R. The information-processing module of the battery was derived from the Sternberg memory search task that yielded scores on measures of speed of memory search and information processing. A variety of self-report measures were also administered, including state and trait anxiety (State-Trait Anxiety Inventory), depression (Center for Epidemiological Studies Depression Scale), hostility (Cook–Medley Hostility Scale), Type A Behavior (Type A Self Rating Inventory), social support (Social Support Questionnaire), health locus of control (Health Locus of Control Scale), and emotional responsiveness to stressors (Emotional Reactivity Scale).

A factor analysis of the cognitive variables obtained in this study yielded three factors: Speed of information processing/immediate memory, verbal memory, and figural memory. Figure 11.2 shows that compared with normotensive individuals, hypertensives performed more poorly on the set of tasks relating to speed of information processing and immediate memory (Digit Symbol, Trails B, Stroop, and Reaction Time [slope]). There were no significant differences between hypertensives and normotensives on the remaining tasks.

A factor analysis of self-report measures also yielded three factors. The first factor related to mood and included state and trait anxiety, depression, social support, hostility, and emotional reactivity. The second factor was comprised of Type A behavior measures. The third factor was health locus of control. Further analysis yielded a significant effect for state anxiety and a trend toward an effect for social support. First, hypertensives reported higher levels of state anxiety relative to normotensives. It should be noted that these differences in anxiety did not statistically account for any observed differences in cognitive performance. These differences in state anxiety, however, may be viewed as a factor impacting on the general quality of life of hypertensive individuals. Second, there was a tendency for hypertensives to report lower levels of social support as compared to normotensives. It was also noted that the effects of hypertension on

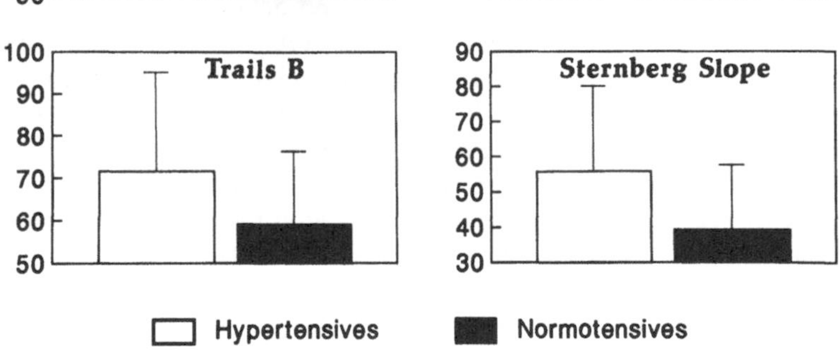

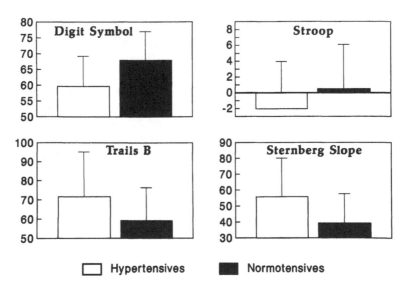

FIG. 11.2. Hypertensive and normotensive performance on various tests representing speed of information processing/immediate memory. Hypertensives completed significantly fewer items on Digit Symbol and Stroop and performed more slowly on Trails B (seconds) and Sternberg Reaction Time (milliseconds), *ps* < .05.

neurobehavioral functioning could not be accounted for on the basis of age or education (see Fig. 11.3).

These data confirmed previous findings that hypertensive individuals exhibit impairments on measures of information processing and neuropsychological functioning compared to normotensive individuals. Moreover, this study was unique in that three performance dimensions emerged from the data. Information processing, in particular, was identified as an area of relative deficits for hypertensives. It was concluded that performance decrements exhibited by hypertensives were relatively specific and appear to primarily involve cognitive processes of a "speeded" nature. They exhibited slower memory search rates, took longer to complete Trails B, and completed fewer symbols on Digit Symbol. It is possible that these timed measures were more sensitive to subtle cognitive impairments than tests not based on speed of processing and performance. Moreover, it was suggested that the tests employed in this study may have greater sensitivity to cognitive deficits than clinically based neuropsychological batteries. The hypertensive-related performance differences observed in this study are reliable; yet, there are no data to suggest that these deficits are associated with any disturbances in activities of daily living. These types of neuropsychological deficits are not known to translate directly into occupational difficulties or problems in performing activities of daily living. However, this issue has not been adequately studied using empirical methods.

Despite some difficulties in interpretation of these data, this study offers unique contributions to the field (Elias & Elias, 1993). Not only did this

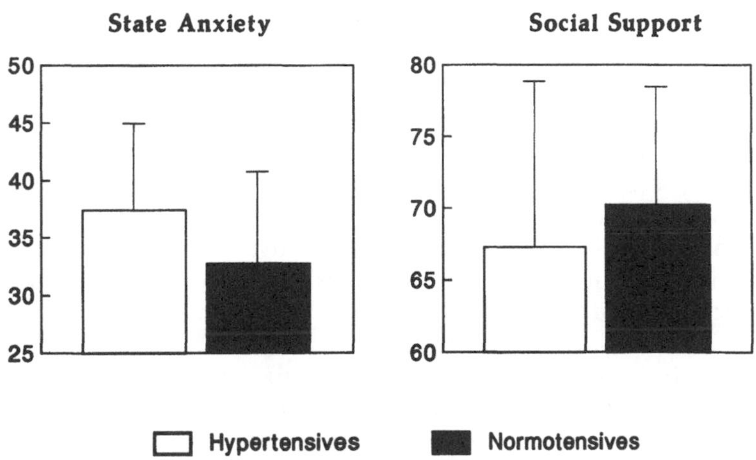

FIG. 11.3. Mean scores for hypertensives and normotensives on state anxiety and social support questionnaires. Statistical analysis revealed that hypertensives reported greater levels of state anxiety during neuropsychological test ($p < .01$), and lower levels of social support ($p < .10$), as compared to normotensives.

study replicate previous findings that hypertensives perform at a lower level than normotensives, but, more important, it made use of an information processing task to determine, on a microanalytic level, which of several important components of memory are affected by hypertension. More global clinical measures permit somewhat less precise analyses of performance as compared to the type of information processing task used in the aforementioned study. Although identified as measuring memory, learning, or other components of mental operations, clinical measures almost always involve multiple and inseparable components. Upon examination of a representative group of studies, it becomes evident that the classification of tests into neuropsychological function categories may be arbitrary and offer fewer insights into mechanisms of altered cognitive function. Furthermore, the information processing approach to assessment of neurobehavioral function is built on a paradigm originating from cognitive theory. Clinical neuropsychological measures generally developed from clinical description of the presence or absence and locus of brain injury. Taken together, both approaches appear to provide different, but potentially complementary, information about cognitive performance. Continued inclusion of both types of assessment may help resolve some of the inconsistencies within the research literature.

FUTURE RESEARCH DIRECTIONS

Although this research area has progressed significantly during the past decade, several issues require further investigation. There is a paucity of research on the impact of neurobehavioral deficits on activities of daily living, quality of life, and job performance. As the performance of hypertensives in studies discussed in this chapter does not reflect brain damage or abnormal performance, impact on quality of life may be quite subtle and occur only in later stages of the disease. Yet, the potential progression of the hypertensive's cognitive performance currently is not understood. Longitudinal tracking of cognitive performance and daily functioning of normotensive and hypertensive samples would be valuable.

The role of moderating variables in the relationship between cognitive functioning and hypertension remains unclear. A variety of factors, besides those directly associated with physiological processes altered by hypertension, may be identified in order to explain more completely the differences in cognitive functioning between normotensive and hypertensive samples. Further investigation into the role of demographic variables, such as age, education, and gender; psychological states, such as anxiety or depression; medications; general health status; alcohol and other substance use; and comorbid conditions, such as coronary artery disease, may provide valuable information and help account for differences noted in the research literature. In addition, the severity and duration of hypertension may help explain variations between studies. Future research should carefully control for these factors and may discover additional variables not yet considered.

Research may also investigate potential mechanisms by which hypertension affects cognition. It is possible that hypertension alters physiological processes related to blood flow in the brain. Hypertension may be associated with small and diffuse cerebral infarctions throughout the brain, causing a generalized decline in cognitive functioning. Hypertension also may interfere with sympathetic activation in the central nervous system, therefore, altering arousal mechanisms throughout the brain. The use of modern technology, such as positron emission tomography (PET) scan studies, may prove to be valuable in identifying physiologic processes responsible for cognitive declines. Magnetic resonance imaging (MRI) may also be useful in the identification of brain regions affected by hypertension. This technique may be used to document changes that occur with reductions in blood pressure.

Future research also may benefit from more comprehensive measurement approaches and conceptual advances. Neuropsychological batteries employed in studies generally lack strong theoretical bases. Rather, they are derived empirically, from clinical observations and test only a few, generalized domains of cognitive functioning. The procedure employed by Blumenthal et al. (1993) is an example of how more specific aspects of cognitive functioning may be measured. Use of more comprehensive neuropsychological test batteries that tap additional dimensions of cognitive function would be worthwhile.

Finally, research may benefit from examination of the impact of antihypertensive treatments on the observed performance deficits. Such research may begin by examining the effect of currently accepted treatment strategies for hypertension, including medications, weight loss, exercise, sodium and alcohol restriction, and stress management, on cognitive function. Beta blockers, which were common antihypertensive agents, have been shown to adversely affect cognition in some studies (see Rosen & Kostis, 1985). The impact of newer antihypertensive medications that work peripherally, such as angiotensin converting enzyme (Ace) inhibitors, may prove to be different than the deficits observed with centrally acting drugs (Blumenthal, Ekelund, & Emery, 1990). Effective management of elevated blood pressure could stabilize or even reverse cognitive deficits associated with hypertension.

REFERENCES

Blumenthal, J., Ekelund, L., & Emery, C. (1990). Quality of life among hypertensive patients with a diuretic background who are taking atenolol and enalapril. *Clinical Pharmacology and Therapeutics, 48*, 447–454.

Blumenthal, J., Madden, D., Pierce, T., Siegel, W., & Appelbaum, M. (1993). Hypertension affects neurobehavioral functioning. *Psychosomatic Medicine, 55*, 44–50.

Elias, M., & Elias, P. (1993). Hypertension affects neurobehavioral functioning: So what's new? *Psychosomatic Medicine, 55*, 51–54.

Elias, M., Robbins, M., & Schultz, N. (1987). Influence of essential hypertension on intellectual performance: Causation or speculation? In J. Elias & P. Marshall (Eds.), *Cardiovascular disease and behavior* (pp.107–135), Washington DC: Hemisphere.

Elias, M., Robbins, M., Schultz, N., & Pierce, T. (1990). Is blood pressure an important variable in research on aging and neuropsychological test performance? *Journal of Gerontology: Psychological Science, 45*, 128–135.

Elias, M., Robbins, M., Schultz, N., & Streeten, D. (1986). A longitudinal study of neuropsychological test performance for hypertensive and normotensive adults: Initial findings. *Journal of Gerontology, 41*, 503–505.

Elias, M., Robbins, M., Schultz, N., Streeten, D., & Elias, P. (1987). Clinical significance of cognitive performance by hypertensive patients. *Hypertension, 9*, 192–197.

Elias, M., Schultz, N., Robbins, M., & Elias, P. (1989). A longitudinal study of neuropsychological test performance by hypertensive and normotensive: A third measurement point. *Journal of Gerontology, 44*, 25–28.

Franceschi, M., Tancredi, O., Smirne, S., Mercinelli, A., & Canal, N. (1982). Cognitive processes in hypertension. *Hypertension, 4*, 226–229.

Friedman, M., & Bennett, P. (1977). Depression and hypertension. *Psychosomatic Medicine, 39*, 134–142.

Joint National Committee on Detection, Evaluation, and Treatment of High Blood Pressure. (1988). *Archives of Internal Medicine, 148*, 1023–1038.

Light, K. (1978). Effects of mild cardiovascular and cerebrovascular disorders on serial reaction time performance. *Experimental Aging Research, 4*, 3–22.

Madden, D., & Blumenthal, J. (1989). Slowing of memory-search performance in men with mild hypertension. *Health Psychology, 8*, 131–142.

Mazzucchi, A., Mutti, A., Poletti, A., Ravanetti, C., Novarini, A., & Parma, M. (1986). Neuropsychological deficits in arterial hypertension. *Acta Neurologica Scandinavia, 73*, 619–627.

Oppenheimer, B., & Fishberg, A. (1928). Hypertensive encephalopathy. *Archives of Internal Medicine, 41*, 264.

Page, I., (1987). *Hypertension mechanisms*. New York: Grune & Stratton.

Rosen, R., & Kostis, J. (1985). Biobehavioral sequellae associated with adrenergic-inhibiting antihypertensive agents: A critical review. *Health Psychology, 4*, 579–604.

Schmidt, R., Fazekas, F., Offenbacher, H., Lytwyn, H., Blematl, B., Niederkorn, K., Horner, S., Payer, F., & Friedl, W. (1991). Magnetic resonance imaging white matter lesions and cognitive impairment in hypertensive individuals. *Archives of Neurology, 48*, 417–420.

Spieth, W. (1964). Cardiovascular health status, age, and psychological performance. *Journal of Gerontology, 19*, 277- 284.

Joint National Committee on Detection, Evaluation, and Treatment of High Blood Pressure. (1988). *Archives of Internal Medicine, 148*, 1023–1038.

Waldstein, S., Manuck, S., Ryan, C., & Muldoon, M. (1991). Neuropsychological correlates of hypertension: Review and methodological considerations. *Psychological Bulletin, 110*, 451–468.

Wilkie, F., Eisdorfer, C., & Nowlin, J. (1976). Memory and blood pressure in the aged. *Experimental Aging Research, 2*, 3–16.

12 Effectiveness of a Combined Behavioral–Drug Intervention for Hypertension: Drug, Personality, and Quality of Life Effects

David Shapiro
Ka Kit Hui
Mark E. Oakley
Jagoda Pasic
University of California, Los Angeles

Larry D. Jamner
University of California, Irvine

In the fifth report of the Joint National Committee on Detection, Evaluation, and Treatment of High Blood Pressure (JNC-V; 1993), certain lifestyle modifications were recommended as definitive or adjunctive therapy of hypertension. These included weight reduction, moderation of alcohol and sodium intake, and increased physical activity. Although their effectiveness has not been conclusively determined, such interventions, the JNC-V Committee concluded, can improve the cardiovascular risk profile and can offer multiple benefits at little cost. Also mentioned as beneficial adjunctive interventions are tobacco avoidance, decreased dietary fats, and adequate potassium intake. Although the report states that stress can raise blood pressure acutely and contribute to the cause of hypertension, it also concluded that the available literature does not support the use of relaxation therapies for definitive therapy of hypertension. This conservative position seems at odds with the wealth of literature on behavioral interventions. There are dozens of studies and extensive reviews, including four major meta-analyses of behavioral interventions (variously labeled nondrug treatments, arousal reduction treatments, and relaxation therapy; Andrews, MacMahon, Austin, & Byrne, 1984; Jacob, Chesney, Williams, Ding, & Shapiro, 1991; Kaufmann et al., 1988; Ward, Swan, & Chesney, 1987).

The results of the meta-analyses have provided support for the potential of behavioral methods, but mainly for unmedicated patients. In studies of combined drug–behavioral treatments, the results have been less encouraging. The conclusions of these meta-analyses seem to vary depending on the number and apparent quality of the studies included in the analysis, most particularly the degree to which the control groups served as adequate comparisons. Perhaps the single most critical general finding in the literature is that the decline in blood pressure in treated patients is generally proportional to pretreatment levels (see Jacob et al., 1991). Therefore, patients with higher levels of blood pressure would appear to be the best candidates for behavioral interventions. As current medical consensus mandates drug treatment for such patients (JNC-V), it is necessary to evaluate the potential benefit of a behavioral intervention as an adjunct to drug therapy in subjects with higher levels of pressure and more severe hypertension. This poses a dilemma, given the methodological complications in differentiating between drug and behavioral effects, which no doubt accounts for the failure to detect a significant improvement in medicated patients who have participated in behavioral interventions (Kaufmann et al., 1988).

Oakley and Shapiro (1989) discussed critical methodological issues in conducting studies of drug-behavioral interactions in treatment studies and laid out a framework of research in this area. We proposed that the reduction in antihypertensive medication level required to maintain blood pressure at controlled levels (e.g., < 90 mmHg diastolic blood pressure) be used as the primary outcome measure rather than reduction in blood pressure. It is this framework that guided the study described in this chapter. In this study, we compared a combined drug-behavioral treatment with a drug-only control condition. We present the major results for reduction in drug requirements and changes in blood pressure over the critical phases of the study. Significant reductions in drug requirements were obtained in both treatment and control conditions with greater benefits achieved in the combined drug-behavioral group. Moreover, clinic, ambulatory, and home blood pressure continued to be maintained at controlled levels after medication requirements were reduced.

Although this study was not directed specifically at the effects of antihypertensive drug therapy on quality of life, periodic assessments were made of individual symptoms related to drug side effects, psychosocial factors, personality characteristics, cognitive function, and health habits. The methods included standardized tests and questionnaires adapted from the extensive quality of life literature (Barnett, 1991; Dimsdale, 1992; Jern & Zanchetti, 1992). The following issues were considered: Are the reductions in drug requirements achieved in the program associated with changes in quality of life? Do these changes differ when relaxation is combined with drug treatment as compared to drug treatment only?

This chapter reviews the data for the initial and treatment phases of the study through a 6-month follow-up period.

METHODS

Key Features of Study

The key features of the study are listed in Table 12.1, and the design and sequence of procedures and measures are outlined in Fig. 12.1.

1. To qualify for participation in the study, subjects had to have an unmedicated diastolic blood pressure (DBP) between 95 and 110 mmHg. Volunteers already on antihypertensive medication were slowly weaned off their current medications prior to evaluation of their eligibility for the study. After being completely withdrawn, they were followed over a 4- to 6-week period. The criterion for entry into the study was based on DBP averaged over three visits over a 2- to 4-week period. About 15% of the volunteer subjects did not qualify in this time period. Discussion of other selection and exclusion criteria follow.

2. After qualification, a minimal drug requirement was established for each subject to achieve blood pressure (BP) at DBP ≤ 90 mmHg. All patients were given the same sequence of drugs in five steps starting with diuretic (Dyazide^{TM}, hydrochlorothiazide 25 mg and triamterene 50 mg) followed by the selective beta blocker atenolol from 25 mg to 100 mg in 25 mg increments. At each step, BP was assessed over three visits over 2 to 3 weeks, until the DBP criterion was achieved.

3. Subjects were then randomized into treatment and control groups. During this phase, which lasted 6 weeks, treatment subjects participated in a stress management program in weekly 2-hour group sessions described later and a brief clinical and BP evaluation. To assure comparable amounts of contact with the project staff, control subjects also visited the clinic at

TABLE 12.1
Key Features of Study

1. Participation based on unmedicated DBP between 95mmHg and 110 mmHg.
2. Minimal drug requirements established prior to randomization of subjects into treatment and control groups using five successive steps of study drugs. Criterion of BP control was DBP ≤ 90 mmHg. If patients were previously on antihypertensive medication, it was withdrawn prior to evaluation.
3. Subjects randomized into treatment and control groups.
4. All subjects (treatment and control) systematically stepped down off medications after major treatment phase.
5. All adjustments of medications followed set rules, based on clinic DBP averaged over three visits.
6. All patients followed for a minimum of 1 year.

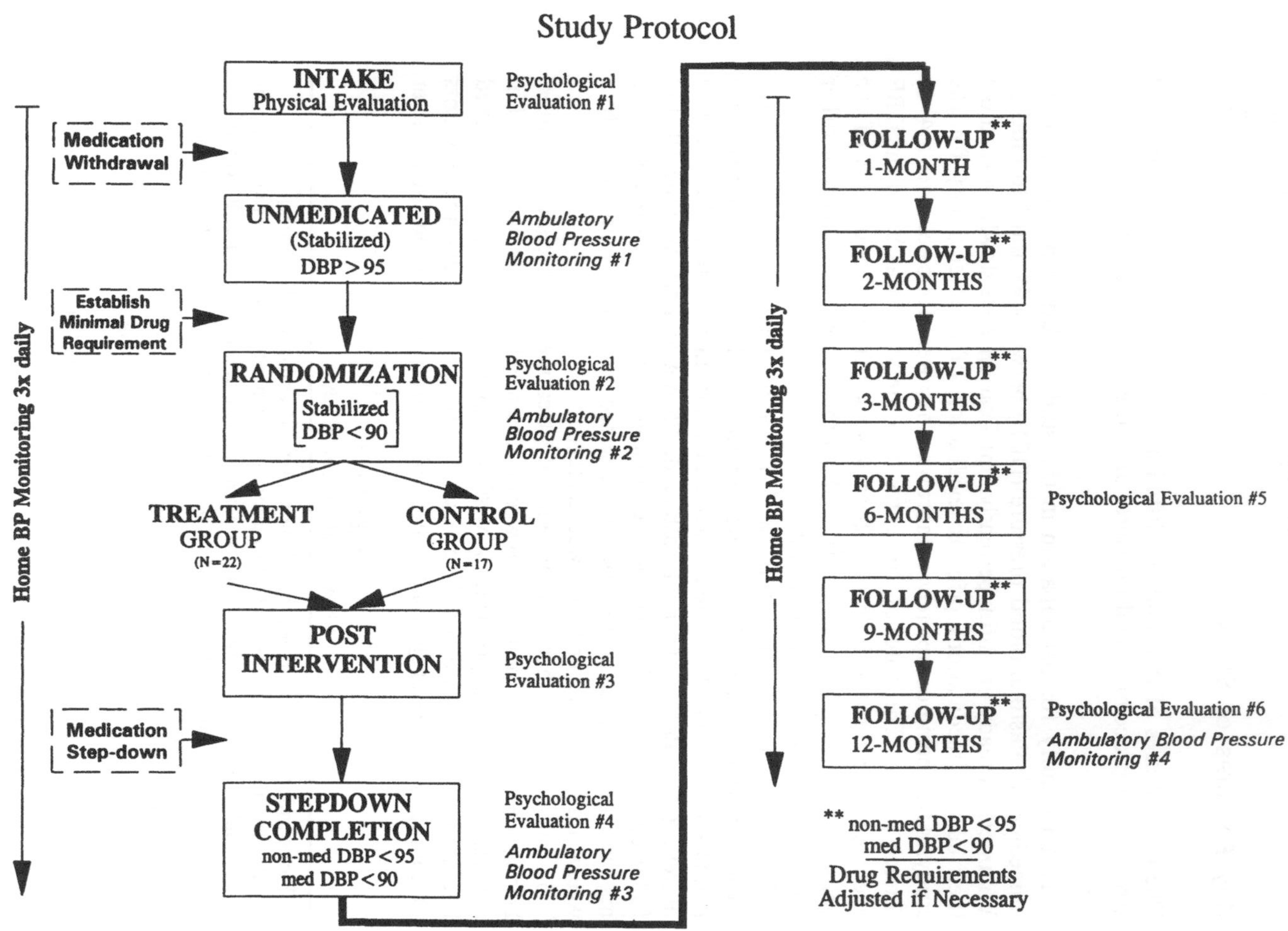

FIG. 12.1. Study protocol showing all phases of the program, procedures for establishing drug requirements, periodic psychological assessments (personality, psychosocial, and quality of life), and multiple clinic and ambulatory blood pressure assessments.

the same times for the clinical and BP evaluation only. No changes in medication were made in this phase of the study.

4. All subjects (treatment and control) then participated in a drug stepdown procedure in which medication level was reduced by one step at a time. This process was begun so long as BP was stable and still under control (< 90 mmHg, DBP) at the end of the 6-week period. After each step down of medication, BP was assessed over three visits in a 2- to 3-week period. Stepdown was considered completed at the lowest step at which DBP remained equal to or below 90 mmHg. For subjects who were able to be stepped off all medication, DBP had to remain below 95 mmHg DBP.

5. The follow-up period was initiated at the completion of the stepdown procedure. During follow-up, all subjects were seen for a BP assessment and brief check-up at 1-month intervals for 3 months and then at 3-month intervals for at least 1 year. Treatment subjects also participated in a 30-minute "booster" session during each follow-up visit along with the BP evaluation in which they discussed problems and reviewed adherence to the various procedures of the intervention. During these visits, if the DBP (three readings) was above criterion, this triggered two more visits to determine if medication had to be stepped up. If so, the next step of medication was added, and a new three-visit evaluation commenced, and so on, as required. Medication adjustments continued throughout the remaining follow-up period, as needed, following strict rules, which were identical for treatment and control subjects.

6. Figure 12.1 indicates the periodic personality, psychosocial, and quality of life evaluations (see following section), and the times at which ambulatory blood pressure monitoring was done. Throughout the program, all subjects were asked to record their own BP three times a day.

Subjects

Subjects were recruited by means of advertisements and announcements in local and community newspapers and by referral from physicians. A stated goal of the project was to determine whether the behavioral intervention was more effective than the control procedure in reducing drug requirements. However, all subjects were told that participation in the various procedures of the program, including home and ambulatory blood pressure monitoring, would be beneficial in the management of their hypertension and in lowering drug requirements. For many subjects, a major incentive in participating was to reduce or get off drugs entirely.

Only subjects with primary hypertension were included in the study, as determined by history and an intake physical examination that included fundoscopy, 12-lead electrocardiography, urinalysis, hematology, and serum chemistry. Exclusion criteria included: secondary hypertension;

hypertension complications (left ventricular hypertrophy, proteinuria, retinopathy); history of cardiovascular disorders, stroke, diabetes, asthma, epilepsy, obstructive valvular disease, malignant hypertension, renal disease, or hepatic disease; pregnancy; severe obesity; drug or alcohol abuse; current medical or psychiatric treatment; and contraindications to the administration of the study medications. Aside from the BP eligibility requirement, subjects had to be willing and able to carry out all the procedures and to commit themselves to the large number of required clinic visits.

Characteristics of the 39 final participants are given in Table 12.2.

Tests and Measurements

Home BP Recording. Subjects were instructed by the nurse on how to take their own BP using an auscultatory sphygmomanometer (Propper Model #214011) following American Heart guidelines. A T-connector and a teaching stethoscope were used to check their procedures and accuracy. Subjects were asked to record their BP three times a day on three occasions at home during the day (i.e., on awakening, before dinner, and at bedtime). Only certain home recordings used in the analyses are presented in this chapter. For the initial major phases prior to the follow-up, we used the readings made on the 3 days parallel to the 3 clinic days used for the clinic BP assessments. For the follow-up visits, we used 3 consecutive days nearest to the clinic visit of the particular follow-up visit.

TABLE 12.2
Subject Characteristics

	Treatment	*Control*
Sample size	22	17
Age	48.4 (9.1)	54.8 (6.1)
Gender	8F	9F
	14M	8M
Years hypertension	6.6 (5.3)	9.6 (6.3)
Ethnicity	5 Asian	2 Asian
	1 Black	5 Black
	16 White	10 White
Education (yrs.)	15.8 (3.0)	16.6 (3.2)
Marital status	14 Married	14 Married
	5 Single	0 Single
	2 Divorced	2 Divorced
	0 Separated	1 Separated
	1 Widowed	0 Widowed
Family history of hypertension	19 Positive	15 Positive
	3 Negative	2 Negative

Note. Standard deviations are given in parentheses following mean values.

Clinic BP Recording. Clinic BP was obtained with a random-zero sphygmomanometer (Hawksley & Sons). Three successive readings were taken at 2-minute intervals after a 10-minute rest period. Means of the three readings were used in the analyses, usually combined with the means obtained on two additional visits.

Ambulatory BP Monitoring (ABPM). ABPM was done at specific phases of the program (see Fig. 12.1), using the ACCUTRACKER II developed by Suntech Medical Instruments of Raleigh, North Carolina. Previous research has established the validity and reliability of this monitoring device (Light, Obrist, & Cubeddu, 1988; White, Schulman, McCabe, & Nardone, 1987). The ambulatory data were downloaded into a computer for subsequent analysis.

Subjects were fitted with the ambulatory blood pressure monitor for 24-hour recording and given verbal and written instructions about the monitor's operation and care. They were instructed to carry on with their usual activities, keep their arm still at their side whenever the recorder operated, and avoid strenuous activities that would impair the operation of the recorder. Test readings were obtained to ensure proper operation of the device. It was programmed to operate at random intervals, three times an hour during waking hours and hourly during sleep. All ambulatory recordings were made on a weekday. Reported in the analyses are mean values per subject for awake and sleep periods at various phases of the program. In the analyses, artifacts were eliminated using methods described elsewhere (Shapiro, Jamner, & Goldstein, 1993).

Personality, Psychosocial, and Quality of Life Assessments. At various phases of the study (see Fig. 12.1), all subjects took a computer-administered battery of personality tests including: (a)Buss–Durkee Hostility Inventory (BDHI), a 75-item true–false questionnaire designed to provide a total score and scores on Assault, Indirect, Resentment, Suspicion, Irritability, Negativism, Guilt, and Verbal Hostility subscales; (b) Marlowe–Crowne Social Desirability Scale, used as a measure of defensiveness; (c) Taylor Manifest Anxiety Scale; (d) State and Trait forms of the Spielberger State-Trait Anxiety Inventory; and (e) Beck Depression Inventory. These personality tests were selected as standardized assessments of psychological characteristics examined in quality of life studies (e.g., Aberg & Tibblin, 1989) and also because of their empirical association with hypertension or with blood pressure variations in healthy subjects (Jamner, Shapiro, Goldstein, & Hug, 1991; Johnson & Spielberger, 1992). The test battery included other brief scales and questionnaires designed to assess various psychosocial factors and quality of life. These included work performance, sleep problems, physical symptoms, drug side effects, and sexual function. Various health habits were assessed: use of caffeine, alcohol, and salt; amount of regular exercise and leisure/recreational activity. A neurophysical test of short-term memory was also administered using the Selective Reminding Test. (Buschke, 1973)

Cognitive-Behavioral Intervention

Subjects in the treatment group participated in six weekly 2 hour sessions in groups of two to four. The sessions were arranged to cover a wide variety of cognitive and behavioral methods designed to facilitate stress and BP reduction. The specific methods ar listed in Table 12.3. A principal component of the program was progressive muscle relaxation training that was taught in the sessions. Subjects were provided with relaxation tapes to practice once a day at home. They were also provided with a digital temperature biofeedback device for home practice in relaxation using this method.

Each subject was given a manual of procedures, describing the basic concepts and methods and laying out the various exercises to be done at home over the 6-week period. The manual provided a rationale for the intervention in general and for each specific procedure. Brief questionnaires were used at the beginning of each session to assess adherence to the home practice and the subject's utilization of the various cognitive and behavioral techniques in everyday situations. Over the course of the study, subjects tended to focus their attention and effort on two or three procedures that they preferred and found useful.

Data Analysis

Changes in drug requirements were analyzed by Fisher's Exact Test and *t* test. Changes in the blood pressure variables were analyzed by repeated

TABLE 12.3
Components of Behavioral Intervention

1. Progressive muscle relaxation training with daily home practice.
2. Cue-controlled relaxation and imagery.
3. Autogenic training.
4. Assertiveness training.
5. Digital temperature biofeedback training with home practice.
6. Time management.
7. Deep diaphragmatic breathing.
8. Cognitive–behavioral therapy.
9. Daily home practice.
10. Manual describing general rationale and explanation of methods, session-by-session topics and exercises, and home practice assignments.

measure analysis of variance with condition (control, treatment) as the between-subject factor and phase as the within-subject factor (e.g., Randomization vs. Stepdown Completion). The same method of analysis was used for the quality of life variables with the addition of amount of medication reduction across phase as a second between-subject factor. In the analyses of variance, we used the MGLH Program of SYSTAT (Version 5.0).

RESULTS

Reduction in Drug Requirements

Table 12.4 presents the number of subjects at each medication step at each of three major phases of the study: Randomization (R), Stepdown (S), and Six-Month Follow-Up (F6). Significant and comparable reductions in medication level were shown in both groups ($p < .0001$) at Stepdown Completion, compared to Randomization. By the 6-month follow-up, some but not all control subjects had regressed to Randomization (pretreatment) levels, although the reduction in medication remained significant for each group looked at separately (treatment, $p < .0001$; control, $p = .03$). At 6 months, almost twice as many subjects were off all medication in the treatment group (64%) compared to the control group (35%). In the treatment group, 17 out of 22 subjects reduced at least one step of medication as compared to 7 out of 17 subjects in the control group ($p = .044$). In addition, using the five steps as a measure of medication level, the treatment group achieved a reduction of 1.2 steps compared to 0.4 steps in the control group ($p = .009$).

In summary, although both treatment and control subjects were able to

TABLE 12.4
Drug Requirements in Three Major Phases of Study

	Treatment			*Control*		
	R	*S*	*F6*	*R*	*S*	*F6*
None		14	14		11	6
Dyazide	10	4	4	11	3	6
Dyazide + 25 mg atenolol	10	4	4	5	3	4
Dyazide + 50 mg atenolol	1			1		1
Dyazide + 75 mg atenolol						
Dyazide + 100 mg atenolol	1					

Note. R = Randomization; S = Stepdown Completion; F6 = Six-Month Follow-Up.

reduce their medications, the reduction in drug requirement was significantly greater in the treatment group. The difference did not occur immediately after treatment at the Stepdown Completion phase, at which time the control subjects were able to show a short-term improvement, but emerged over the ensuing 6 months. The fact that 20 patients out of the sample of 39 (51%) were able to be withdrawn completely from medication and remain free of medication for 6 months is remarkable given the fact that all that patients, most of whom had been medicated prior to enrollment in the study, had been withdrawn from medication during their initial evaluation for eligibility and had all shown increases in BP to 95 mmHg and over at that time. In addition, the reductions occurred in subjects with carefully and systematically established minimal drug requirements.

Blood Pressure Findings

Clinic Blood Pressure. The clinic BP data for the four major phases (Randomization, Post-Intervention, Stepdown completion, and Six-Month Follow-Up) are given in Table 12.5. Table 12.5 also presents the unmedicated clinic BP levels for both groups. Administration of medications at minimal drug requirement levels produced sizeable reductions in both clinic SBP ($p < .0001$) and DBP ($p < .0001$) from unmedicated to randomization phase. By definition, subjects had to be below 90 mmHg DBP to be randomized into the treatment or control group. Comparable reductions were achieved in both groups.

Table 12.5 shows the progression of clinic BP change over the major phases of the study. From Randomization to Post-Intervention, during which time medications were not changed, a small nonsignificant decrease in DBP occurred in both groups. At the same time, SBP increased a small

TABLE 12.5
Clinic SBP and DBP (mmHg) at Unmedicated (U), Randomization (R), Post-Intervention (P), Stepdown Completion (S), and Six-Month Follow-Up (F6) in Treatment and Control Groups

	U	*R*	*P*	*S*	*F6*
Treatment					
SBP	145.8	127.3	129.7	135.2	133.3
DBP	98.9	85.4	83.6	89.3	87.4
Control					
SBP	149.5	131.4	128.4	141.2	136.3
DBP	97.0	85.5	82.1	88.8	85.4

Note. Each value shown is the mean of three visits, three readings per visit.

amount in the treatment group and decreased a small amount in the control group (p = .017). From Randomization to Stepdown Completion, during which considerable and comparable reductions were made in medications in both groups, both treatment and control subjects increased to the same degree in both SBP (p = .002) and DBP (p = .004). DBP appears to be close to pretreatment levels (R), whereas SBP is somewhat elevated. For all subjects, the mean increase from Randomization to Six-Month Follow-UP was 5.5 mmHg in SBP and 1.1 in DBP. DBP remained under control despite the significant reduction in medication level, particularly in the treatment group, although SBP became slightly elevated in both groups. Moreover, about half of the sample were free of medication at this time. It is also notable that clinic SBP and DBP did not differ significantly between groups at any phase whether medication levels were comparable or different for the two groups.

Home Blood Pressure. From Unmedicated to Randomization phases, establishment of minimal drug requirements produced sizable reductions in home SBP (p < .0001) and home DBP (p = .0001), comparable to those obtained in the clinic measures. The pattern of values for the three following phases was similar to that shown for clinic BP, a rise in both SBP and DBP from Randomization to Stepdown Completion (p = .005 and p = .025, respectively), which was comparable for both groups. At the Six-Month Follow-Up, SBP and DBP were reduced somewhat and were at levels that were not significantly different from the pretreatment Randomization phase. The considerable reduction in medication in the treatment group in particular was associated with little change in DBP. Thus, the home BP data support the clinic BP findings in showing that reduction in drug requirements can be accomplished while maintaining BP at controlled levels.

ABPM. Significant reductions in awake SBP (p < .0001), sleep SBP (p < .001), and in awake DBP (p < .0001) and sleep DBP (p < .0001) occurred with the administration of study drugs (change from Unmedicated to Randomization). From Randomization to Stepdown Completion for all subjects, there were significant increases in awake DBP (p < .001), sleep SBP (p = .041), sleep DBP (p < .001), but not for awake SBP. The changes were comparable in both groups. Compared to the Unmedicated values, the Stepdown Completion values were lower in all comparisons, statistically significant for awake SBP (p = .029), awake DBP (p = .009), and sleep DBP (p = .005). ABPM data were not obtained at the Six-Month Follow-up. In general, the ABPM data appear to parallel the clinic and home BP findings.

Personality, Psychosocial, Health Habits, and Quality of Life Effects

For simplicity of presentation, we present analyses of changes in the various measures from the time of randomization to subsequent assessments.

Randomization to Post-Intervention. In this 6-week period, treatment subjects participated in the cognitive-behavioral intervention, and control subjects visited the clinic at the same times for a clinical and BP evaluation. Medication levels were not changed. One significant change occurred: a reduction in Verbal Hostility in the treatment group (4.7 to 3.9) and a slight increase in Verbal Hostility in the control group (4.3 to 4.6; $p = .04$). This effect may reflect a focus in the behavioral intervention on assertiveness as a means of dealing with hostile situations. In this comparison, with the exception of Verbal hostility, the behavioral intervention by itself had no effect on personality, psychosocial, cognitive, or quality of life variables.

Randomization to Stepdown Completion. In this period, highly significant reductions in medication level occurred that were comparable in both treatment and control groups. Independent of treatment condition, Defensiveness (scores on the Marlowe–Crowne Social Desirability scale) decreased as a function of amount of medication reduction ($p = .021$), as shown in Fig. 12.2 (left panel). The greater the reduction in medication from Randomization to Stepdown Completion, the greater the decrease in Defensiveness. A similar interaction was observed between Assault Hostility and medication reduction ($p = .021$), as shown in Fig. 12.3 (left panel). Independent of treatment condition, the greater the reduction in medication, the greater the decrease in Assault Hostility. Finally, a significant three-way interaction was obtained between phase, group (treatment, control), and medication reduction for Verbal Hostility ($p = .037$) (Fig. 12.4). The greater the individual amount of reduction in medication, the greater the increase in Verbal Hostility in the treatment group subjects. An opposite but nonsignificant relationship was observed in the control group. Note that, in general, treatment subjects as a group showed a slight decrease in Verbal Hostility, whereas control subjects as a group showed a slight increase in Verbal Hostility. This is the same pattern observed over the 6-week treatment phase, as discussed previously.

In summary, several personality characteristics changed from Randomization to Stepdown Completion that are generally independent of whether or not subjects participated in the behavioral intervention and that appear to be related to the medication reduction in this period. Defensiveness and

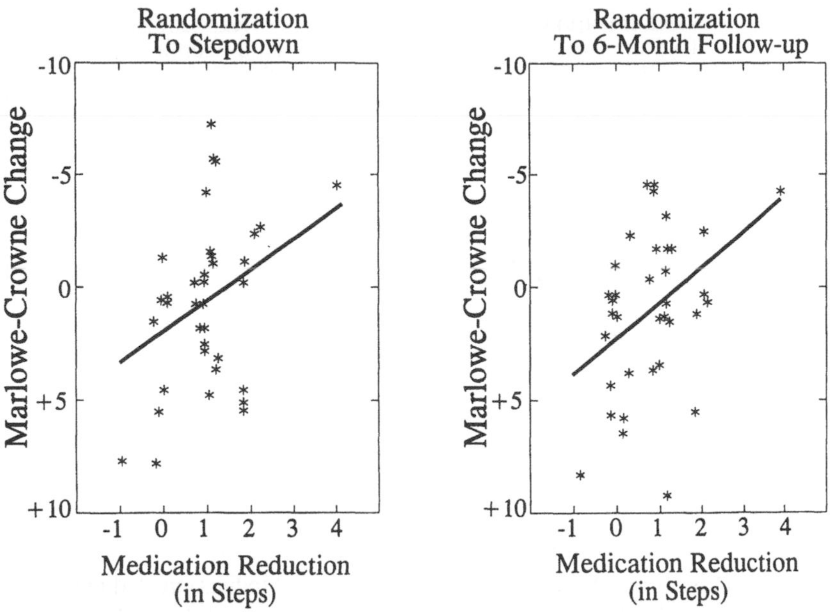

FIG. 12.2. Relation between change in scores on the Marlowe-Crowne Social Desirability scale (a measure of Defensiveness) and medication reduction from Randomization to Stepdown Completion and from Randomization to Six-Month Follow-Up. Note that the points at each level of medication reduction are slightly dispersed so that multiple subjects appearing at a given X-Y coordinate can be shown. This procedure was also used in plotting the points in Figs. 12.3 and 12.4.

Assault Hostility were shown to decrease as a function of individual differences in amount of medication reduction. Verbal Hostility also changed as a function of medication reduction and treatment condition, the only effect having an apparent association with the behavioral intervention. No other personality, psychosocial, cognitive, or quality of life effects were obtained.

Randomization to Six-Month Follow-Up. Some of the same effects shown for Randomization to Stepdown Completion were maintained at the Six-Month Follow-Up. The previously described effect for Defensiveness and drug reduction was also obtained in this analysis ($p = .004$), as shown in Fig. 12.2 (right panel). As before, independent of treatment condition, the greater the reduction in medication, the greater the reduction in Defensiveness. As previously described, Assault Hostility was reduced as a function of medication reduction ($p = .006$; see Fig, 12.3, right panel). A significant reduction in Anxiety (TMAS) was shown from Randomization to Six-Month Follow-Up, independent of group (6.5 to 5.3, $p = .005$). This

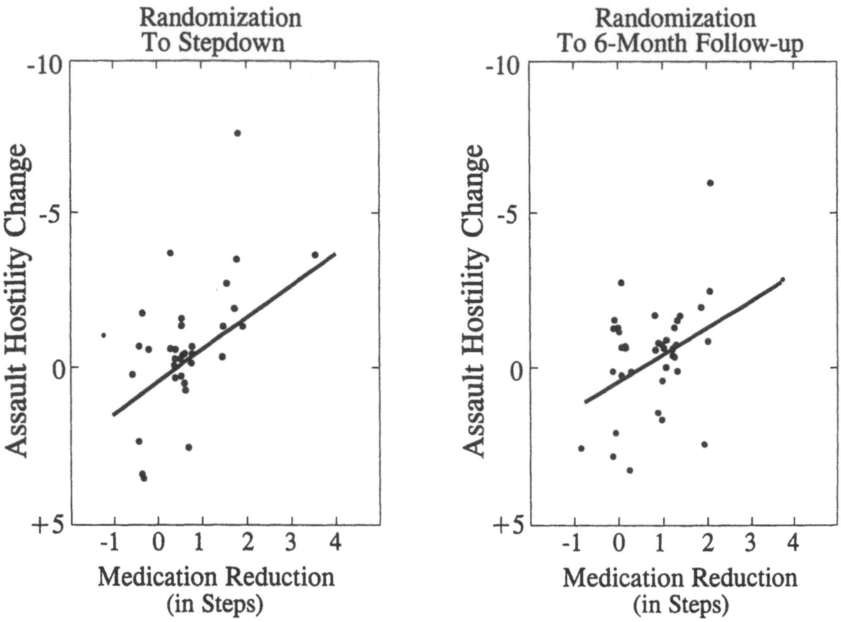

FIG. 12.3. Relation between change in scores on the Assault Hostility subscale of the Buss-Durkee Hostility Inventory and medication reduction from Randomization to Stepdown Completion and from Randomization to Six-Month Follow-Up.

reduction was general and not tied to individual differences in medication reduction.

In summary, in comparison of changes from Randomization to Six-Month Follow-Up, during which there was a considerable reduction in medication level, particularly in the treatment group, one overall change was a reduction in Anxiety for all subjects. Reductions in Assault Hostility and Defensiveness depended on the degree of medication reduction, effects that were independent of whether or not subjects participated in the behavioral intervention. No other personality, psychosocial, cognitive, or quality of life effects were obtained in this comparison.

In all of these analyses, few significant effects were obtained for other personality, psychosocial, cognitive, health habits, or quality of life measures. After the establishment of minimal drug requirements, participation in this drug-behavioral program, whether as a treatment or as a control subject, was not associated with changes in any physical symptoms, sleep problems, work performance, or sexual function. Thus, reductions in medication were generally not associated with changes in customary quality of life variables.

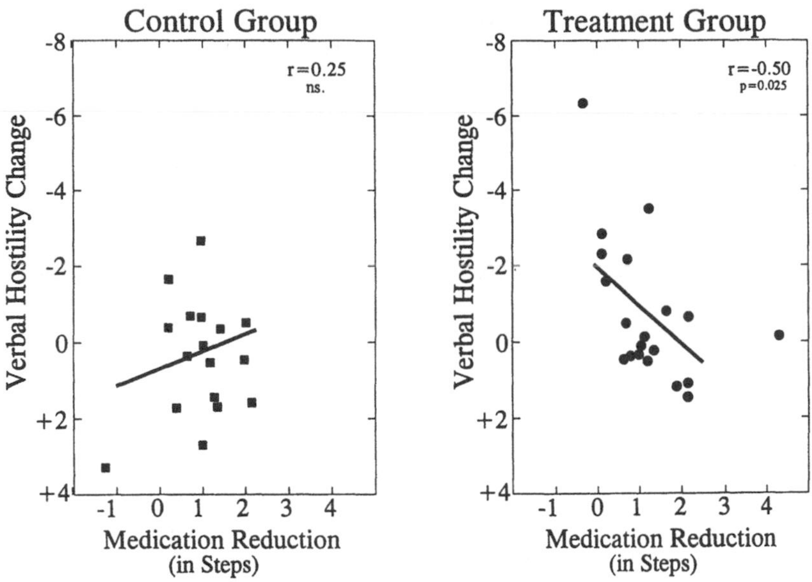

FIG. 12.4 Relation between change in scores on the Verbal Hostility subscale and medication reduction from Randomization to Stepdown Completion in Control and Treatment groups.

GENERAL DISCUSSION AND CONCLUSIONS

The addition of a cognitive–behavioral intervention to the antihypertensive drug treatment of mild-to-moderate hypertension proved effective in reducing drug requirements. This intervention was about twice as effective in reducing drug requirements in the behavioral treatment intervention as compared to the control group. Six months after the posttreatment stepdown was completed, 64% of the treatment group remained completely free of medication as compared to 35% of the control group. The significance of the medication reduction can be viewed in relation to the pattern of blood pressure change associated with the program. Consider the 14 patients in the treatment group who were off all medications at the 6-month follow-up. At the time of initial qualification (Unmedicated), their clinic BP averaged 145/97 mmHg. At the time of the 6-month follow-up when they were also free of medications, their clinic BP averaged 137/88 mmHg. The reduction of 8/9 mmHg can be considered an index of the BP lowering effect of the program in these subjects.

Results of the present study are consistent with the findings reported by Glasgow, Engel, and D'Lugoff (1989), the best example of a similar attempt to determine the extent to which a behavioral intervention might supplement or replace antihypertensive drug treatment of hypertension. As in the present study, the investigators used a standardized protocol for adjusting drug requirements in a combined behavioral and drug treatment of hypertension. However, the Glasgow et al. study differed in several major respects. First, the behavioral treatment was a stepped sequence of behavioral methods, beginning with self-monitoring only and continuing with systolic blood pressure feedback and then with relaxation therapy. The total duration was about 7 months, compared to 6 weeks (plus periodic "booster" sessions) in the present study. Second, the control subjects were assigned to a Referred Care protocol, but no attempt was made to titrate their drugs or to attempt stepdown after treatment as was the case in the present study. Thus, there is no way to know for sure whether a stepdown of medications might not have been as effective for the control group as it was in the Stepped Care group. Third, unlike the present study in which specific study drugs were employed and administered in a stepwise fashion, the patients in the Glasgow et al. study continued on drugs that they had used just prior to the study. Fourth, patients were not evaluated off medications prior to intake into the study. In comparing the two sets of findings, one can see that the Referred Care control group in the Glasgow et al. study either increased in their usage of such medications as diuretics (150% increase) or stayed about the same throughout the program. In the present study, in which we stepped down the control subjects, a definite decrease in drug requirements was observed. In the treatment group of Glasgow et al., reductions of medications occurred, which were generally greater in the diuretics-only patients than in those on combined therapy. The maximum decrease was to 30% of initial level for the diuretics-only group and to 60% in two other groups involving other drug therapies (including beta blockers and vasodilator). We can compute a similar percentage in the present study using the five drug steps as a 5-point scale. For the treatment group, at the time of the 6-month follow-up, subjects were on the average at 29% of their initial level, whereas the control group was at 68% of their initial medication level. The figure for our treatment group matches that reported by Glasgow and colleagues for their best condition; the figure for the control group is far superior to their control subjects, which was never lower than 90%. The Glasgow et al. study does not indicate how many subjects were completely free of medications, so in this respect we have no way to compare our data with theirs. In general, however, the present study reinforces the conclusion drawn by Glasgow et al. that a behavioral intervention can be an effective supplement or replacement for antihypertensive drug therapy.

The benefits of the behavioral intervention of this study appear to be much more substantial than those reported in the National Heart, Lung, and Blood Institute Pooling Project (Kaufmann et al., 1988). In fact, their meta-analysis did not yield any evidence of the superiority of combined drug–behavioral treatments over control procedures. The question is to what can we attribute the apparent benefits obtained in this study of a combined drug and behavioral treatment? One possibility is the quality of the intervention itself, which included a large variety of methods of stress reduction, ranging from cognitively focused approaches to perception of and coping with stress and emotional response to behaviorally and physiologically oriented relaxation and biofeedback methods. The variety of treatment components may have allowed individual subjects to utilize those methods they found most congenial or effective, for whatever reasons. Second is the close, personal, and frequent contact between a key member of the project staff and the patient. This key staff member was the same person throughout the study, usually a nurse/practitioner. The nature and extent of the contact was the same for both treatment and control groups. It probably facilitated adherence to the behavioral procedures in the treatment group and no doubt also facilitated reduction of drug requirements in the control group, which was likely a function of their self-monitoring of blood pressure and greater attention to their hypertension.

A critical question is what did the treatment subjects learn and how did they incorporate what they learned into their daily life? In considering the paucity of results on the various assessments of personality and psychosocial variables, it does not appear that subjects in the treatment group changed very much in their characteristic response dispositions or in their general adaptation to everyday life stress. It seems likely, however, that they did learn ways of reducing or modifying their reactivity to situations, which in turn served to reduce their blood pressure and hence need for medication. This learning was probably facilitated by an increase in subjects' awareness of their blood pressure and its day-by-day and week-by-week fluctuations, most likely a byproduct of the recording of their own blood pressure at home, and the many blood pressure assessments made in frequent clinic visits. Stress reduction methods can therefore be translated into the learning of different ways of reducing one's own blood pressure, abetted by an increased awareness of changes in one's blood pressure and one's characteristic ways of responding to stress and to emotional stimulation. The careful titration of drugs at the beginning of the program and in the stepdown process later on may have also induced a greater sensitivity to factors leading to variations in one's blood pressure. This process may have in part helped some of the control group subjects to reduce their medication requirements. In the case of the treatment group, this process was likely useful in combination with learning various methods of reducing blood pressure. Given that blood pressure levels were at controlled and relatively low levels, subjects could orient themselves to momentary fluctuations, particularly increases, in their blood pressure, and to ways of bringing their pressure back to controlled levels. Perhaps a focus on what might make blood pressure increase in a person in whom it is already controlled and on what might be done to return it to a controlled level may be of greater benefit than a focus on what might make blood pressure decrease in a person whose blood pressure is already elevated.

Despite the wide range of psychological and quality of life assessments, only one variable was found to be sensitive to differences between groups. Verbal Hostility tended to decrease more in the treatment than in the control group, although the degree to which Verbal Hostility decreased was a function of medication reduction. Apparently, the treatment by itself served to decrease Verbal Hostility overall. However, the more a subject reduced medication, the more Verbal Hostility tended to increase. An incidental effect of the medication itself may be to decrease Verbal Hostility, and reducing medication thereby may return it to higher levels. The subjects who showed more than one step of medication reduction were on combined therapy of diuretic and atenolol, with the possibility that the beta blocker served to reduce Verbal Hostility, whereas its removal served to increase it again.

Medication reduction, independent of treatment group, was associated with changes in Defensiveness and Assault Hostility. In this case, degree of medication reduction was associated with a decrease in both of these characteristics, implying that the medication (probably the addition of a beta blocker) served to increase these characteristics. The design of this study, however, does not allow a definite conclusion about the nature of these drug effects on psychological characteristics. All patients were placed on the same sequence of drugs, and stepped off in reverse sequence. Nonetheless, the results are suggestive of hypotheses for future study about possible differential effects of diuretic and beta blockers on Defensiveness and on various components of hostility.

Finally, the paucity of quality of life findings related to drug reduction deserves further comment. The present study employed either diuretic or diuretic combined with atenolol. Neither drug has been associated with major negative quality of life findings, with the exception of sexual dysfunction associated with diuretics in males (Chang et al., 1991). Moreover, the literature in general on quality of life in hypertension is not without controversy, and there is no real consensus about the magnitude and direction of quality of life effects. Major uncertainties remain in attempts to arrive at definite conclusions about the quality of life consequences of antihypertensive medications (Barnett, 1991; Dimsdale, 1992; Jern & Zanchetti, 1993). A recent meta-analysis could not identify negative effects with treatment (Beto & Bansal, 1992). Another important consideration is the fact that minimal drug requirements were established and individualized for each patient in the present study rather than randomized as in usual clinical drug trials. This may have served to minimize quality of life effects. Moreover, stepdown of medication was also individualized for each subject.

What are the practical implications of the results of this research? Addition of a relatively simple and inexpensive group-administered intervention appears to be beneficial in reducing drug requirements or in providing an alternative to drug treatment for some patients. In an era of increasing attention to alternatives to usual medical therapy and to prevention, behavioral interventions of this kind have their place in the treatment of hypertension. Their focus need not be on restructuring an individual's personality characteristics, but rather should probably emphasize what one can do to keep one's blood pressure under control or to return it to controlled levels in the face of circumstances that tend to elevate it. Monitoring one's own pressure regularly is one simple and inexpensive method of enhancing awareness of changes in one's own blood pressure and facilitating control. The combination of drug and behavioral interventions may have definite advantages in that the drug treatment by itself reduces blood pressure, thereby eliminating any risk associated with interventions designed for patients off antihypertensive medications. At the same time, the behavioral intervention can facilitate continued control as medication is no longer needed. The present study was carried out in mild-to-moderate hypertension. Future research is needed to apply the same approach in patients with more severe hypertension and on other drug regimens and to adapt the procedures for general application in the management of hypertension.

ACKNOWLEDGMENTS

This research was supported by Research Grant HL-40584 from the National Heart, Lung, & Blood Institute. Our thanks to Marci Lovett and Jill Foster for their many contributions to this research.

REFERENCES

Aberg, H., & Tibblin, G. (1989). Addition of non-pharmacological methods of treatment in patients on antihypertensive drugs: Results of previous medication, laboratory tests and life quality. *Journal of Internal Medicine, 226*, 39–46.

Andrews, G., MacMahon, S. W., Austin, A., & Byrne, D. G. (1982). Hypertension: comparison of drug and non-drug treatments. *British Medical Journal, 284*, 1523–1526.

Barnett, D. B. (1991). Assessment of quality of life. *The American Journal of Cardiology, 67*: 41C–45C.

Beto, J. A., & Bansal, V. K. (1992). Quality of life in treatment of hypertension: A meta-analysis of clinical trials. *American Journal of Hypertension, 5*, 125–133.

Buschke, H. (1973). Selective reminding for analysis of memory and learning. *Journal of Verbal Learning and Verbal Behavior, 12*, 543–550.

Chang, S. W., Fine, R., Siegel, D., Chesney, M., Black, D., & Hulley, S. B. (1991). The impact of diuretic therapy on reported sexual function. *Archives of Internal Medicine, 151*, 2402–2409.

Dimsdale, J. E. (1992). Reflections on the impact of antihypertensive medications on mood, sedation, and neuropsychologic functioning. *Archives of Internal Medicine, 152*, 35–40.

Fifth report of the Joint National Committee on Detection, Evaluation, and Treatment of High Blood Pressure. (1993). *Archives of Internal Medicine, 153*, 154–183.

Glasgow, M. S., Engel, B. T., & D'Lugoff, C. (1989). A controlled study of standardized behavioral stepped treatment for hypertension. *Psychosomatic Medicine, 51*, 10–26.

Jacob, R. G., Chesney, M. A., Williams, D. M., Ding, Y., & Shapiro, A. P. (1991). Relaxation therapy for hypertension: Design effects and treatment effects. *Annals of Behavioral Medicine, 13*, 5–17.

Jamner, L. D., Shapiro, D., Goldstein, I. B., & Hug, R. (1991). Ambulatory blood pressure and heart rate in paramedics: Effects of cynical hostility and defensiveness. *Psychosomatic Medicine, 53*, 393–406.

Jern, S., & Zanchetti, A. (1993). The issue of quality of life in antihypertensive therapy. *Journal of Human Hypertension, 7*, S46–S49.

Johnson, E. H., & Spielberger, D. C. (1992). Assessment of the experience, expression, and control of anger in hypertension research. In E. H. Johnson, W. D. Gentry, & S. Julius (Eds.), *Personality, elevated blood pressure, and essential hypertension* (pp. 3–24). Washington, DC: Hemisphere.

Kaufmann, P. G., Jacob, R. G., Ewart, C. K., Chesney, M. A., Muenz, L. R., Doub, N., Mercer, W., & HIPP Investigators. (1988). Hypertension Intervention Pooling Project. *Health Psychology, 7*(Suppl.), 209–224.

Light, K. C., Obrist, P. A., & Cubeddu, L. X. (1988). Evaluation of a new ambulatory blood pressure monitor (Accutracker 102): Laboratory comparisons with direct arterial pressure, stethoscopic auscultatory pressure and readings from a similar monitor (Spacelabs Model 5200). *Psychophysiology, 25*, 107–117.

Oakley, M. E., & Shapiro, D. (1989). Methodological issues in the evaluation of drug-behavioral interactions in the treatment of hypertension. *Psychosomatic Medicine, 51*, 269–276.

Shapiro, D., Jamner, L. D., & Goldstein, I. B. (1993). Ambulatory stress psychophysiology: The study of "compensatory and defensive counterforces" and conflict in a natural setting. *Psychosomatic Medicine, 55*, 309–323.

Ward, M. M., Swan, G. E., & Chesney, M. A. (1987). Arousal-reduction treatments for mild hypertension: A meta-analysis of recent studies. In S. Julius & D. R. Bassett (Eds.), *Behavioral factors in hypertension. Handbook of Hypertension* (Vol. 9, pp. 285–302). Amsterdam: Elsevier.

White, W. B., Schulman, P., McCabe, E. J., & Nardone, M. B. (1987). Clinical validation of the accutracker, a novel ambulatory blood pressure monitor using R-wave gating for Korotoff sounds. *Journal of Clinical Hypertension, 3*, 500–509.

13 Health-Related Quality of Life in HIV-Infected Persons: A Conceptual Model

Paul D. Cleary
Harvard Medical School

Ira B. Wilson
New England Medical Center

Floyd J. Fowler, Jr.
Center for Survey Research

Increasingly, researchers, clinicians, and policymakers are recognizing that the measures traditionally used to assess the efficacy and effectiveness of medical treatment, such as physiologic function and mortality, do not adequately reflect the ways many people monitor and evaluate their health. Because of work in the social and clinical sciences, there is an emerging consensus that it is more appropriate to adopt a broader and more comprehensive focus on health-related quality of life (HQL; Bombardier et al., 1986; Canadian Erythropoietin Study Group [CESG], 1990; Cleary, Epstein et al., 1991; Croog et al., 1986; McDowell & Newell, 1987; Thier, 1992).

In essence, HQL refers to the various aspects of a person's life that are affected strongly by changes in health status (health related) and that are important to the person (quality of life). Although there are many definitions of HQL, most people agree that it encompasses dimensions such as physical functioning, social functioning, role functioning, sexual functioning, and mental health. These types of measures are particularly important in the evaluation of chronic conditions, such as human immunodeficiency virus (HIV) infection, where the principal goals of care often are improvements in domains that are not captured by biologic or physiologic data.

A major advantage of this approach is that it is more comprehensive and focuses on things that are of value to recipients of support and health care.

The term *quality of life* has an intuitive meaning to most people and there is a consensus that a major goal of health care is to maximize quality of life.

Measuring HQL, however, is complex, and widespread adoption of these health outcomes was hindered for some time by a lack of consensus about several methodologic, practical, and conceptual issues (Deyo & Patrick, 1989). The emergence of substantial evidence that existing measures are reliable and valid (McDowell & Newell, 1987) has allayed many methodologic concerns, and the development of shorter, easier to administer instruments has removed some practical barriers to measuring HQL. There remains some confusion, however, about a key conceptual issue: How are different measures of HQL related to each other? How do they complement or supplement traditional clinical measures (Feinstein, 1992; Patrick, 1992; Patrick & Bergner, 1990)?

In this chapter, we describe a model for categorizing and differentiating different types of measures typically subsumed under the category of HQL and suggest how this conceptual framework would help both clinicians and social scientists develop more specific, testable hypotheses about the relationships among different measures of health and HQL. We propose that distinct theoretical models may be needed to explain variation in different types of outcomes that traditionally have been subsumed under the term HQL. Another benefit of adopting such a model is that it can help to clarify the conceptual and empirical links between more traditional clinical measures of health status and more comprehensive measures of HQL. We have presented this model in more detail elsewhere (Wilson & Cleary, in press). Here we provide an overview of its main characteristics and use some data from a recent study of persons with acquired immune deficiency syndrome (AIDS; Cleary et al., 1993) to illustrate its potential usefulness.

Traditional Model for HQL

Traditionally, researchers who study HQL have measured the multiple dimensions of HQL thought to be most salient for the study population and treated them as multiple measures of a single construct. Articles describing how to interpret results of studies using multiple HQL measures have focused on how to analyze multiple endpoints to get a global statistic (Tandon, 1990) and not on the theoretical relationships among measures.

The implicit model in these types of analyses is that all HQL subscales measure a single construct, and all clinical and background factors and therapeutic interventions have a comparable influence on each dimension of HQL. If asked explicitly about these issues, almost no clinician or researcher in this area would agree with these assumptions, but this is what is implied by many published analyses of HQL data.

Proposed Model

We think that measures of health can be thought of as on a continuum of increasing biologic, social, and psychologic complexity (Wilson & Cleary, in press). At one end of the continuum are biologic measures, and at the other are more complex and integrated measures, such as physical functioning and general health perception (Fig. 13.1).

Biologic/Physiologic Factors. The most basic or fundamental determinants of health status are molecular and genetic factors, but biologic and physiologic factors are most commonly assessed and monitored in routine clinical practice. Examples are laboratory values such as serum hemoglobin and CD4 counts, measures of physiologic function such as pulmonary function tests, physical exam findings, comorbid illnesses, and medications. These types of factors are influenced primarily by biological characteristics of the patients and biological processes.

Symptoms. Symptom status is the next level in our model. We define a *symptom* as a patient's perception of an abnormal physical, emotional, or cognitive state. When symptoms are evaluated, the assessment is at the level of the organism as opposed to the level of specific cells or organs. Examples of symptoms are fever, nausea, pain, fatigue, and emotional symptoms associated with anxiety and depression. These are the feelings and experiences that a patient typically describes to a physician.

Symptoms often are thought of as predictable responses to a particular pathophysiological condition and as such, are used to diagnose certain

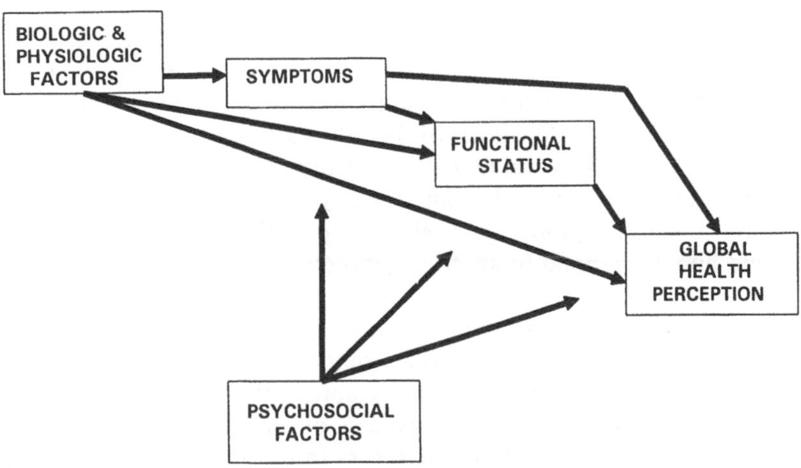

FIG. 13.1. Model of health-related quality of life.

diseases. When thinking about the assessment of HQL, however, it is important to distinguish between very specific and independently measured indicators of cellular and organic function, such as serum hemoglobin, and more general and patient reported indicators, such as pain and fatigue.

An important differences between these classes of measures is that the latter are influenced by a much wider array of determinants. Specifically, patient symptom reports are influenced by complicated interactions of biologic, physiologic, psychological, and social factors. For example, symptom reports are influenced not only by underlying pathophysiological processes, but also by the way the individual reacts to and processes bodily sensations, factors that are difficult to measure, likely to vary greatly from person to person, and unlikely to be changed by an intervention by a physician or health-care system (Barsky, Cleary, & Klerman, 1992; Cleary, 1986). Thus, reported symptoms represent the distillation and summary of a large quantity of complex information, the source of which is necessarily, and exclusively, the patient.

The relationship between biologic and physiologic variables and symptoms is complex (Deyo, 1991). Certain critical biologic and physiologic variables can show profound abnormality without the patient having any symptoms. For example, the CD4 counts of a patient infected with HIV may be below 200 before symptoms of HIV infection develop. Although such an abnormality has definite prognostic significance and should provoke specific clinical responses if discovered, it would not directly influence the patient's quality of life until symptoms became manifest.

The relationships between physiologic condition and symptom reports are similarly complex in several other medical conditions. For patients with back problems, for example, patients with clearly abnormal physiology may report no pain, whereas it may be impossible to detect a physiological reason for some patients who report severe disabling pain. Although such inconsistencies are well known to clinicians and social scientists alike, it is important to recognize such relationships when modeling the associations between physiological indicators of health state and symptom reports. Explicitly trying to assess and model the factors that may account for such discrepancies should help to elucidate the psychosocial processes related to the expression of symptoms, as well as help clinicians understand better when and how to respond to specific symptoms.

Functioning. The next level in our model is functional status, and like symptom status, it is an important point of integration. Among the determinants of functional status are symptom state, social factors, and psychological characteristics. Many aspects of an individual's social environment, such as social support and access to medical care, may have an important effect on his or her functioning. Also, patient-specific factors, such as personality and motivation are likely to be important determinants of functioning. (Greenfield & Nelson, 1992; Patrick, 1987)

Many studies have included both clinical and functional status measures among the outcomes examined (Alonso et al., 1992; Bombardier & Raboud, 1991; Bombardier et al., 1986; CESG, 1990; Cleary, Epstein et al., 1991; Cleary, Greenfield, Mulley et al., 1991; Croog et al., 1986; Fowler et al., 1988; Gelber, Goldhirsch, & Cavalli, 1991; Kaplan et al., 1989; Laupacis, Wong, & Churchill, 1991; Lurie, Ward, Shapiro, & Brook, 1984; Meenan et al., 1984; Nerenz, Repasky, Whitehouse, & Kahkonen, 1992; Tugwell et al., 1990; Wachtel et al., 1992; Wassertheil et al., 1991). These studies, many of which are clinical trials, show convincingly that measures of HQL can be as sensitive to clinically important changes as traditional clinical variables.

Only a few of these studies, however, look at the relationships among different measures of HQL. (Alonso et al., 1992; CESG, 1990; Cleary et al., 1993; Kaplan et al., 1989; Laupacis et al., 1991; Meenan et al., 1984; Nerenz et al., 1992; Wachtel et al., 1992).

One advantage of modeling the associations among specific symptoms, physiological indicators of heath status, and functional status is that the model makes explicit that factors other than health status affect functioning. A related issue is that these associations may vary for different types of patients. For example, one of the most direct and simplest measures of functional status is one's ability to work. Ability to work clearly is affected by health status, but it is also strongly determined by the demands and expectations associated with one's job. For example, some jobs have high demands for cognitive skills whereas other jobs have high physical demands. Early symptoms of AIDs dementia complex (Price et al., 1988) may have very little, if any impact on a person's ability to continue in a job that requires mainly general physical activity (i.e., no fine motor skills). Such symptoms might have a devastating impact, on the other hand, on someone in a highly cognitive job, such as air traffic control or research. Conversely, physical impairment may have little impact on the performance of a primarily cognitive task but have a dramatic impact on one's ability to do physical work.

Global Health Perceptions

We view global health perceptions as individuals' synthesis of other information about their health. That is, our premise is that people implicitly or explicitly review and synthesize the features of their current condition that they use to define the construct of health when asked to evaluate their general health. This could include information, such as reported by a physician (e.g., CD4 count), symptoms (e.g., fatigue), or perceived difficulties performing physical, social, or work activities. It also may reflect information that we normally would not include under the construct of health status. For example, we recently have conducted in-depth interviews to refine global health measures and have found that many respondents base their health ratings partly on behaviors presumed related to their health (e.g., drinking too much) even though they currently are not experiencing any adverse consequences of those behaviors.

Thus, a single rating of overall health probably is a complex integration of information across many domains. Interestingly, very little is known about the types of information patients use to develop such summary ratings, or the salience or weights they attach to different indicators of health. We do know that the psychological processes affecting the way individuals combine information and express ratings or preferences are extraordinarily complex (Fischhoff, 1991; Kleinmuntz, 1990). We hope that by explicitly modeling the associations among symptoms, functional status, and global ratings we can begin to explain some of these processes and develop a better understanding of the multitude of factors affecting such global ratings.

As is true when discussing functional status, a related task is to understand how these associations differ in different subgroups of the population. For example, in a study of patients undergoing prostatectomy (Fowler et al., 1988) we found that among patients with severe symptoms, 32% reported no day-to-day limitations because of their prostate condition, and 19% reported no worry about their health due to their prostate. Among patients who had already had an episode of acute retention, 47% reported no day-to-day limitations, 19% no discomfort from the prostate, and 42% no worry about health due to their prostate. Clearly, the relationship between severity of symptoms and patients' concern about the symptoms is complex, and has important implication for treatment (Fowler, 1991; Fowler et al., 1988). Until we learn more about measuring and modeling these preferences for individuals or particular populations, our ability to interpret changes in overall health perceptions will be limited.

Summary of Model

Our model emphasizes that biological and physiological measures, symptom status, functional status, and general perceived health can be thought of as existing on a continuum of increasing biological, social, and psychological complexity. There are several ways in which this model differs from earlier efforts to articulate these relationships. This model divides these various outcomes into levels and allows one to specify the key variables that influence the outcome at that level. We also emphasize the importance of symptoms as a critical link between biologic/physiologic variables and measures of function. As one moves from left to right in the model one moves outward from the cell to the individual to the interaction of the individual with society. The concepts at each level are increasingly integrated and synthetic and increasingly difficult to define and measure. At each level there are an increasing number of inputs that cannot be controlled by physicians or the health care system as it is traditionally defined.

Implications for Interpreting HQL Measures

Complex concepts such as role functioning or HQL will be easier for clinicians to understand and interpret when their relationship to simpler, more familiar concepts is made clear (Patrick & Bergner, 1990; Ware & Sherbourne, 1992). For example, in the HIV-infected patient, understanding the meaning and significance of a decrement in role functioning will be easier if we understand how role functioning relates to clinical variables such as CD4 counts, specific opportunistic infections, depression, and pain.

Implications for Clinical Diagnosis and Treatment

As noted earlier, decline in important physiologic parameters such as CD4 counts or the spread of metastatic tumor all can be clinically silent. Measuring HQL in combination with disease specific parameters may help detect such decline, particularly if the goal is to detect the slow progression of an existing chronic symptom. Obtaining such diagnostic information is inexpensive and not burdensome to the patient. Experienced clinicians use this approach intuitively; they often know when something is "not right" with a patient and initiate further evaluation.

Several studies have shown, however, that physicians do not assess patient-perceived function and HQL accurately (Calkins, et al., 1991; Nelson, Conger, Douglass, 1983; Nerenz et al., 1992) which emphasizes the need to measure HQL using standardized instruments. Developing more information about the associations between physiologic phenomena and HQL should increase the usefulness of such an approach to clinical diagnosis.

There currently is no clear linkage between the diagnosis and treatment of HQL "problems," although creative efforts are being made in this area (Wasson et al., 1992). Several studies suggest that assessment of HQL can lead to improvements in HQL (Applegate et al., 1990; Lefton, Bonstelle, & Frengley, 1983; Liem, Chernoff, & Carter, 1986; Rubenstein et al., 1984).

A clear formulation of the relationships specified in this, or a more elaborated model could help clinicians and researchers decide which health status endpoints to use in monitoring a response to a therapy. The endpoints of interest to physicians and researchers may not be identical with those most important to patients. Complex and integrated measures, although appealing because of their scope and breadth, may be insensitive to clinically important changes.

AN ILLUSTRATION USING DATA ON QUALITY OF LIFE IN PERSONS WITH AIDS

We recently developed a new quality of life measure for persons with HIV infection and used it in face-to-face interviews with 189 AIDS patients in the Boston area. Following the model described previously, we think of symptoms as the most specific patient-reported measures of health status. Measures that are less specific but assess a broader range of consequences of illness include measures of disability and functional status. The least specific and most comprehensive measures of health status are patients' global evaluations. In this study we grouped our measures in this way and assessed: (a) which symptoms are most predictive of functional impairment and (b) which symptoms and which aspects of functional impairment best predict patients' overall perception of their health and their life satisfaction.

METHODS

We conducted the study at three sites: an academic group practice based at a private teaching hospital; a specialized ambulatory care clinic at a public teaching hospital; and a health maintenance organization. Patients were eligible for this study if they were diagnosed with CDC-defined AIDS and were current patients at one of the three study sites.

There were 293 eligible patients during the study period. Thirty-three patients died before they could be contacted. Of the remaining 260 patients, 13 were too sick to interview, 30 could not be contacted, and 28 refused to participate. We successfully interviewed 189 patients, representing 65% of eligible patients. Respondents were not significantly different from the total eligible population with respect to age, gender, risk group, or race/ethnicity (Fowler, et al., 1992).

Most study participants were male, under the age of 35, white, and well educated. About 70% of the sample were men who said they considered themselves gay or bisexual. About 7% of the sample were women, and 25% of all respondents said they had used illegal intravenous drugs. We have described the rationale and methods for the study and subject characteristics in detail elsewhere (Cleary et al., 1993; Fowler et al., 1992).

Measures

To assess HQL, we developed a comprehensive set of subscales for assessing the symptoms and functioning of persons with HIV infection that includes HIV-specific measures of symptoms. The interview included: measures of life satisfaction (Andrews & Withey, 1976); three items asking patients to rate their health at its best and worst during the preceding four months and how they felt, on average, during the previous month and on the day of the interview (on a scale ranging from 0 to 100); measures of basic and intermediate activities of daily living (e.g., "During the past month, about how many days did the way you felt make you unable to walk one block or climb one flight of stairs?"; Cleary, Greenfield, & McNeil, 1991; Jette & Cleary, 1987; Jette et al., 1986); emotional well-being (e.g., "How much of the time during the past month have you felt so down in the dumps nothing could cheer you up?"; Cleary, Greenfield, & McNeil, 1991; Cleary, Greenfield, Mulley, et al., 1991; Jette et al., 1986); fatigue (e.g., "How much of the time during the past month did you feel worn out?"; Stewart, Hays, & Ware, 1988); disability (National Center for Health Statistics, 1987); pain ("How much of the time during the past month have you been in extreme pain?"); and several neuropsychological tests to assess cognitive deficits (Price et al., 1988). As part of the interview, we also asked respondents two questions about their memory from the Memory Assessment Clinic Self-Rating Scale (e.g., "In the last month, compared to the best your memory has ever been, how would you describe the speed with which you remember things?"; Winterling, Crook, Salama, & Gobert, 1986). These items were the best predictors of clinical assessments of HIV-related cognitive deficits in a study of 129 patients evaluated for AIDS dementia complex (data available from authors).

We also asked respondents how much of the time in the previous month they had experienced each of 18 symptoms. To develop the list, we first compiled items from several unpublished AIDS symptom inventories. We then revised this list, based on advice from a panel of clinical consultants, to include symptoms thought to be especially important for HIV-infected persons. The final scale included seven symptoms related to neurological complications of HIV infection, three sleep-related symptoms, three fever-related symptoms, and five other general symptoms.

SUMMARY OF RESULTS

We described the results from this study in more detail elsewhere (Cleary et al., 1993), but we review here several findings that illustrate the importance of differentiating among HQL measures. For example, although some

HQL scales combine symptom and functioning measures, our results emphasize the importance of separating them as we have described, when developing both theoretical and statistical models of the associations.

Our first step in developing such a model was to examine the extent to which symptoms predicted limitations in functioning. One instructive finding from these analyses is that every symptom measure was more strongly correlated with limitations in intermediate activities of daily living (IADL) than with basic activities of daily living (BADL). The standard deviation of the IADL scores is higher than for the BADL score, so we do not think this is an artifact of the variances of the scales. It is likely that symptoms have little effect on one's ability to carry out basic activities, but are related to more complex functions.

A second important finding was that the patterns of associations were not consistent with some of our clinical predictions. For example, we thought that specific symptoms such as fever, nausea, and diarrhea would be better predictors than more diffuse symptoms, such as fatigue. Surprisingly, diarrhea and fever had among the lowest correlations with IADL scores and fatigue had one of the highest correlations with the IADL score. The variable with the highest correlation with the IADL score was a summary score that represented the sum of the individual physical symptom scores.

In a regression model, the only symptom measure that was an independent predictor of problems with basic ADLs was the physical symptom score. The physical symptom score and reported fatigue were independent predictors of both limitations in intermediate ADLs and disability days.

Predictors of Summary Variables

Another implication of the model outlined in Fig. 13.1 is that it is important to distinguish overall health perception from symptom and functioning measures. Although most HQL scales include both, little attention generally is given to the associations between these different levels of measurement.

Again, analyzing the data in this way yields several unanticipated findings and raises important theoretical questions. For example, our initial hypothesis was that health perceptions would be influenced most by variables most proximate in our model, such as the limitations in IADL.

Surprisingly, the strongest correlate was the measure of fatigue. The next strongest correlates were limitations in IADLs and the summary physical symptom score. The weakest correlates were reported sleep problems, diarrhea, and limitations in basic ADLs. As expected, the symptom and functioning measures had weaker correlations with the rating of life satisfaction than with the rating of physical health.

This is consistent with our assumption that many factors besides symptoms and functional status influence life satisfaction. The strongest correlates of life satisfaction were fatigue and the physical symptom score. The other symptom and functioning measures were moderately correlated with life satisfaction.

When the rating of average health in the previous month was regressed on the symptom and functioning measures, the significant predictors were bed disability days, fatigue, and the physical symptom score. The significant predictors of the mental health score were the IADL score, the measure of fatigue, and the physical symptom score.

A linear regression in which life satisfaction was a dependent variable showed that the summary health rating and the mental health score explained 27% of the variance in life satisfaction and that none of the other symptom or functioning measures were significant predictors of life satisfaction.

CONCLUSIONS

We have presented a hierarchical model of the relationships among different measures of health that disaggregates or decomposes various measures into what we hypothesize are its component parts, emphasizing its usefulness in conceptualizing these relationships. The preliminary data we have presented highlight the potential benefits of such a model.

Measures of HQL have the potential to influence not only the diagnosis, prognosis, and treatment of individual patients, but also the assessment of quality of care, cost-effectiveness research, and the assessment of the health of populations. (American College of Physicians, 1988; Lohr, 1989; Patrick & Bergner, 1990; Thier, 1992; Ware & Sherbourne, 1992) The relationships among traditional clinical variables and health status measures have not been adequately conceptualized in much of the work done to date, and an explicit model, such as the one described here, will facilitate the understanding of these associations. Such a model should be useful in the formulation of strategies to improve function and HQL.

ACKNOWLEDGMENTS

This work was supported by grant #1-R01-HS06239 from the Agency for Health Care Policy and Research. The authors thank Arnold Epstein, MD, Constantine Gatsonis, PhD, Lisa Iezzoni, MD, Michael P. Massagli, PhD, Barbara J. McNeil, MD, PhD, George R. Seage, III, DSc, and Joel Weissman, PhD for their numerous contributions to the model and study described in this chapter.

REFERENCES

Alonso, J., Anto, J. M., Gonzalez, M., Fiz, J. A., Izquierdo, J., & Morera, J. (1992). Measurement of general health status of non-oxygen-dependent chronic obstructive pulmonary disease patients. *Medical Care, 30*, MS125-MS135.

American College of Physicians. (1988). Comprehensive functional assessment for elderly patients. *Annals of Internal Medicine, 109*, 70-72.

Andrews, F. M., & Withey, S. B. (1976). *Social indicators of well-being: Americans' perceptions of life quality*. New York: Plenum.

Applegate, W. B., Miller, S. T., Graney, M. J., Elam, J. T., Burns, R., & Akins, D. E. (1990). A randomized, controlled trial of a geriatric assessment unit in a community rehabilitation hospital. *New England Journal of Medicine, 322*, 1572-1578.

Barsky, A. J., Cleary, P. D., & Klerman, G. L. (1992). Determinants of perceived health status of medical outpatients. *Social Science Medicine, 34*, 1147-1154.

Bombardier, C., & Raboud, J. (1991). A comparison of health-related quality-of-life measures for rheumatoid arthritis research. *Controlled Clinical Trials, 12*, 243S-256S.

Bombardier, C., Ware, J., Russell, I. J., Larson, M., Chalmers, A., Read, J. L., & the Auranofin Cooperating Group. (1986). Auranofin therapy and quality of life in patients with rheumatoid arthritis. *The American Journal of Medicine, 81*, 565-578.

Calkins, D. R., Rubenstein, L. V., Cleary, P. D., Davies, A. R., Jette, A. M., Fink, A., Kosecoff, J., Young, R. T., Brook, R. H., & Delbanco, T. L. (1991). Failure of physicians to recognize functional disability in ambulatory patients. *Annals Intern Medicine, 114*, 451-454.

Canadian Erythropoietin Study Group. (1990). Association between recombinant human erythropoietin and quality of life and exercise capacity of patients receving haemodialysis. *British Medical Journal, 300*, 573-578.

Cleary, P. D. (1986). Illness behavior: A multidisciplinary model. In S. McHugh, T. M. Vallis (Ed's.), *New directions in illness behavior research*. (pp. 119-149). New York: Plenum.

Cleary, P. D., Epstein, A. M., Oster, G., Morrissey, G. S., Stason, W. B., Debussey, S., Plachetka, J., & Zimmerman, M. (1991). Health-related quality of life among patients undergoing percutaneous transluminal coronary angioplasty. *Medical Care, 29*, 939-950.

Cleary, P. D., Fowler, F. J., Weissman, J., Massagli, M. P., Wilson, I., Seage, G. R., Gatsonis, C., & Epstein, A. (1993). Health-related quality of life in persons with AIDS. *Medical Care, 31*, 569-580.

Cleary, P. D., Greenfield, S., & McNeil, B. J. (1991). Assessing quality of life after surgery. *Controlled Clinical Trials, 12*, 189S-203S.

Cleary, P. D., Greenfield, S., Mulley, A. G., Pauker, S. G., Schroeder, S. A, Wexler, L., & McNeil, B. J. (1991). Variations in length of stay and outcomes for six medical and surgical conditions in Massachusetts and California. *Journal of the American Medical Association, 266*, 73-79.

Croog, S. H., Levine, S., Testa, M. A., Brown, B., Bulpitt, C. J., Jenkins, C. D., Klerman, G. L., & Williams, G. H. (1986). The effects of antihypertensive therapy on the quality of life. *New England Journal of Medicine, 314*, 1657-1664.

Deyo, R. A. (1991). The quality of life, research, and care. *Annals of Internal Medicine, 114*, 695-697.

Deyo, R. A., & Patrick, D. L. (1989). Barriers to the use of health status measures in clinical investigation, patient care, and policy research. *Medical Care, 27*, S254-S268.

Feinstein, A. R. (1992). Benefits and obstacles for development of health status assessment measures in clinical settings. *Medical Care, 30*, MS50–MS56.

Fischhoff, B. (1991). Value elicitation: Is there anything in there? *American Psychologist, 46*, 835-847.

Fowler, F. J. (1991). Patient reports of symptoms and quality of life following prostate surgery. *European Urology, 20*, 44–49.

Fowler, F. J., Massagli, M. P., Weissman, J., Seage, G. R., III., Cleary, P. D., & Epstein, A. (1992). Some methodological lessons for surveys of persons with AIDS. *Medical Care, 30*, 1059–1066.

Fowler, F. J., Wennberg, J. E., Timothy, R. P., Barry, M. J., Mulley, A. G., & Hanley, D. (1988). Symptom status and quality of life following prostatectomy. *Journal of the American Medical Association, 259*, 3018–3022.

Gelber, R. D., Goldhirsch, A., & Cavalli, F. (1991). Quality-of-life adjusted evaluation of adjuvant therapies for operable breast cancer. *Annals of Internal Medicine, 114*, 621–628.

Greenfield, S., & Nelson, E. C. (1992). Recent developments and future issues in the use of health status assessment measures in clinical settings. *Medical Care, 30*, MS23–MS41.

Jette, A. M., & Cleary, P. D. (1987). Functional disability assessment. *Physical Therapy, 67*, 1854–1859.

Jette, A. M., Davies, A. R., Cleary, P. D., Calkins, D. R., Rubenstein, L. V., Fink, A., Kosecoff, J., Young, R. T., Brook, R. H., & Delbanco, T. L. (1986). The functional status questionnaire: Its reliability and validity when used in primary care. *Journal of General Internal Medicine, 1*, 143–149.

Kaplan, R. M., Anderson, J. P., Wu, A. W., Mathews, W. C., Kozin, F., & Orenstein, D. (1989). The Quality of Well-Being Scale. Applications in AIDS, cystic fibrosis, and arthritis. *Medical Care, 27*, 27–43.

Kleinmuntz, B. (1990). Why we still use our heads instead of formulas: Toward an integrative approach. *Psychological Bulletin, 107*, 296–340.

Laupacis, A., Wong, C., & Churchill, D. (1991). The use of generic and specific quality-of-life measures in hemodialysis patients treated with erythropoietin. *Controlled Clinical Trials, 12*, 168S–179S.

Lefton, E., Bonstelle, S., & Frengley, J. D. (1983). Success with an inpatinet geriatric unit: A controlled study of outcome and follow-up. *Journal of the American Geriatric Society, 31*, 149–155.

Liem, P. H., Chernoff, R., Carter, W.J. (1986). Geriatric rehabilitation unit: A 3-year outcome evaluation. *Journal of Gerontology, 41*, 44–50.

Lohr, K.N. (Ed.) Advances in health status asessment: Conference proceedings. *Medical Care*, 1989; 27 (suppl):S1.

Lurie, N., Ward, N. B., Shapiro, M. F., & Brook, R. H. (1984). Termination from Medi-Cal—Does it affect health? *New England Journal of Medicine, 311*, 480–484.

McDowell, I., & Newell, C. (1987). *Measuring health: A guide to rating scales and questionnaires*. New York: Oxford University Press.

Meenan, R. F., Anderson, J. J., Kazis, L. E., Egger, M. J., Altz-Smith, M., Samuelson, C. O., Jr., Willkens, R. F., Solsky, M. A., Hayes, S. P., Blocka, K. L., Weinstein, A., Guttadauria, M., Kaplan, S. B., & Klippel, J. (1984). Outcome assessment in clinical trials. Evidence for the sensitivity of a health status measure. *Arthritis and Rheumatism, 27*, 1344–1351.

National Center for Health Statistics. (1987). *National Health Interview Survey, 1986: Interviewer's manual*, (HIS Rep. No. 100). Hyattsville, MD: National Center for Health Statistics.

Nelson, E. C., Conger, B., & Douglass, R. (1983). Functional health status levels of primary care patients. *Journal of the American Medical Association, 249*, 3331–3338.

Nerenz, D. R., Repasky, D. P., Whitehouse, F. W., & Kahkonen, D. M. (1992). Ongoing assessment of health status in patients with diabetes mellitus. *Medical Care, 30*, MS112–MS124.

Patrick, D. L. (1987). Commentary: Patient reports of health status as predictors of physiologic health in chronic disease. *Journal of Chronic Diseases, 40*, 37S–40S.

Patrick, D. L. (1992). Strategies for improving and expanding the application of health status measures in clinical settings: Discussion. *Medical Care*, 30, MS198–MS201.

Patrick, D. L., & Bergner, M. (1990). Measurement of health status in the 1990's. *Annual Review of Public Health, 11*, 165–183.

Price, R. W., Brew, B., Sidtis, J., Rosenblum, M., Scheck, A. C., & Cleary, P. (1988). The brain in AIDS: central nervous system HIV-1 infection and AIDS dementia complex. *Science, 239*, 586–592.

Rubenstein, L. Z., Josephson, K. R., Wieland, G. D., English, P. A., Sayre, J. A., & Kane, R. L. (1984). Effectiveness of a geriatric evaluation unit: A randomized clinical trial. *New England Journal of Medicine, 311*, 1664–1670.

Stewart, A. L., Hays, R. D., & Ware, J. E. Jr. (1988). The MOS short-form General Health Survey: Reliability and validity in a patient population. *Medical Care, 26*, 724–735.

Tandon, P. K. (1990). Applications of global statistics in analyzing quality of life data. *Statistics in Medicine, 9*, 819–827.

Thier, S. O. (1992). Forces motivating the use of health status assessment measures in clinical settings and related clinical research. *Medical Care, 30*, MS15-MS22.

Tugwell, P., Bombardier, C., Buchanan, W. W., Goldsmith, C., Grace, E., Bennett, J. K., Williams, H. J., Egger, M., Alarcon, G. S., Guttadauria, M., Yarboro, C., Polisson, R. P., Szydlo, L., Luggen, M. E., Billingsley, L. M., Ward, J. R., Marks, C. (1990). Methodtrexate in rheumatoid arthritis: impact on quality of life assessed by traditional standard-item and individualized patient preference health status questionnaires. *Archives of Internal Medicine, 150*, 59–62.

Wachtel, T., Piette, J., Mor, V., Stein, M., Fleishman, J., & Carpenter, C. (1992). Quality of life in persons with human immunodeficiency virus infection: Measurement by the Medical Outcomes Study Instrument. *Annals of Internal Medicine, 116*, 129–167.

Ware, J. E., & Sherbourne, C. D. (1992). The MOS 36-item short-form health survey (SF–36) 1. conceptual framework and item selection. *Medical Care, 30*, 473–483.

Wassertheil-Smoller, S., Blaufox, D., Oberman, A., Davis, B. R., Swencionis, C., O'Connell-Knerr, Hawkins, C. M., & Langford, H. G. (1991). Effect of antihypertensives on sexual function and quality of life: The TAIM study. *Annals of Internal Medicine, 114*, 613–620.

Wasson, J., Keller, A., Rubenstein, L., Hays, R., Nelson, E., Johnson, D., & The Dartmouth Primary Care COOP Project. (1992). Benefits and obstacles of health status assessment in ambulatory settings: The clinician's point of view. *Medical Care, 30*, MS42–MS49.

Wilson, I. B., & Cleary, P. D. (in press). The relationship between clinical measures and quality of life: A model. *Journal of The American Medical Association, 272.*

Winterling, D., Crook, T., Salama, M. & Gobert, J. (1986). *A self-rating scale for assessing memory loss*. Bethesda, MD: Memory Assessment Clinics Inc.

14 Psychosocial Interventions and Quality of Life Changes Across the HIV Spectrum

Susan Lutgendorf
Michael H. Antoni
Neil Schneiderman
Gail Ironson
Mary Ann Fletcher
University of Miami

When acquired immune deficiency syndrome (AIDS) was first diagnosed in this country, individuals frequently learned their human immunodeficiency virus (HIV) serostatus only in the advanced symptomatic stages of disease progression. Under these circumstances, with relatively short latencies between diagnosis and death, quality of life assumed less importance in HIV treatment than it does today. Currently, with increased emphasis on early HIV antibody testing of individuals in high-risk groups and increased medical options for treatment, individuals may now live with known HIV infection for up to 12 to 15 years (Pantaleo, Graziosi, & Fauci, 1993). Within this frame, patients are commonly infected with the virus for 6 to 10 years before the onset of AIDS-defining symptoms (Fauci, 1991; Pantaleo et al., 1993). As such, HIV-infected individuals are now being faced with a chronic, degenerative, progressive disease, which at this time still has no cure. When HIV infection is viewed as a chronic disease, a myriad of quality of life issues emerge.

QUALITY OF LIFE

Quality of life is a term that has inspired countless articles, a variety of measurement scales, and even conferences, and yet it has evaded consensual definition (Spitzer, 1987). The significance of quality of life was recognized by Karnofsky, Abelmann, Craves, and Burchenal (1948) at least 45 years ago, when Karnofsky developed a measure of quality of functioning for cancer patients to accompany the more traditional statistic "length of survival time" as a measure of treatment success. About the same time, the World Health Organization (WHO) adopted a broad definition of health in its Constitution stating, "Health is not only the absence of infirmity and disease, but also a state of physical, mental and social well-being" (WHO, 1947, p. 29). Quality of life has been defined as a multidimensional construct that includes "a wide range of capabilities, limitations, symptoms, and psychosocial characteristics that describe an individual's ability to function and derive satisfaction from a variety of roles" (Wenger, Mattson, Furberg, & Elinson, 1984a, p. 908). According to Wenger, Mattson, Furberg, & Elinson (1984b) there are three major facets of quality of life in medical conditions: (a) functional capacity, or the ability to perform activities of daily life, and to function socially, intellectually, emotionally, and economically; (b) perceptions of well-being and satisfaction with life; and (c) physical manifestations of disease, such as symptomatology and impairment.

A more phenomenological approach to quality of life stresses the importance of people's subjective perception of current ability to function as compared with their own internalized standards of what is possible or ideal (Cella & Tulsky, 1990; Ziller, 1974), or, alternately, with their ability to achieve their life ambitions (Cohen, 1982). Lipowski (1969), in an earlier argument, proposed a similar emphasis, stating that an individual's experience of the disease process, its personal meaning, and the impact of this meaning on his behavior and interaction with others are all important factors in the disease process, which should be viewed as "a total human response." It is noteworthy in this regard that the relative importance of different functions varies with the individual. For example, loss of function of lower extremities might affect an athlete much more than a painter. Patients do change their own standards and expectations, however, in accordance with their disease status. For example, in a study in which healthy subjects, postmyocardial infarction (MI) patients and bronchial carcinoma patients were asked to rate their general satisfaction with the quality of their life, a much larger proportion of MI and carcinoma patients than healthy patients rated themselves as "very satisfied," presumably due to their altered expectations of what might be possible for them (Muthny, Koch, & Stump, 1990). This underlines the importance of subjective perception and expectation in measuring quality of life. It has been suggested that the construct of quality of life encompasses both a cognitive and an affective component (Campbell, Converse, & Rodgers, 1976; de Haes & van Knippenberg, 1985). Appraisal of one's condition is a cognitive operation, whereas reaction to that appraisal and consequent emotional functioning is affectively influenced.

Another interpretation of the construct of quality of life highlights the psychosomatic interconnection of mind and body. Fava (1990) stressed that psychosocial factors related to a patient's appraisal of the disease process and how it is affecting the patient's life will themselves affect the course of the disease and its symptomatology. For example, in the cardiovascular literature, post-MI psychosocial difficulties such as depression, pessimism, maladaptive coping strategies, social isolation, and high levels of life stress have been shown to be predictive of less successful cardiac outcomes. In these studies, outcome measures have included increased hospital readmissions, diminished work, and poorer sexual functioning (Stern, Pascale, & Ackerman, 1977), greater self-reported pain (Pancheri et al., 1978), and increased mortality rates over 2- to 3-year periods (Obier, MacPherson, & Haywood, 1977; Ruberman, Weinblatt, Goldberg, & Chaudhary, 1984). Psychosocial factors may serve as mediators of disease course via their positive or negative effect on wellness behaviors, self-care, and sense of control (Ewart, Taylor, Reese, & Devusk, 1983; Follick et al., 1988; Krantz, 1980). In addition, there are likely to be direct pathways between the experience of stress and physiological endpoints. For example, mental stress has been shown to be causally related to myocardial ischemia in patients with coronary artery disease (Rozanski et al., 1988). It has been proposed that stress exerts its influence by lowering the threshold of cardiac vulnerability to ventricular fibrillation (Ruberman et al., 1984). Thus it may indeed be possible that quality of life factors such as mental and emotional well-being, satisfaction, and general life stress may influence disease course and symptomatology.

Quality of Life Variables in HIV

Until recently there have been few studies of quality of life in HIV infection. Nevertheless, for comprehensive evaluation of pharmacological interventions, determination of appropriate targets of psychosocial interventions, and evaluating efficacy of such interventions, assessment of impact on quality of life is critical. We discuss here some of the relevant HIV-related quality of life studies and review psychosocial factors relevant to an understanding of quality of life issues in HIV.

Among descriptive studies examining quality of life in HIV infection, it has been demonstrated, not surprisingly, that HIV infection creates a great disruption in quality of life (Ragsdale & Morrow, 1990; Wachtel et al., 1992). The impact of the infection, as one would expect, is relative to the stage of the disease, with HIV-infected individuals who are still asymptomatic having much less diminution in quality of life than patients with full-blown AIDS (Kaplan, Anderson, & Patterson, 1991; Ragsdale & Morrow, 1990). In addition, Kaplan and colleagues (1991) demonstrated significant correlations in HIV-infected individuals between scores on the Quality of Well-Being scale (QWB; Kaplan & Anderson, 1988), CD4 counts, neuropsychological status, and the vigor and depression scales of the Proflile of Mood States. Ellerman (1989) used the Spitzer Quality of Life Index (Spitzer et al., 1981) to assess the quality of daily living in men with AIDS or AIDS-related complex (ARC). He found that these men spent a substantial part of their day (an average of 5.9 hours) in health-care related activities, including time spent on personal medical care, paperwork, and extra hours of sleep. The average Spitzer Index of his sample was 6.8, indicating even greater compromise in quality of life than published normative scores for cancer patients and patients with other chronic illnesses.

Wu and colleagues (1991) validated a health status questionnaire (MOS-HIV) specific to individuals with early HIV infection. Starting with core items from the Medical Outcomes Study Short-form General Health Survey (Stewart, Hays , & Ware, 1988), they added items relevant to HIV infection such as cognitive function, energy level and fatigue, health distress, and a single item assessing quality of life in general. The resultant questionnaire was shown to differentiate between physical function, overall health, cognitive function, pain, and role function between subjects with asymptomatic HIV infection and those with early ARC. However, reliable discrimination between the groups was not found on subscales assessing social function, mental health, energy level and fatigue, and health distress (Wu et al., 1991). This type of instrument represents an important step in the development of a quality of life outcome measure for AIDS clinical trials, but does not offer a clear enough differentiation of the psychosocial factors most relevant to early HIV infection.

HIV infection has a multifaceted effect on quality of life. Although HIV spectrum disease is affecting increasing proportions of the heterosexual population, the majority of the individuals diagnosed with HIV infection are still homosexual men, a trend projected to continue through 1994 Centers for Disease Control [CDC], (1993). Current estimates of AIDS cases among African Americans and Hispanics run as high as 51% of all AIDS cases, and the disease is spreading more rapidly among at-risk members of these groups than among the population at large (CDC, 1993). Many AIDS patients are young, with 69% of AIDS cases in this country in individuals under 40 and 91% under age 50 (Hoffman, 1991). As such, these patients are faced with a terminal diagnosis at a point in their lives in which developmentally they still have many aspirations regarding careers, relationships, and life goals. This causes even a greater sense of loss and alienation than would a disease occurring later in life when an individual might expect to fall ill as part of the normal aging process (Hoffman, 1991).

The physical and psychosocial complications of HIV-related disease often present as an overlay on a lifestyle already associated with stigmas, such as job discrimination, racial prejudice, and social stigmatization. Diagnosis of HIV seropositivity may result in exposure of an individual's sexual orientation and lifestyle, requiring the person to face previously avoided ostracism. The association of AIDS with already stigmatized groups such as gay men and intravenous drug users, and the common attribution that becoming HIV infected is the person's own fault has led to added stigmitization of people with AIDS. This, combined with a large wave of sentiment toward the identification and possible isolation of infected persons (Blendon & Donelan, 1988; Walkey, Taylor, & Green, 1990) has resulted in social stigma and derogation of the victims of the disease (Hoffman, 1991).

Because HIV is a debilitating, progressive disease, infected individuals frequently experience multiple uncontrollable stressors along with the onset and progression of the disease. These may include loss of work, social isolation, increased medical costs, financial problems, difficulties with self-care, and death of members in the social support system (Blendon & Donelan, 1988; Bloom & Carliner, 1988; Ginzburg & Gostin, 1986; Redfield & Burke, 1988; Walkey et al., 1990). These issues compound the many issues normally accompanying diagnosis and progression of any chronic disease, including loss of self-esteem, independence, and reorientation of identity (McDaniels, Hepworth, & Doherty, 1992) as well as physical and emotional withdrawal of individuals making up the infected person's social support systems (Dunkel-Schetter & Wortman, 1982; Glasser & Strauss, 1965). Hoffman (1991) poignantly stated, "At its simplest, AIDS is about loss. It is about the loss of one's health, vitality, sensuality, and career—and most profoundly, the letting go of the future as one had envisioned it" (p. 468).

Such multifaceted difficulties provide a formidable challenge to even the most well adjusted individuals, and may lead to a diminished sense of self-efficacy, feelings of despair, anxiety, and depression, accompanied by increases in maladaptive attempts at coping, such as denial, avoidance, substance abuse, and unprotected sex (Antoni, 1991).

In Miami, we have been working with men who are showing emotional distress, but do not yet show functional impairment. Thus we have utilized other scales than traditional quality of life scales to enable us to measure more subtle multidimensional impairments in quality of life. We felt that use of a variety of psychosocial instruments, rather than a single quality of life instrument, would provide greater specificity in the domains of interest. Thus we have chosen to operationalize quality of life in terms of (a) emotional functioning, including depression and anxiety; (b) social functioning and role functioning, including social support systems and quality of relationships; and (c) physical functioning, including symptoms of disease progression. Based on previous findings (Ellerman, 1989; Kaplan et al., 1991; Ragsdale & Morrow, 1990), we operated with the assumption that in the population we are studying, disease progression can be thought of as one preliminary indicator of physical functioning and impairment and that to the extent that the onset of HIV-related symptoms can be delayed, we are forestalling functional impairments in the quality of life.

We now look at some of the important determinants of quality of life in HIV infection, such as coping, appraisals of stressors, self-efficacy, ability to elicit social support, and immune functioning, and describe how we have seen these factors modulated by psychosocial interventions as illustrated in Table 14.1.

TABLE 14.1
Quality of Life Issues for HIV-1 Disease Stages

Stage	*CD4+ Categories*	*Physical Indicators*	*Moderators of Quality of Life*	*Quality of Life Issues*
Asymptomatic HIV infection	≥ 500/μL	May have persistent generalized lymphadenopathy	*Appraisals:* Anticipatory grieving, catastrophizing and other cognitive distortions; changed expectations of future; identity and self-esteem issues; reassessment of spiritual and existential issues *Coping:* Dealing with present and future uncertainties; at risk for denial, disengagement, substance abuse, risky sex, suicidality. Issues of eliciting social support	*Emotional functioning:* Depression, anxiety, anger; often increasing at diagnosis and diminishing and recycling as individual confronts realities of living with HIV disease *Role functioning:* Often able to work; possible decrements in job mobility and career opportunities; job loss *Social functioning:* Fear, isolation, issues of trust in relationships; stigmatization; changes in social support networks due to deaths; relationship and sexual changes; isolation, withdrawal *Physical functioning:* Normal but may be altered due to depression or anxiety; may have hypervigilance regarding all physical symptoms
Symptomatic HIV infection	200–499/μL	Emergence of symptoms such as thrush, night sweats, low-grade fevers, oral hairy leukoplakia, peripheral neuropathy; commonly taking antiretroviral drugs and/or PCP prophylaxis	*Appraisals:* Anticipatory grieving, catastrophizing and other cognitive distortions; changed expectations of future; identity and self-esteem issues related to threats to occupational and functional abilities; reassessment of spiritual and existential issues	*Emotional functioning:* Depression, anxiety, anger, often increasing on emergence of symptoms, and then fluctuating with challenges and threats to present and future functioning. *Role functioning:* Often able to work. May take on new roles as part of HIV support-related network.

			Coping: Dealing with present and future uncertainties; at risk for denial, disengagement, substance abuse and risky sex	*Social functioning:* Changes in social support networks due to deaths; isolation; withdrawal; relationship and sexual changes; stigmatization *Physical functioning:* May have reduced energy levels; moderate symptomatology; possible cognitive deficits; pain; wasting
AIDS	<200 or <14% of T-lymphocytes	• Opportunistic infections such as extensive candidiasis, cryptococcal meningitis • Kaposi's sarcoma • tuberculosis • pneumocystis carinii pneumonia • lymphomas Commonly taking antiretroviral drugs, chemotherapy, antibiotics, etc.	*Appraisals:* Facing chronic illness and death; grieving about current and anticipated losses; catastrophizing and other cognitive distortions; reassessment of spiritual and existential issues *Coping:* Coping strategies may be overwhelmed in dealing with current difficulties such as financial losses, medical costs, treatment and side effects, housing; may lose some traditional coping strategies such as recreational outlets	*Emotional functioning:* Depression, anxiety, anger may cycle according to fluctuations in disease status and appraisals; relief from uncertainty *Role functioning:* Diminished capacity for work; role changes—often need care instead of being a caretaker *Social functioning:* May have diminished social networks due to lack of mobility, illness, as well as deaths among friends *Physical functioning:* Self-care difficulties; fatigue; wasting; much time spent in medical care; debilitation from infection and treatments; possible cognitive deficits

PHASES OF PSYCHOSOCIAL RESPONSE TO HIV

HIV Diagnosis

HIV diagnosis is often seen as a sentence for premature death, preceded by a period of unpleasant decline and dependency, due to decreasing physical and psychological competence. As mentioned, seropositivity is further stigmatized due to an association with sex, drugs, and public confusion regarding contagion. Understandably, diagnosis is most frequently perceived as a catastrophic event, and as a stressor of sufficient magnitude that it would result in distress for almost anyone in such a situation (Hoffman, 1991).

Notification of an HIV seropositive diagnosis has been associated with an increased incidence of *DSM-IIIR* Axis I affective and adjustment disorders, most notably adjustment disorder with depressed mood (Goodkin, 1988; Jacobsen, Perry, & Hirsch, 1990; Ostrow et al., 1989; Perry et al., 1990; Rundell, Paolucci, & Beatty, 1988; Woo, 1988). The sustained emotional distress accompanying diagnosis is highlighted by Namir's (1986) finding that 81% of HIV positive homosexual respondents reported an interest in psychological interventions, although only 28% were receiving psychosocial services. The extent of depression may be seen in the increased suicide rate among HIV-infected men, which may be as much as 36 times the rate of age-matched uninfected men (Kizer, Green, & Perkins, 1988; Marzuk et al., 1988; Rundell et al., 1988). Other common reactions to a seropositive diagnosis are anger, anxiety, hypervigilance about physical symptoms, feelings of doom, and a sense of pressure to undertake sweeping lifestyle changes (Christ & Weiner, 1985; Hoffman, 1991; Kaisch & Anton-Culver, 1989; Viney, Henry, Walker, & Crooks, 1989).

Early Asymptomatic Infection

Previously resolved issues regarding internalized homophobia and related self-esteem issues may resurface and threaten a fragile emotional stability as individuals struggle to deal with diagnosis and early HIV infection (Hoffman, 1991). For HIV-infected gay men, the stressors found to be most closely associated with emotional distress and maladaptive coping are the HIV-related deaths of loved ones and the anticipation of one's own future illness and death due to HIV infection (Martin, Dean, Garcia, & Hall, 1989). Frequently reported social complaints in early phases of the infection include problems such as difficulties forming new romantic relationships and friendships, telling friends and family about one's diagnosis, and problems with employment, such as diminished job mobility and compromised career opportunities due to health insurance difficulties and reported discriminatory hiring practices. Wu and colleagues (1991) found that although many patients with early HIV infection felt capable of working, quite a few had lost their jobs. Although no external symptoms are observed at this stage, with the exception of chronic lymphadenopathy, dimunition of energy, distress over health symptoms, and mental distress are frequently endorsed complaints in asymptomatic HIV infection (Wu et al., 1991).

Because the course of asymptomatic HIV infection can last as long as 10 years (Fauci, 1991; Pantaleo et al., 1993) infected individuals may have time to come to terms with an HIV-positive diagnosis and to develop new, more adaptive coping strategies. Although initially an HIV-positive person appears to be healthy, there is often a significant drop in CD4 cell counts and other immunological changes, even in asymptomatic individuals, which signals a decline in immune functioning. Eventually most, if not all, infected persons become symptomatic. As CD4 cell counts drop below 500, symptoms such as thrush, night sweats, and viral and fungal infections begin to occur. These infections may result in altered self-image and energy levels (Redfield & Burke, 1988). Frank AIDS occurs when the person has a CD4 count of below 200 or less than 14% of their total lymphocyte count, or develops opportunistic infections such as *pneumocystic carinii* pneumonia or cryptococcal meningitis (CDC, 1992).

Emergence of Symptoms

The next major crisis affecting psychosocial as well as physical functioning is the emergence of HIV-related symptoms. Although an individual may have re-established psychological equilibrium by employing denial as a coping strategy during the asymptomatic phase of the disease, this stance is no longer possible when symptoms start to appear (Bury, 1982; McDaniels et al., 1992). During this phase the individual may once again have to face the discomforting uncertainties that had been anticipated at the time of diagnosis, but this time with an increased sense of inevitability and urgency. Uncertainty related to the unpredictable course of HIV infection may be responsible for the finding that individuals with symptomatic HIV infection (prior to onset of AIDS defining symptoms) often experience greater psychological distress than do individuals once they have received a diagnosis of full-blown AIDS (Dilley, Ochitill, Perl, & Volberding, 1985). The anticipation of recurring, uncontrollable, and unpredictable stressors such as new symptoms, medical costs, uncertain medical treatments, and impaired autonomy (Blendon & Donelan, 1988; Ginzburg & Gostin, 1986; Redfield & Burke, 1988; Walkey et al., 1990) may result in an increased risk for depression, distress, and increased sexual risk behaviors and substance abuse as methods of avoiding this distress (Antoni, 1991). This risk may be compounded in situations where social support is compromised due to HIV-related deaths, social withdrawal, and avoidance by acquaintances and significant others who may have difficulty dealing with the disease (Beckett & Rutan, 1990; Christ & Weiner, 1985; Gambe & Getzel, 1989; Martin, 1988).

In addition, some HIV-infected individuals report feeling "toxic" and deliberately isolate themselves from relationships due to fear of rejection and concern about infecting others (Beckett & Rutan, 1990; Gambe & Getzel, 1989). Thus the unique characteristics of this illness lead to a situation in which individuals sorely need social support, but are afraid of reaching out to others, and thus feel isolated with unmet needs for social support (Hoffman, 1991). One study found that although HIV seropositivity itself was not associated with depressive symptomatology, as more symptoms emerged, the extent of reported depressive symptomatology was directly related to the number of self-reported HIV-related symptoms (Ostrow et al., 1989). In addition in HIV-related illness, self-perceptions of poorer physical health as well as increased objectively measured medical symptoms have been strongly related to perceived absences of social support, especially sources of instrumental social support (Namir, Alumbaugh, Fawzy, & Walcott, 1989). In assessing quality of life in early ARC, Wu et al. (1991) found that their subjects reported the greatest suffering in the areas of fatigue, distress over health, emotional distress, and pain. Thus the emergence of symptoms, in addition to compromising physical functioning, appears to greatly increase the amount of distress in the lives of HIV-positive symptomatic individuals.

Quality of life takes on new overtones as more AIDS-specific treatments are developed, and benefits as well as side effects of treatments must be evaluated. For example, antiretroviral medications such as zidovudine (AZT) are routinely recommended at this time for asymptomatic and early symptomatic HIV infection for individuals with less than 500 CD4 cells (Hamilton et al., 1992; Volberding et al., 1990). However, AZT has been shown to have side effects including headache, insomnia, malaise, nausea, gastrointestinal upset, confusion, and occasional hematologic toxicity with anemia and neutropenia (Fischl et al., 1990). Zidovudine given at an early stage (200 to 500 CD4 cells/mm^3) appears to delay disease progression to AIDS, and at least one study has reported that patients receiving AZT had higher levels of physical functioning and well-being than a matched placebo control group (Wu et al., 1990). However, once AIDS symptoms do manifest, disease progression may be more rapid and symptoms more debilitating in people who have been taking AZT for some time than in persons who started receiving AZT later in the disease process (Hamilton et al., 1992). Because of the variability in statistics such as these, and because the side effects of many contemporary medications used to treat AIDS vary so much in type and severity, quality of life variables assume great importance as a means of evaluating the effectiveness of HIV treatment regimens (Burgess & Catalan, 1991; de Haes & van Knippenberg, 1985).

Barker and colleagues (Barker, Tindall, & Carballo, 1990), in a discussion of 14 double-blind placebo-controlled clinical trials in HIV disease published between June 1982 and June 1989, found that only three included even a brief measurement of quality of life, the Karnofsky Performance Index. More recently, the Quality of Well Being Scale (QWB) has been used along with the Karnofsky scale to assess quality of life in a placebo-controlled trial of AZT in patients with AIDS and ARC (Wu, Matthews, et al., 1990). Findings indicated a general decline in functional status of patients over the course of the study. When mortality was controlled in statistical analyses, Karnofsky scores were higher for the AZT group at the end of the 19-week blinded study, but at 1 year no significant differences were observed between groups on either quality of life measure. Although the authors stressed the importance of quality of life assessment as a component of AIDS treatment evaluation, they questioned whether the QWB was sensitive enough to discriminate functional status in patients with such advanced disease.

In a further study, Wu and colleagues (Wu, Rubin, et al., 1990) used the Medical Outcome Study-HIV scale (Wu et al., 1991) and the QWB to assess early ARC patients in a randomized trial of AZT. Findings indicated that although AZT was associated with initial decrements in quality of life, after 1 year there were no differences in functional status between the treatment and control groups. A second study (Gelber, Lenderking, Corron, Fischl, & Testa, 1991) examining quality of life in a randomized trial of AZT in early ARC patients, used adverse health reports, such as increased symptoms, as a quality of life measure. This group found that the AZT group reported more adverse health effects as compared to the placebo group, but that the placebo group showed faster disease progression and more severe symptomatology when it did occur. Again, because this study used such coarse and likely, insensitive measures, it is difficult to draw firm conclusions about the effects of such treatments on quality of life from this line of work.

Progression to AIDS

As individuals develop full-blown AIDS, there is some indication that the onset of AIDS may be accompanied by a lessening of psychological distress from the levels experienced by symptomatic (without AIDS) HIV-infected men (Dilley et al., 1985; Tross & Hirsch, 1988). This may reflect a relief from the unpredictability of not knowing if and when the first signs of

AIDS may occur. Adjusting to long-term progressive illness including changes in self-image, autonomy, expectations of self, and preparation for death are issues that must be addressed in this stage (Hoffman, 1991). Employment status often changes dramatically at this point in the disease. Several studies have found that a majority of men diagnosed with AIDS in their samples had become unemployed (Chuang, Devins, Hunsley, & Gill, 1989; Dilley et al., 1985). One study reported that the average monthly income of patients with AIDS or ARC had fallen by an average of $1,000 per month and that unemployment was common since their diagnosis (Ellerman, 1989). Even intermittent episodes of *pneumocystis carinii* pneumonia are highly associated with diminished abilities to maintain employment (Wachtel et al., 1992). Change in employment status is often accompanied by devastation on many fronts—loss of sources of social support, identity, income, and medical insurance.

It has been noted that with progression of HIV infection from asymptomatic to symptomatic, individuals go through a continual process of emotional crises, recycling through the stages that Kubler-Ross (1969) originally enumerated as part of the dying process (Hoffman, 1991). These stages have since been identified as expected responses to any significant stressor (Horowitz, 1976): denial, anger, bargaining, depression, and acceptance. Moreover, it has been observed that HIV-infected patients have reactions that are more intense and labile than those described by Kubler-Ross (Hoffman, 1991). The high percentage of seropositive individuals diagnosed with adjustment disorders is a testimony to the difficulties encountered as individuals struggle to come to terms with their illness and its impact on their often young lives (Hoffman, 1991).

Previous theoretical models looking at responses to life transitions have highlighted the importance of individual differences as well as environmental factors in determining whether particular life events result in growth or deterioration (Lazarus & Folkman, 1984; Schlossberg, 1981, 1989). Although HIV diagnosis may be perceived as universally catastrophic, differences in appraisals, sense of control, potential for growth or deterioration, attributions of causality, and social support may make a difference in how an individual feels about the disease and how the person is able to cope with it. The ability of attitude to affect the impact of a seropositive diagnosis is highlighted by a study examining global, nonspecific changes in social functioning following a seropositive diagnosis. Although a majority of the sample of asymptomatic seropositive gay men reported that seropositivity had a negative effect on their social functioning, 32% reported a positive effect on their social interactions (Kaisch & Anton-Culver, 1989). Thus, attitudes and coping skills may have a major impact on quality of life after HIV diagnosis.

USE OF PSYCHOSOCIAL INTERVENTIONS TO IMPROVE QUALITY OF LIFE

Given that psychosocial factors can be important to many aspects of quality of life among HIV-infected persons, scientists have tried to develop interventions designed to improve those factors that optimize quality of life for these individuals. Specifically, psychosocial interventions that enhance an individual's sense of control, teach adaptive coping strategies, improve ability to elicit social support, and modify ways that individuals think about stressors, may enhance psychological adjustment in HIV-infected individuals, thereby improving the quality of their lives. In the cardiovascular literature it has been shown that interventions that increase patients' sense of control and predictability may facilitate recovery and lead to lower morbidity and mortality risks due to coronary heart disease (Follick et al., 1988; Krantz, 1980). Similarly a study with HIV-infected men found that individuals who believed they could positively influence their health status through life-style changes showed less distress (Moulton, Sweet, Temoshok, & Mandel, 1987). To the extent that psychological responses to the disease affect disease progression, survival time or symptomatology may be affected as well.

In contrast, indirect coping strategies such as substance abuse and high-risk sexual behaviors may accelerate disease progression and ultimately have a pejorative influence on physical functioning. This can occur by these behaviors interfering with host resistance (Brown, Stimmel, Taub, Kochwa, & Rosenfeld, 1974; Glassmen, Bennett, & Randall, 1985; Roe, 1979; Tisman, Herbert, Go, & Brenner, 1971) as well as introducing other pathogens that may (a) serve as co-factors in the progression of the disease (Ciobanu, 1989; Esterling et al., 1992; Rinaldo, 1989) or (b) introduce new strains of the virus and reinfection (Martin & Vance, 1984; Penkower et al., 1991). Such maladaptive coping strategies also contribute to disease spread in the population (Kelly & St. Lawrence, 1988).

Our work has looked at some of the important determinants of quality of life that are affected by HIV infection: factors such as coping, ability to elicit social support, cognitive appraisals, and immune function. These factors impact the components of quality of life previously enumerated: emotional functioning and well-being, social functioning and role functioning, as well as physical functioning. These quality of life factors are affected both by the discovery that a person is HIV positive, and later on, by the progression of the disease. Initially, we directed our efforts toward developing an intervention to improve some of these quality of life factors in gay men who were first learning that they were HIV seropositive. Group cognitive behavioral stress management (CBSM), which can help improve both appraisals and adaptive coping strategies, encourage emotional expression, provide social support, and teach relaxation skills, seemed to be an appropriate intervention strategy for this population.

In a model delineating hypothesized effects of this intervention on an HIV population, Antoni (1991) suggested that as individuals begin to feel they can cope more effectively, they feel more confident, as well as less depressed and anxious. They may also be more likely to reduce risk behaviors such as substance use and unprotected sex. In addition, improved social support can also decrease depression and anxiety. Overall diminutions in distress are thought to result in more normalized neuroendocrine function, less stress-related impairments in cell-mediated immunity, more normalized immunologic surveillance of herpes viruses, and possible decreases in HIV replication. This model has been modified to show how our intervention aims are thought to lead to changes in quality of life outcome measures (see Fig. 14.1).

PHASES OF OUR RESEARCH PROGRAM

Our HIV research in Miami has involved three different phases. Initially we worked with gay men who were anticipating receipt of a HIV diagnosis, and we examined factors affecting quality of life, coping strategies, self-efficacy, and social support before, during, and after the men received their diagnosis. We also examined the effect of a CBSM intervention on these variables. In a subsequent study, we worked with men who knew they were HIV seropositive, but who were still asymptomatic. Again we assessed variables related to quality of life before, during, and after a CBSM intervention. In our current studies we are working with men who are HIV positive and symptomatic. These men fit into CDC categories B1 and B2 (CDC, 1992), but without AIDS defining criteria. We are evaluating the effects of a group CBSM intervention on improving their quality of life. Changes in clinical symptoms and immunological measures were also evaluated in each protocol.

HIV-1 Serostatus Notification

In the first phase of our work, we studied 47 healthy gay men between the ages of 18 and 40 who were symptom free and had chosen to learn their HIV status for the first time. HIV+ men had mean baseline CD4 counts of 484 cmm (Antoni et al., 1991). The average age of these subjects was about 30 and the majority were White, college-educated, and employed, with an annual income of $20,000 to $30,000 (Antoni, August et al., 1990). Once accepted into the study they were randomly assigned to a 10-week CBSM

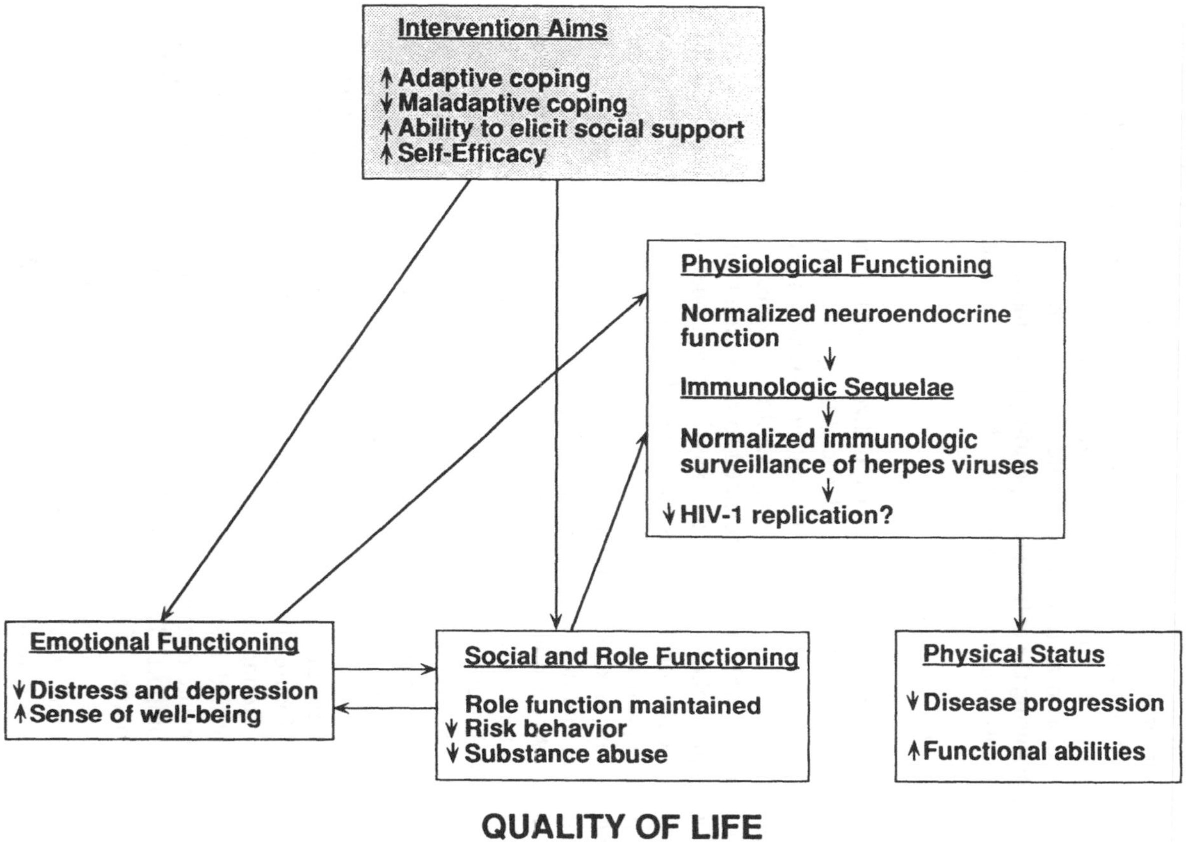

FIG. 14.1. Model describing hypothesized effects and related physiological processes of our cognitive behavioral intervention on quality of life in HIV-infected individuals. Adapted with permission from Antoni (1991).

group, an aerobic exercise group, or an assessment-only control group. This discussion focuses on the effects of the CBSM group and not the exercise training condition. Psychological and immunological assessments were conducted at study entry, and at 4, 6, 8, and 10 weeks into the study. Notification of serostatus occurred between Weeks 5 and 6, and was given by a licensed clinical social worker, who had received extensive training in pre- and posttest counseling. The goal of this intervention was to test if cognitive behavioral techniques could be used to attenuate anxiety and depression during the anticipatory period preceding serostatus notification, and in the early stages of coping with the impact of the diagnosis.

Intervention Components

Our intervention was designed to utilize CBSM techniques to impact appraisals, coping strategies, and social support (Antoni, 1991; Antoni, Baggett, et al., 1991). The intervention lasted for 10 weeks, and met semiweekly, with one of the weekly sessions devoted to CBSM strategies, and the other weekly session dedicated to relaxation training. Our intervention with this cohort combined a psychoeducational model with CBSM strategies. Educational modules included information on the psychological and physiological aspects of the stress response, AIDS and the immune system, sexual risk behaviors and behavioral change, preparing for HIV notification, and different types of social support.

Initially we introduced subjects to an appraisal-based model demonstrating the relationship of appraisal to the experience of stress (Beck & Emery, 1985), using HIV-related examples, such as effects of appraisal on distress related to receiving a seropositive HIV status. This was followed by identification of frequently used cognitive distortions (Beck, Rush, Shaw, & Emery, 1979) and use of personal examples from homework to identify each individual's most commonly used cognitive distortions. Subsequently participants were taught how to refute and replace cognitive distortions. The next unit focused on behavioral change and coping skills training, with the goal of altering maladaptive and indirect coping strategies. These modules identified maladaptive coping, taught more direct methods of coping to alleviate distress, and assertiveness training. Finally we emphasized social support. This came about through group interaction and by identifying sources of social support and problems with social support systems. We have found in our experience that the common nature of experiences faced, both in relation to HIV and in relation to gay lifestyle, enhanced group cohesion. We felt the homogeneity of a uniform stressor that was being faced was important in enhancing social support. The model of a homogeneous support group has been successful in other interventions with populations with chronic illnesses such as breast cancer patients

(Spiegel, Bloom, Kraemer, & Gottheil, 1989), melanoma patients (Fawzy, Cousins, et al., 1990), and seropositive gay men (Coates, McKusick, Stites, & Kuno, 1989).

Throughout this protocol subjects also learned progressive muscle relaxation (Bernstein & Borkevec, 1973) once weekly. In addition to weekly training sessions, subjects were requested to practice at least twice daily at home, and to monitor their at-home relaxation frequency on practice cards.

We hypothesized that whereas the control group would demonstrate post-HIV diagnosis increases in depression and anxiety—which have been commonly reported in the literature (e.g., Goodkin, 1988; Hoffman, 1991; Ostrow et al., 1989)—the CBSM group, because of their training, would be more equipped to deal with their distress, and would show much smaller increases in depression or anxiety accompanying seropositivity notification. Second, we hypothesized that these psychosocial changes would run in tandem with immune changes, such that the CBSM group would show no change or increments in both phenotypic and functional immune measures, whereas the control group would show decrements in these measures pre- to postdiagnosis.

Initial Impact of HIV Seropositivity

We found that members of the control group who were notified of their HIV seropositivity showed significant increases in anxiety and depression scores as assessed by the Profile of Mood States (POMS; McNair, Lorr, & Droppleman, 1981) in the 2 weeks following notification. In contrast, among men participating in the CBSM group who received seropositivity notification, there were no significant changes in anxiety or depression during the short-term postnotification period. In fact, their depression scores following notification did not differ significantly from norms for college students (Antoni, Baggett, et al., 1991; see Fig. 14.2).

We were further interested in identifying important factors within the CBSM group related to this psychological buffering. One factor that stood out was the variation between subjects in compliance with the relaxation homework. On the basis of self-monitoring diary data maintained by subjects in the CBSM condition, we found that the mean frequency of progressive muscle relaxation home practice per week was 4.94 sessions per week in the week preceding notification, 6.35 in the week of notification, and 4.47 in the week following notification. However, the extent of any individual's relaxation practice for any given week ranged from 0 to 14 sessions (Antoni, Baggett, et al., 1991). Interestingly, we found that the subjects who had most prepared themselves for anxiety management by actively practicing relaxation during the 5-week prenotification period showed lower postnotification POMS distress and depression scores, as

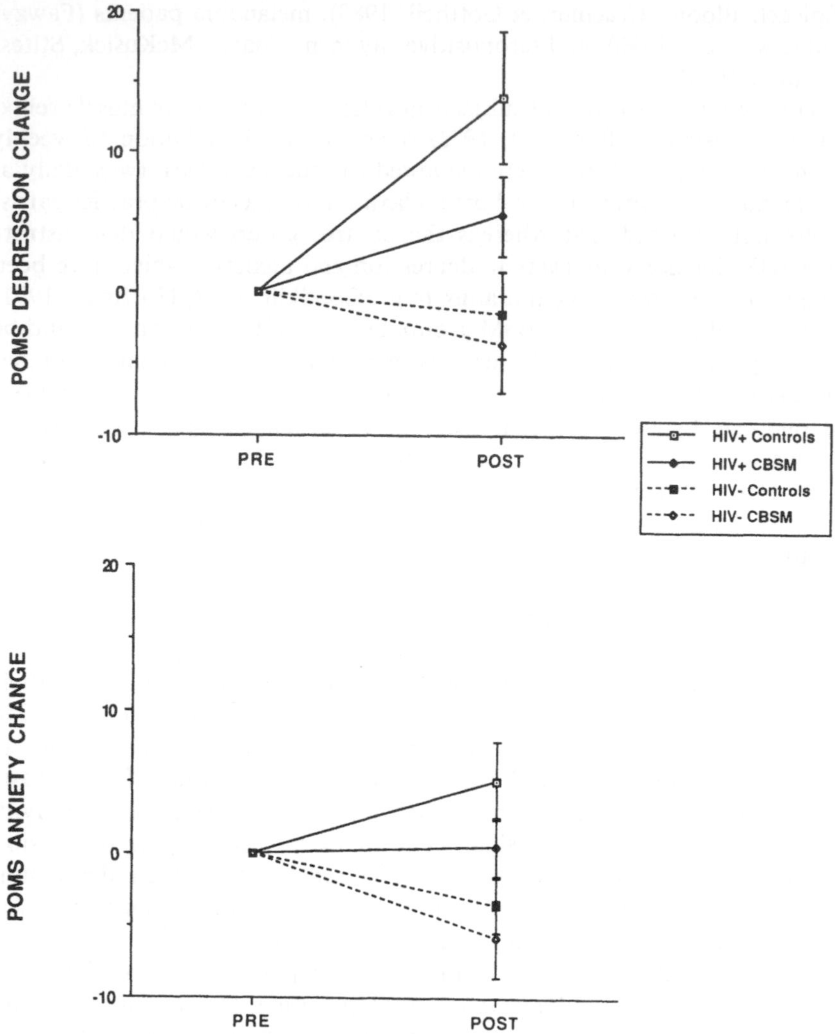

FIG. 14.2. Effects of CBSM intervention on POMS depression and anxiety score changes following notification of HIV-1 antibody status among gay men (Antoni, Baggett et al., 1991). Reprinted by permission.

indicated by correlations with frequency of relaxation practice (Antoni, Baggett, et al., 1991) In the high anxiety period of seropositivity notification, it appeared that relaxation practice gave the men a concrete skill they could utilize for anxiety reduction.

These psychological changes were also paralleled by immunological changes. The men in the control group who were notified of their seropositivity showed slight decrements in natural killer cell cytotoxicity

(NKCC), CD4, and NK (CD56) cell counts, and decreased responsivity to stimulation with the mitogen phytohemagglutinin (PHA) over the 2-week pre- to postnotification period. In contrast, CBSM subjects who were notified of their seropositivity displayed significant increases in CD4 and NK cell counts as well as slight increases in NKCC and in proliferative response to PHA during this period. Those subjects who had practiced home relaxation more frequently over the initial 5 weeks of the study not only showed lower POMS distress and depression scores following notification, but also demonstrated higher CD4 and NK (CD56) cell counts and greater proliferative responses to PHA, even after covarying prenotification distress levels (Antoni, Baggett, et al., 1991). Those individuals who continued their practice of relaxation as a method of dealing with the difficult emotions that emerged during the postnotification period (Weeks 5–7) also showed significantly higher numbers of CD4 and NK cells during this time.

Postnotification Adjustment

We had hypothesized that during the 5-week adjustment period following diagnosis, HIV-seropositive CBSM intervention group members would show improvements in social support utilization and adaptive coping skills as compared to the HIV seropositive men in the control group. Simultaneously we expected to see decreases in maladaptive coping strategies such as denial, disengagement, and substance use in the CBSM group as compared to the control group. We expected these findings to be paralleled by immune decrements in the control group and maintenance of immune functioning or enhancement in the CBSM group. We found that during this period, men in the control group showed both significant decrements in social support received, measured on the Social Provisions Scale (Cutrona & Russell, 1987), and decreases in coping strategies involving seeking out of social support. In contrast the men in the CBSM group maintained their prenotification social support levels and continued to actively seek social support in the weeks following notification (Friedman et al., 1990). The CBSM group members also showed significant decreases in behavioral disengagement (helplessness) over this period (Antoni, Ironson, et al., 1991). Relaxation frequency during the entire 10-week CBSM period was also correlated with decreases in depression over this period. These findings suggest that this 10-week stress management intervention may soften the impact of HIV seropositivity notification by enabling study participants to maintain or more fully utilize social support and to enhance their adaptive coping strategies.

Over the 10-week period of the study, we found that control group members showed significant decrements in lymphocyte proliferation to PHA and in several measures of NK activity. However, these men showed little change in CD4 counts or proliferative responses to pokeweed mitogen (PWM) over the same time period. On the other hand, those men in the CBSM group showed increases in responsivity to PHA and increases or maintenance in measures of NK activity. Again we looked at the importance of frequency of relaxation within the CBSM condition among those men who found out they were seropositive. After controlling for pretreatment immune values, we found that frequency of relaxation practice predicted higher posttreatment NKCC, PHA, and PWM values for these subjects (Antoni, Ironson, et al., 1991).

Previous work has shown that higher Epstein-Barr virus viral capsid antigen (EBV-VCA) antibody titers are commonly seen in asymptomatic HIV-1 seropositive individuals and in those with AIDS, suggestive of latent viral reactivation (Esterling et al., 1992; Rosenberg & Fauci, 1991). There is some evidence that EBV serves as a cofactor in the development of AIDS by allowing HIV entry into EBV-transformed B lymphocytes via expression of the CD4 receptor on these cells (Rosenberg & Fauci, 1991; Sumaya, Boswell, & Ench, 1986). Other work has related EBV-VCA antibody titers in healthy college students to stress levels (Esterling, Antoni, Kumar, & Schneiderman, 1990; Glaser et al., 1991; Glaser et al., 1987) and has shown that these latent herpes virus antibody titers are modifiable with relaxation-based interventions (Kiecolt-Glaser et al., 1985).

Because of the possible importance of EBV-VCA in HIV-related disease progression, as well as the possibility of increasing host control over the expression of this latent virus by stress reduction, we thought it important to assess the impact of the CBSM intervention on EBV-VCA antibody titers in our subjects. We found that over the course of the intervention, HIV-positive CBSM subjects showed significant decreases in both EBV-VCA and human herpesvirus-type 6 (HHV-6) antibody titers as compared to the control group whose antibody titers remained constant over the 10-week period. We controlled for nonspecific polyclonal activation by determining that there were no changes in total IgG, nor in Forssman antibodies over the course of the intervention (Esterling et al., 1992). In addition, no differences between groups were observed either at baseline or over time in antibody to EBV early antigen, which arises in association with recent EBV infection.

Thus, in this group of seropositive asymptomatic men, we found that a CBSM intervention appeared to attenuate the distress responses associated with the stressor of notification of a positive HIV status by enhancing the participants' coping strategies and utilization of social support and by helping the participants modulate their mood. These psychosocial changes were also accompanied by moderate enhancement of immune functioning in the experimental group as compared to decrements in the same measures for the control group.

Given, as described earlier, that receipt of HIV diagnosis is accompanied by high rates of distress and even suicide (Goodkin, 1988; Hoffman, 1991; Jacobsen, et al., 1990; Kizer et al., 1988; Marzuk et al., 1988; Ostrow et al., 1989; Perry et al. 1990; Rundell et al., 1988; Woo, 1988) our finding that a cognitive behavioral intervention at the time of diagnosis seems to enable individuals to maintain emotional equanimity and to utilize positive coping strategies has important implications for the quality of life of these men. Ability to utilize successful coping skills, nondistorted appraisals, and ability to elicit social support may be critical determinants of the men's ability to maintain emotional balance, a sense of well-being, and integrated social functioning in what otherwise may seem to be an overwhelming situation. Our CBSM intervention in the short run appears to have the ability to enable individuals to mobilize their strengths and supports to deal with the trauma of diagnosis. The fact that immunological functioning was also buffered in the short run is an indication that these emotional changes do have physiological concomitants that may have important implications for disease progression and functional capacity for these men in the long run. In fact, our next step was to see what implications these short-term changes had for long-term functioning and physical symptomatology.

Longer Term Follow-Up

One- and 2-year follow-ups were undertaken with these individuals to examine which individual psychosocial characteristics predicted more successful outcomes. We found that coping strategies used to deal with HIV-1 antibody status notification were important predictors of both emotional functioning and immune status immediately following intervention and 1 year later. Specifically, maladaptive coping strategies including denial and disengagement were associated with greater depression at the end of the intervention as well as 1 year later (Antoni, Goldstein, et al., 1991). Conversely, positive coping skills such as active coping, planning, and positive reappraisal were related to less depression at these time points. Not only were coping strategies during the time of the intervention related to depression 1 year after the intervention, but importantly, these factors were also related to immune functioning 1 year later. We found that extent of denial at the end of the intervention, increase in denial following the diagnosis, and greater frequency of relaxation practice during the 10-week intervention period predicted higher CD4 counts and greater PHA responsivity 1 year later (Ironson et al., 1994).

In assessing the contribution of psychosocial factors to quality of life, relating psychological symptoms and immunological findings to longer term clinical symptoms and disease status is crucial. We conducted 2-year follow-ups on 21 HIV seropositive subjects for whom physical exams and hospital records were available. In our initial assessment these HIV seropositive men were asymptomatic. Two years later 5 of the 21 men had developed AIDS, and 4 more had developed HIV-related symptoms (thrush, fevers, and leukoplakia). Even controlling for CD4 cell count at study entry, several important psychological predictors of disease progression emerged. These included extent of distress at the time of diagnosis, denial still remaining at the end of the intervention, increase in denial over the course of the study, and poor adherence to the protocol, both in group attendance and relaxation practice frequency. The greater the denial and distress, the poorer the prognosis (Ironson et al., 1994). Thus psychosocial factors may be capable of not only influencing emotional functioning and well-being over time, but also may contribute to symptomatology, which directly impacts the individual's functional status, and in turn is one of the most important determinants of overall quality of life (Ragsdale & Morrow, 1990).

COPING WITH THE CHRONIC BURDEN OF HIV-1

From the first phase of our study we had learned that CBSM can attenuate the psychological distress accompanying diagnosis in the short run. We also learned that some of the ways people cope with stress may be predictive of psychological adjustment, immune status, and health over longer periods. However, as many HIV seropositive individuals are beyond the initial crisis of diagnosis we needed to ascertain whether CBSM could do more than buffer the acute stressor of diagnosis. Could a CBSM intervention be used to help individuals manage the chronic burdens of being HIV seropositive and in so doing, optimize quality of life for those affected? Second, we wondered whether CBSM could either boost or help maintain immune status in those with a declining immune system. Third, would the improvements in coping and quality of life be paralleled by improvements (i.e., normalization) or maintenance of immune status?

Early HIV Infection

As mentioned earlier, even asymptomatic HIV disease is accompanied by wide-ranging psychosocial challenges as well as a great many uncertainties. These arise in relation to the unpredictable course of the HIV infection as well as with respect to anticipated stressors that are potentially uncontrollable, such as impaired occupational and social functioning, decreased earning power, high costs of medical care, complex medical treatments, difficulties with self-care, and declining social supports (Blendon & Donelan, 1988; Ginzburg & Gostin, 1986; Redfield & Burke, 1988; Walkey et al.,

1990). Dealing with anticipatory grief is another important issue (Hoffman, 1991).

In a second study, our subjects were gay men who knew of their HIV-positive status, but were still asymptomatic. Although their physical functioning had not yet been affected by the virus, knowledge of their positive serostatus and its eventual implications had permeated their consciousness, behavior, and sense of well-being. Many were carrying the burden of this knowledge and its implications without having disclosed it to their family, acquaintances, or work associates. For several this led to an increased sense of isolation as well as feelings of duplicity, a sense of living a double life in which some people knew the truth about them and some did not. In addition to the psychological stress arising from such nondisclosure, recent studies on trauma have indicated that carrying undisclosed emotionally laden information may have negative health and immune consequences as well (Esterling et al., 1990; Pennebaker, Barger, & Tiebout, 1989; Pennebaker & Beall, 1986; Pennebaker, Kiecolt-Glaser, & Glaser, 1988; Pennebaker & Susman, 1988).

Although without evident HIV-related symptoms, quite a few of the men we interviewed were vigilant regarding possible symptomatology and treated any new cold or flu symptom with dread until the symptoms were proven innocuous. As one subject intimated, "When you notice a mark on your body or start to come down with a cold, you wonder if it is the beginning of the end or just a normal bruise, cold, or whatever." These men had all known their HIV status from 6 months to 5 years. Interestingly, some were still dealing with leftover anger regarding the manner in which they had been told they were positive. Several were quite angry about being seropositive, and about friends or partners who had left them after finding out they were infected.

Some subjects expressed reluctance to terminate relationships, even when they were problematic or dysfunctional, for fear of not finding a new partner, not living long enough to form another long-term relationship, or for fear of being sick and dying alone. Other relationship problems included how and when to tell prospective lovers or sexual partners of their seropositivity, and dealing with fears of rejection. Some men reported being reluctanct to have sex with someone who was uninfected for fear of infecting him, whereas others expressed fear of getting close to someone who was positive to avoid going through a loss when that person got sick. Another concern was whether to and how to disclose HIV status to family members who did not know that a subject was gay, much less seropositive. This type of issue typically involved facing issues of loss and grieving all over again through the eyes of someone they cared about, who would be finding out their status for the first time. Employment issues included concerns about making job transitions because of not wanting to jeopardize health insurance and yet wanting to maximize the quality of their professional lives while they still had the opportunity. Thus some of the predominant issues facing these men included anger, fear, loss, and uncertainty.

Given the complexity of these issues and the attendant difficulties with control and predictability, we felt that these men were especially at risk for depression and helplessness, accompanied by feelings of low self-efficacy. In addition, we were concerned that the normal coping strategies of these men might be overwhelmed, putting these men at risk for maladaptive coping stragies such as escaping through fantasy, substance abuse, risky sexual behaviors, denial, and disengagement. We were also concerned about social withdrawal.

The cognitive behavioral intervention for these asymptomatic men was specifically adapted to address these issues. Again, it was a 10-week, group-based intervention that included a weekly cognitive behavioral session as well as a weekly progressive muscle relaxation session. This group had a much different flavor from the first cohort because the men already knew their diagnosis, and the anxiety regarding impending notification was absent. The early part of the intervention maintained its psychoeducational focus, with sessions on HIV and the stress response, cognitive appraisals, refuting and replacing cognitive distortions. For this cohort, the group sessions discussing impending notification and postnotification concerns were replaced with a session dealing with unfinished issues related to seropositivity notification and notification of others regarding one's seropositivity. Behavior change, assertiveness, and social support were also addressed in group sessions. Strategies for eliciting social support and changing patterns of social support were specifically addressed. Examples used and issues brought up by these men focused on current and future adjustment in dealing with the chronic stressors of HIV infection, as outlined earlier. Although the men in the first phase of the study were dealing with existential and relationship issues especially with respect to diagnosis, this intervention focused more on day-to-day living issues such as how to deal with the daily anxieties and uncertainties related to seropositivity.

In pilot work with 11 asymptomatic gay men with known HIV-1 infection, we found that following the 10-week CBSM intervention, subjects reported decreases in POMS scores for anxiety, depression, anger, fatigue, and confusion, as well as increases in vigor. Subjects reported increases in adaptive coping strategies as well as significant decreases in several maladaptive coping strategies as related to the threat of AIDS in their life. Specifically this included decreases in mental disengagement and denial as well as increases in active coping, planning, and acceptance. Because of the small number of subjects, these findings did not reach statistical significance, but do point in the direction of adaptive psychosocial changes. Preliminary findings at this point indicate that these results are paralleled by immune status changes, but we do not yet know how this intervention affected development of physical symptomatology and disease progression in these men.

Thus, with individuals facing the chronic stressor of HIV infection, a CBSM intervention appears to help individuals improve their emotional well-being by decreasing levels of distress, and may further act to enhance their positive coping abilities. These findings were similar to those obtained by Fawzy and colleagues using a similar intervention with early stage primary melanoma patients (Fawzy, Cousins et al., 1990). Mobilization of coping abilities is essential for maximization of health-enhancing behaviors, and minimization of risk behaviors such as substance abuse and risky sexual activities.

Having had such promising results with men in the early stages of HIV-1 spectrum disease, we wondered how generalizable these findings would be to men in more advanced stages of the disease, whose issues and capacities would be somewhat different. Would CBSM be useful for helping men deal with symptomatic HIV-1 infection when overt signs of the infection made denial less feasible, yet distractions (work, hobbies, entertainment) might be less available or unrealistic? Would the immunomodulating effects of the CBSM intervention that we observed in early HIV-1 infection in individuals with more intact immune systems generalize to individuals whose immune systems may be accelerating downwards? These questions are crucial to understanding whether a psychosocial intervention can impact both psychological and physiological quality of life factors in more advanced stages of the disease.

DEALING WITH SYMPTOMS

The psychological issues affecting emotional functioning at this stage of HIV-1 infection include a breakdown of denial regarding of HIV-1 infection and its implications coupled with a re-emerging anxiety about facing chronic, uncontrollable, and unpredictable stressors in the future (Antoni, 1991; Dilley, et al., 1985; Hoffman, 1991; Schneiderman, Antoni, Ironson, LaPerriere, & Fletcher, 1992). These stressors may include disease progression, treatment responsiveness and side effects, financial uncertainties, medical costs (Bloom & Carliner, 1988), social stigmatization (Blendon & Donelan, 1988; Ginzburg & Gostin, 1986), and loss of familiar sources of social support (Christ & Weiner, 1985; Dilley et al., 1985; Gambe & Getzel, 1989; Martin, 1988). At this stage there is often a resurgence of existential issues, and individuals are again at risk for hopelessness and despair, social isolation, and maladaptive coping strategies (Antoni, 1991; Hoffman, 1991). Maintenance of a sense of well-being depends on being able to address these issues and maximizing the individual's coping strategies. This was our goal in working with men at this stage of the disease.

In the current phase of our research, we are working with known HIV-infected gay men who are at least mildly symptomatic, but do not meet CDC AIDS defining criteria. These men have symptoms such as thrush, night sweats, persistent lymphadenopathy, and fungal infections, among a host of others. For some of them, HIV-related symptoms have taken on a kind of immediacy, and participation in the group represented an active attempt to change their lifestyle as a way of bolstering their health. For many, creating a low-stress lifestyle in the midst of their daily activities is a priority. For some subjects, sources of self-esteem and identity have shifted from former occupations to participation or leadership in AIDS-related activities, such as an HIV information hotline, or fund-raising events. For some subjects, joining our study was a way of contributing to the cause.

With this group of men we altered our intervention protocol to respond to their needs at this stage of disease. Overall, we downplayed the didactic tone of the modules to include much greater experiential participation. Initially we directed our efforts toward increasing participants' awareness of stress in their lives (Beck & Emery, 1985). This included both emotional and physical manifestations of stress, the types of situations most likely to create stress for them, and the types of responses they were most likely to have to the experienced stress. Next we focused on the appraisal process, with sessions covering automatic thoughts, refuting, and replacing automatic thoughts (Beck, Rush, Shaw, & Emery, 1979). We used examples more specific to this population, for example, analyzing one's automatic thoughts on finding out knowledge of dropping CD4-cell counts. We have also expanded our instruction of coping strategies to include discussions of different kinds of coping strategies (Lazarus & Folkman, 1984), personal preferences of coping styles, matching preferential coping styles with life situations, and obstacles to adaptive coping. Finally we discussed social support and social support utilization, especially directed at the issues of this population, including social withdrawal, death, loss, and changing priorities in relationships. We expanded our relaxation protocol to give the subjects a variety of active stress reduction strategies from which they can select. To this end we now include progressive muscle relaxation (Bernstein & Borkevic, 1973), breathing techniques (Smith, 1985, 1988, 1990), autogenic training (Luthe, 1963, 1969), and meditative techniques (LeShan, 1974; Smith, 1985, 1988, 1990). Subjects were still instructed to practice twice a day, but they can select the techniques that they like the best.

With this cohort we found that different types of issues tended to arise in group discussions. Relationship issues now included dealing with long-term lovers who were ailing from HIV or had frank AIDS. This gave rise to concerns as to whether our subjects themselves would be next to decline, and if so, who would take care of them. Dealing with one's own needs for independence without feeling guilty, and at the same time caring for an ailing partner caused conflict for several individuals. Several had been faced with moral dilemmas: Should one stay with or leave a partner who was dying with a bad attitude, thus making the subject's life miserable, and possibly influencing the subject's health as well.

Some felt grateful for their own support system but expressed concern about family members who had no one to confide in regarding the illness. For several, the immediacy of symptoms gave rise to a re-evaluation of life meaning in response to a more impending life threat. Several members had given up substance abuse and reported a new or renewed sense of spirituality in their lives. Others had lost their faith in God following HIV infection. Participants expressed emotions such as wanting to be as happy as possible while things were good; fears of dying, being sick, losing independence; fears of the unknown—wondering when the boom would fall; feeling the clock ticking away. Many had deep seated stores of anger—anger about being gay, about being mistreated because of being gay, about yet another friend dying, about being HIV positive, having their lives stolen, their dreams cut out from under them, and about the unfairness of the disease. Some members of our groups had seen more than 30 people die— lovers, friends, mentors. Almost every week had a fresh reminder of the ruthlessness of the disease with someone else sharing the news that a friend had died. Feelings varied from loss of interest in life to a sense of gratitude for being taught how to live a fuller life from their HIV infection. Some members, in fact, expressed the feeling that their quality of life had improved since their HIV diagnosis because they were no longer taking things for granted, but that they instead wanted to get the most out of every moment. For those who were still working, an ever present question was how to keep a stressful job, and at the same time take care of oneself and one's health.

At this point, while we have not yet analyzed data from this group, qualitative feedback from the participants indicates that the intervention has been successful in improving dysfunctional cognitions and in enhancing mood, thus indicating that emotional well-being may be positively impacted by this intervention. Sometimes these changes are expressed in ways that are more subtle than can be captured by change scores on psychosocial scales. One subject perhaps summed this up best when he announced 6 weeks into the group that he was "no longer waking up every day with a sense of dread." In fact, he reported that over the remainder of the intervention, his sense of dread did not return. Instead he felt renewed energy, and felt the strength to make several important life decisions regarding business investments and career directions. In each of these decisions, he described the importance of personal integrity as paramount, in having chosen to live the remainder of his life in accordance with what he perceived to be the deepest level of personal truth. A second subject reported that he could now allow his ailing lover to get angry, because he no longer felt personally threatened when his lover got angry. Each of these subjects described the sense of a burden having been lifted as these changes emerged in their lives.

In summary, our findings suggest that behavioral interventions such as CBSM may enhance coping and social support, which contribute to improvement of quality of life factors such as emotional functioning, social functioning, and sense of well-being for HIV-infected men during several phases of HIV spectrum disease. These phases include the acutely stressful period immediately following notification of HIV-positive status, the adjustment period following this news, and the process of dealing with chronic symptomatic HIV infection. Normalization of some aspects of immunological status were found to accompany some of these psychosocial changes in the short run. Longer term follow-up indicated relationships between psychosocial factors and improved immunological status and physical functioning up to 2 years later. Factors such as increased use of active coping strategies, including relaxation exercises, use of more functional appraisals and elicitation of social support, and decreased use of denial/avoidance coping strategies may be key predictors of longer term emotional well-being, social functioning, and physical functioning in HIV-infected populations.

FUTURE DIRECTIONS

As we work more with symptomatic men, our research will increasingly need to incorporate assessments of daily functioning and physical illness burden, as well as the assessments of emotional and social functioning that we have used in earlier phases of our research. The HIV-adapted MOS (Wu et al., 1991) represents a preliminary step in addressing the impact of HIV infection on daily living, and further refinement of instruments such as this will be important in addressing issues of daily functioning in quality of life research with HIV populations. Development of instruments that effectively assess quality of life factors in men at all stages of HIV disease is an important priority in upcoming research. Because many symptomatic men are taking antiretroviral drugs at this time and will be participating in new drug protocols as they emerge, assessment of the quality of life impact of these pharmacological agents, and how they interface with psychosocial intervention strategies will be increasingly important.

Special issues need to be addressed in emerging models of quality of life assessment in HIV populations. For example, the way resurgence of stigmatization and self-doubt affects sense of identity and well-being need to be addressed in quality of life research as well as in psychosocial interventions. Loss of employment and its financial and existential consequences are also factors that impact sense of self and well-being and need to be addressed both in research as well as in interventions. The effect of repeated HIV-related bereavements on an individual's social network and the emotional, social, and physical sequelae of bereavement have implications for HIV quality of life research as well. Finally, the way an individual comes to terms with the current and anticipated changes in their life and concomitant attitidinal and spiritual changes may have tremendous impact on sense of well-being (e.g., Hoffman, 1991), and this aspect of the individual's functioning must not be ignored in future research.

In HIV infection quality of survival time has become a paramount issue. Probing the relationships among coping strategies, social support, emotional well-being, realistic appraisals of one's functioning in comparison to their aspirations, and the influence of psychosocial functioning on disease course are central missions of our research program. Through behavioral interventions specifically tailored to the life concerns of our participants, our aim has been to enhance the quality of life of HIV-infected persons, and possibly, to turn this illness into a challenge for continued growth and development.

ACKNOWLEDGMENTS

This work was supported by grants MH18917-07 and MH40106.

REFERENCES

Antoni, M. (1991). Psychosocial stressors and behavioral interventions in gay men with HIV infection. *International Review of Psychiatry, 3*, 383–399.

Antoni, M., August, S., Baggett, L., Ironson, G., Saab, P., & Schneiderman, N. (1988). *Cognitive-behavioral stress management intervention manual for HIV high risk groups.* Unpublished manuscript, University of Miami, Department of Psychology, Miami, FL.

Antoni, M. H., August, S., LaPerriere, A., Baggett, H. L., Klimas, N., Ironson, G., Schneiderman, N., & Fletcher, M. A. (1990). Psychological and neuroendocrine measures related to functional immune changes in anticipation of HIV-1 serostatus notification. *Psychosomatic Medicine, 52*, 496–510.

Antoni, M. H., Baggett, L., Ironson, G., LaPerriere, A., August, S., Klimas, N., Schneiderman, N., & Fletcher, M. (1991). Cognitive-behavioral stress management intervention buffers distress responses and immunologic changes following notification of HIV-1 seropositivity. *Journal of Consulting and Clinical Psychology, 59*, 906–915.

Antoni, M. H., Esterling, B., Lutgendorf, S., Fletcher, M., & Schneiderman, N. (in press). Psychosocial stressors, herpesvirus reactivation and HIV-1 infection. In Baum A. & Stein M. (Eds.), *Chronic Diseases*. Hillsdale, NJ: Lawrence Erlbaum Associates.

Antoni, M. H., Goldstein, D., Goodkin, K., Fletcher, M. A., & Schneiderman, N. (1991). Coping responses to HIV-1 serostatus notification predict short and longer-term affective distress. *Psychosomatic Medicine, 53*, 227.

Antoni, M., Ironson, G., Helder, L., LaPerriere, A., Schneiderman, N., & Fletcher, M. A.

(1991). *Cognitive-behavioral stress management intervention reduces social isolation and maladaptive coping behaviors in gay men adjusting to an HIV-1 seropositive diagnosis.* Manuscript submitted for publication.

Barker, S., Tindall, B., & Carballo, M. (1990). Quality of life and clinical trials in HIV infection [letter], *Lancet, 335*, 1045.

Beck, A., & Emery, G. (1985). *Anxiety disorders and phobias: A cognitive perspective.* New York: Basic Books.

Beck, A., Rush, A.J., Shaw, B.F., & Emery, G. (1979). *Cognitive therapy of depression.* New York: Guilford Press.

Beckett, A., & Rutan, J.S. (1990). Treating persons with ARC and AIDS in group psychotherapy. *International Journal of Group Psychotherapy, 40*, 19–29.

Bernstein, D., & Borkovec, T. (1973). *Progressive relaxation training: A manual for the helping professions.* Champaign, IL: Research Press.

Blendon, R. J., & Donelan, K. (1988). Discrimination against people with AIDS: The public's perspective. *New England Journal of Medicine, 319*, 1022–1026.

Bloom, P., & Carliner, G. (1988). The economic impact of AIDS in the United States. *Science, 239*, 604–609.

Brown, S. M., Stimmel, B., Taub, R. N., Kochwa, S., & Rosenfeld, R. E. (1974). Immunologic dysfunction in heroin addicts. *Archives of Internal Medicine, 134*, 1001.

Burgess, A., & Catalan, J. (1991). Health-related quality of life in HIV infection. *International Review of Psychiatry, 3*, 357–364.

Bury, M. (1982). Chronic illness as a biographic disruption. *Sociology of Health and Illness, 4*, 167–182.

Campbell, A., Converse, P. E., & Rodgers, W. L. (1976). *The quality of American life.* New York: Sage.

Cella D. F., & Tulsky, D. S. (1990). Measuring quality of life today: Methodological aspects. *Oncology, 4*, 29–38.

Centers for Disease Control. (1992). 1993 revised classification system for HIV infection and expanded surveillance case definition for AIDS among adolescents and adults. *Morbidity and Mortality Weekly Report, 41* (RR-17), 1–19.

Centers for Disease Control. (1993). Projections of the number of persons diagnosed with AIDS and the number of immunosuppressed HIV-infected persons— United States 1992–1994. *Morbidity and Mortality Weekly Report, 41* (RR-18), 1–29.

Christ, G., & Weiner, L. (1985). Psychosocial issues for AIDS. In V. Devita, Jr., S. Hellman, & S. Rosenberg (Eds.), *AIDS* (pp. 275–297). Philadelphia: Lippincott.

Chuang, H. T., Devins, G. M., Hunsley, J., & Gill, M. J. (1989). Psychosocial distress and well-being among gay and bisexual men with human immunodeficiency virus infection. *American Journal of Psychiatry, 146*, 876–880.

Ciobanu, N. (1989) The role of Epstein-Barr infection in the pathogenesis of AIDS. In R. R. Watson (Ed.), *Co-factors in HIV-1 infection and AIDS* (pp. 34–45). Boca Raton, FL: CRC Press.

Coates, T., McKusick, L., Stites, D., & Kuno, R. (1989). Stress management training reduced number of sexual partners but did not improve immune function in men infected with HIV. *American Journal of Public Health, 79*, 885–887.

Cohen, C. (1982). On the quality of life: Some philosophical reflections. *Circulation, 66* (Suppl. 3.), 29–33.

Corbin, J. M., & Straus, A. (1991). A nursing model for chronic illness management based upon the trajectory framework. *Scholarly Inquiry for Nursing Practice: An International Journal, 5*(3), 155–174.

Cutrona, C., & Russell, D. (1987). The provisions of social relationships and adaptation to stress. In W. H. Jones & D. Perlman (Eds.), *Advances in personal relationships* (Vol. 1, pp. 37–67). Greenwich, CT: JAI Press.

de Haes J. C. J. M., & van Knippenberg, F. C. E. (1985) The quality of life of cancer patients: A review of the literature. *Social Science in Medicine, 20*, 809–817.

Dilley, J. W., Ochitill, H. N., Perl, M., & Volberding, P. A. (1985). Findings in psychiatric consultations with patients with acquired immune deficiency syndrome. *American Journal of Psychiatry, 142*, 82–86.

Dunkel-Schetter, C. A., & Wortman, C. (1982). The interpersonal dynamics of cancer: Problems in social relationships and their impact on the patient. In H. S. Friedman & M. R. Di Mateo (Eds.), *Interpersonal issues in health care* (pp. 69–100). New York: Academic Press.

Ellerman, D. (1989). *Quality of life of persons with AIDS/ARC*. Poster Presented at 5th International Conference on AIDS, Montreal.

Esterling, B. A., Antoni, M. H., Kumar, M., & Schneiderman, N. (1990). Emotional repression, stress disclosure responses, and Epstein-Barr viral capsid antigen titers. *Psychosomatic Medicine, 52*, 397–410.

Esterling, B., Antoni, M. H., Schneiderman, N., LaPeriere, A., Ironson, G., Klimas, N., & Fletcher, M. A. (1992). Psychosocial modulation of antibody to Epstein-Barr viral capsid antigen and human herpes virus-type 6 in HIV-1 infected and at-risk gay men. *Psychosomatic Medicine, 54*, 496–510.

Ewart, C. K., Taylor, C. B., Reese, L. B., & Devusk, R. F. (1983). Effects of early post myocardial infarction exercise testing on self-perception and subsequent physical activity. *American Journal of Cardiology, 51*, 1076–1080.

Fauci, A. S. (1991). Immunopathogenic mechanisms in human immunodeficiency virus (HIV) infection. *Annals of Internal Medicine, 114*, 678–693.

Fava, G. A. (1990). Methodological and conceptual issues in research on quality of life. *Psychotherapy and Psychosomatics, 54*, 70–76.

Fawzy, F. I., Cousins, N., Fawzy, N., Kemeny, M., Elashoff, R., & Morton, D. (1990). A structured psychiatric intervention for cancer patients. I. Changes over time in methods of coping and affective disturbance. *Archives of General Psychiatry, 47*, 720–725.

Fawzy, F. I., Kemeny, M. E., Fawzy, N., Elashoff, R., Morton, D., Cousins, N., & Fahey, J. L. (1990). A structured psychiatric intervention for cancer patients. II. Changes over time in immunological measures. *Archives of General Psychiatry, 47*, 729–735.

Fischl, M., et al., (1990). The safety and efficacy of zidovudine (AZT) in the treatment of subjects with mildly symptomatic human immunodeficiency virus type 1 (HIV) infection. *Annals of Internal Medicine, 112*, 727–737.

Follick, M. J., Gorkin, L., Smith, T., Capone, R. J., Visco, J., & Stablein, D. (1988). Quality of life post-myocardial infarction: Effects of a transtelephonic coronary intervention system. *Health Psychology, 7*, 169–182.

Friedman, A., Antoni, M. H., Ironson, G., La Perriere, A., Schneiderman, N., & Fletcher, M.A. (1990, March). *Behavioral interventions, changes in perceived social support and depression following notification of HIV-1 seropositivity*. Poster presented at Society of Behavioral Medicine Annual Meeting, Washington, DC.

Gambe, R., & Getzel, G. S. (1989). Group work with gay men with AIDS. *Social Casework, 70*, 172–179.

Gelber, R. D., Lenderking, W. R., Corron, D., Fischl, M. A., & Testa, M. A. (1991). Severe adverse events influencing quality of life in a randomized clinical trial of zidovudine vs. placebo (ACTG 016). Poster presented at *7th International Conference on AIDS, WB2112*, Florence.

Ginzburg, H. M., & Gostin, L. (1986). Legal and ethical issues associated with HLTV-III diseases. *Psychiatric Annals, 16*, 180–185.

Glaser, R., Pearson, G.P., Jones, J.F., Hillhouse, J., Kennedy, S., Mao, H., & Kiecolt-Glaser, J. (1991). Stress-related activation of Epstein–Barr virus. *Brain, Behavior and Immunity, 5*, 219-232.

Glaser, R., Rice, J., Sheridan, J., Fertal, R., Stout, J., Speicher, C., Pinshy, D., Kotur, M., Post, A., Beck, M., & Kiecolt-Glaser, J. (1987). Stress-related immune suppression: Health implications. *Brain, Behavior and Immunity, 1*, 7–20.

Glasser, B., & Strauss, A. L. (1965). *Awareness of dying*. London: Weisfield & Nicholson.

Glassmen, A., Bennett, C., & Randall, C. (1985). Effects of ethyl alcohol on human peripheral lymphocytes. *Archives of Pathology and Laboratory Medicine, 109*, 540.

Goodkin, K. (1988). Psychiatric aspects of HIV infection. *Texas Medicine, 84*, 55–61.

Hamilton, J., et al. (1992). A controlled trial of early versus late treatment with zidovudine in symptomatic human immunodeficiency virus infection. *The New England Journal of Medicine, 326*, 437–443.

Hoffman, M. A. (1991). Counseling the HIV-infected client: A psychosocial model for assessment and intervention. *The Counseling Psychologist, 19*, 467–542.

Horowitz, M. (1976). *Stress response syndromes*. New York: Jacob Aronson.

Ironson, G., Friedman, A., Klimas, N., Antoni, M., Fletcher, M. A., LaPerriere, A., Simoneau, J., & Schneiderman, N. (1994). Distress, denial, and low adherence to behavioral interventions predict faster disease progression in gay men infected with human immunodeficiency virus. *International Journal of Behavioral Medicine, 1*, 90–105.

Jacobsen, P. B., Perry, S. W., & Hirsch, D. A. (1990). Behavioral and psychological responses to HIV antibody testing. *Journal of Consulting and Clinical Psychology, 58*, 31–37.

Kaisch, K., & Anton-Culver, H. (1989). Psychological and social consequences of HIV exposure: Homosexuals in Southern California. *Psychology and Health, 3*, 63–75.

Kaplan, R. M., & Anderson, J. P. (1988). The quality of well-being scale: Rationale for a single quality of life index. In C. S. Walker (Ed.), *Quality of life: Assessment and application* (pp. 51–77). London: MTP Press.

Kaplan, R. M., Anderson, J. P., Patterson, T. L. (1991). *Quality of life measurement for persons with HIV infection*. Poster presented at the 7th International Conference on AIDS, TuD61 Florence.

Karnofsky, D. A., Abelmann, W. H., Craver, L. F., & Burchenal, J. H. (1948). The use of the nitrogen mustards in the palliative treatment of carcinoma. *Cancer, 1*, 634–652.

Kelly, J., & St. Lawrence, J. S. (1988). AIDS prevention and treatment: Psychology's role in the health crisis. *Clinical Psychology Review, 8*, 255–284.

Kiecolt-Glaser, J. K., & Glaser, R. (1988). Methodological issues in behavioral immunology research with humans. *Brain, Behavior, and Immunity, 2*, 67–78.

Kiecolt-Glaser, J. K, Glaser, R., Williger, D., Stout, J., Messick, G., Sheppard, S., Ricker, D., Romisher, S. C., Briner, W., Bonnell, G., & Donnerberg, R. (1985). Psychosocial enhancement of immunocompetence in a geriatric population. *Health Psychology, 4*, 25–41.

Kizer, K., Green, M., & Perkins, C. (1988). AIDS and suicide in California [letter]. *Journal of the American Medical Association, 260*, 1981.

Krantz, D. S. (1980). Cognitive processes and recovery from heart attack: A review and theoretical analysis. *Journal of Human Stress, 6*, 27–38.

Kubler-Ross, E. (1969). *On death and dying*. New York: Macmillan.

Lazarus, R. S., & Folkman, S. (1984). *Stress, appraisal and coping*. New York: Springer.

LeShan, L. (1974). *How to meditate*. New York: Bantam Books.

Lipowski, Z. J. (1969). Psychosocial aspects of disease. *Annals of Internal Medicine, 71*, 1197–1206.

Luthe, W. (1963). Autogenic training: Method, research and application in medicine. *American Journal of Psychotherapy, 17*, 174–195.

Luthe, W. (Ed.). (1969). *Autogenic therapy*. New York: Grune & Stratton.

Martin, J. (1988). Psychological consequences of AIDS-related bereavement among gay men. *Journal of Consulting and Clinical Psychology, 56*, 856–862.

Martin, J., Dean, L., Garcia, M., & Hall, W. (1989). The impact of AIDS on a gay community: Changes in sexual behavior, substance use, and mental health. *American Journal of Community Psychology, 17*, 269–293.

Martin, J. L., & Vance, C. S. (1984). Behavioral and psychosocial factors in AIDS: Methodological and substantive issues. *American Psychologist, 39*, 1303-1307.

Marzuk, P. M., Tierney, H., Tardiff, K., Gross, E. M., Morgan, E. B., Hsu, M. A., & Mann, J. J. (1988). Increased risk of suicide in persons with AIDS. *Journal of the American Medical Association, 259*, 1333–1337.

McDaniels, S., Hepworth, J., Doherty, W. J. (1992). *Medical family therapy: A biopsychosocial approach to families with health problems*. New York: Basic Books.

McNair, D. M., Lorr, M., & Droppleman, L. F. (1981). *EITS Manual for the profile of mood states*. San Diego, CA: Educational and Industrial Testing Service.

Moulton, J. M., Sweet, D. M., Temoshok, L., & Mandel, J. S. (1987). Attributions of blame and responsibility in relation to distress and health behavior change in people with AIDS and AIDS-related complex. *Journal of Applied Social Psychology, 17*, 493–506.

Muthny, F. A., Koch, U., & Stump, S. (1991). Quality of life in oncology patients. *Psychotherapy and Psychosomatics, 54*, 145–160.

Namir, S. (1986). Treatment issues concerning persons with AIDS. In L. McKusick (Ed.), *What to do about AIDS* (pp. 87–94). Berkeley: University of California Press.

Namir, S., Alumbaugh, M. J., Fawzy, F. I., & Walcott, D. L. (1989). The relationship of social support to physical and psychological aspects of AIDS. *Psychology and Health, 3*, 77–86.

Obier, K. M., MacPherson, M., & Haywood, J. L. (1977). Predictive value of psychosocial profiles following acute myocardial infarction. *Journal of the National Medical Association, 69*, 59–61.

Ostrow, D. G., Monjan, A., Joseph, J., Van Raden, M., Fox, R., Kingsley, L., Dudley, J., & Phair, J. (1989). HIV-related symptoms and psychological functioning in a cohort of homosexual men. *American Journal of Psychiatry, 146*, 737–742.

Pancheri, P., Matteoli, S., Pollizzi, C., Bellaterra, M., Cristofari, M ., & Puletti, M. (1978). Infarct as a stress agent: Life history and personality characteristics in improved versus non-improved patients after a severe heart attack. *Journal of Human Stress, 4*, 16–42.

Pantaleo, G., Graziosi, C., & Fauci, A. S. (1993). The immunopathogenesis of human immunodeficiency virus infection. *The New England Journal of Medicine, 328*, 327–335.

Penkower, L., Dew, M. A., Kingsley, L., Becker, J. T., Satz, P., Schaerf, F. W., & Sheridan, C. (1991). Behavioral, health, and psychosocial factors and risk for HIV infection among sexually active homosexual men: The Multicenter AIDS cohort study. *American Journal of Public Health, 81*, 2194–2196.

Pennebaker, J. W., Barger, S. D., & Tiebout, J. (1989). Disclosure of traumas and health among holocaust survivors. *Psychosomatic Medicine, 51*, 577–589.

Pennebaker, J. W., & Beall, S. K. (1986). Confronting a traumatic event: Toward an understanding of inhibition and diseases. *Journal of Abnormal Psychology, 95*, 274–281.

Pennebaker, J. W., Kiecolt-Glaser, J. K., & Glaser, R. (1988). Disclosure of traumas and immune function: Health implications for psychotherapy. *Journal of Consulting and Clinical Psychology, 56*, 239–245.

Pennebaker, J. W., & Susman, J. R. (1988). Disclosure of traumas and psychosomatic processes. *Social Science and Medicine, 26*, 327–332.

Perry, S., Jacobsberg, L., Fishman, B., Frances, A., Bob, J., & Jacobsberg, G. (1990). Psychiatric diagnosis before serological testing for the human immunodeficiency virus. *American Journal of Psychiatry, 147*, 89–93.

Ragsdale, D., & Morrow, J. R. (1990). Quality of life as a function of HIV classification. *Nursing Research, 39*, 335–359.

Redfield, R., & Burke, D. (1988). HIV infection: The clinical picture. *Scientific American, 259*, 90–98.

Rinaldo, C. R. (1989). Cytomegalovirus as a cofactor in HIV infection and AIDS. In R. R.

Watson (Ed.), *Co-factors in HIV-1 infection and AIDS* (pp. 151-185). Boca Raton, FL: CRC Press.
Roe, D. A. (1979). *Alcohol and the diet*. Westport, CT: AVI Publishing.
Rosenberg, Z. F., & Fauci, A. S. (1991). Activation of latent HIV infection. *Journal of National Institutes of Health Research, 2*, 41–45.
Rozanski, A., Barey, C. N., Krantz, D. S., Friedman, H. J., Ressler, K. J., Morell, M., Hilton-Chalfen, S., Hestrin, L., Bietendorf, H., & Berman, D. S. (1988). Mental stress and the induction of silent myocardial ischemia in patients with coronary artery disease. *The New England Journal of Medicine, 318*, 1005–1011.
Ruberman, W., Weinblatt, E., Goldberg, J. D., & Chaudhary, B. S. (1984). Psychosocial influences on mortality after myocardial infarction. *New England Journal of Medicine, 311*, 552–559.
Rundell, J., Paolucci, S., & Beatty, D. (1988). Psychiatric illness at all stages of human immunodeficiency virus infection [letter]. *American Journal of Psychiatry, 145*, 652–653.
Schlossberg, N. K. (1981). A model for examining human adaptation to transition. *Counseling Psychologist, 9*, 2–39.
Schlossberg, N. K. (1989). *Overwhelmed: Coping with life's ups and downs*. Lexington, MA: Lexington.
Schneiderman, N., Antoni, M. H., Ironson, G., LaPerriere, A., & Fletcher, M. A. (1992). Applied psychological science in HIV-1 research. *Journal of Applied Preventative Psychology, 1*, 67–82.
Smith, J. C. (1985). *Relaxation dynamics: A cognitive-behavioral approach to relaxation*. Champaign, IL: Research Press.
Smith, J. C. (1988). Steps toward a cognitive-behavioral model of relaxation. *Biofeedback and Self-regulation, 13*, 307–329.
Smith, J. . (1990). *Cognitive-behavioral relaxation training: A new system of strategies for treatment and assessment*. New York: Springer.
Spiegel, D., Bloom, J. R., Kraemer, H. C., & Gottheil, E. (1989). Effect of psychosocial treatment on survival of patients with metastatic breast cancer. *Lancet, 2*, 888–891.
Spitzer, W. O. (1987). State of Science 1986: Quality of life and functional status as target variables for research. *Chronic Diseases, 40*, 465–471.
Spitzer, W. O., Dobson, A. J., Hall, J. , Chesterman, E. , Levine, J., Shepherd, R., Battista, R. N., & Catchlove, B. R. (1981). Measuring the quality of life of cancer patients: A concise QL index for use by physicians. *Journal of Chronic Diseases, 34*, 585–597.
Stern, M. J., Pascale, L., & Ackerman, A. (1977). Life adjustment post-myocardial infarction. *Archives of Internal Medicine, 137*, 1680–1685.
Stewart, A. L., Hays , R. D., & Ware, J. E. (1988). The MOS short-form general health survey: Reliability and validity in a patient population. *Medical Care, 26*, 724–735.
Sumaya, C. V., Boswell, R. N., & Ench, Y. (1986). Enhanced serological and virological findings of Epstein–Barr virus in patients with AIDS and AIDS-related complex. *Journal of Infectious Disease, 154*, 864–870.
Tisman, F., Herbert, V., Go, L., & Brenner, L. (1971). In vitro demonstration and immunosuppression without bone marrow supression by alcohol and biomycin. *Clinical Research, 19*, 730.
Tross, S., & Hirsch, D. A. (1988) . Psychological distress and neuropsychological complications of HIV infection and AIDS. *American Psychologist, 43*, 929–934.
Viney, L., Henry, R., Walker, B., & Crooks, L. (1989). The emotional reactions of HIV antibody positive men. *British Journal of Medical Psychology, 62*, 153–161.
Volberding, P. et al. (1990). Zidovudine in asymptomatic human immunodeficiency virus infection. *The New England Journal of Medicine, 322*, 941–949.
Wachtel, T., Piette, M.S., Mor, V., Stein, M., Fleishman, J., & Carpenter, C. (1992). Quality

of life in persons with human immunodeficiency virus infection: Measurement by the Medical Outcomes Study instrument. *Annals of Internal Medicine, 116*, 129–137.

Walkey, F.H., Taylor, A.J., & Green, D. E. (1990). Attitudes to AIDS: A comparative analysis of a new and negative stereotype. *Social Science Medicine, 30*, 549–552.

Welch, D. (1982). Anticipatory grief: Reactions in family members of adult patients Issues in Mental Health Nursing, 4, 149–158.

Wenger, N. K., Mattson, M. E., Furberg, C. D., & Elinson, J. (Eds.). (1984a). *Assessment of quality of life in clinical trials of cardiovascular therapies.* New York: LeJaq.

Wenger, N. K., Mattson, M. E., Furberg, C. D., & Elinson, J. (1984b). Assessment of quality of life in clinical trials of cardiovascular therapies. *American Journal of Cardiology, 54*, 908–913.

Woo, S. K. (1988). The psychiatric and neuropsychiatric aspects of HIV disease. *Journal of Palliative Care, 4*, 50–53.

World Health Organization. (1947). Constitution of the World Health Organization. *WHO Chronicles, 1*, 29.

Wu, A. W., Matthews, W. C., Brysk, L. T., Atkinson, J. H., Grant, I., Abramson, E., Kennedy, C. J. McCutchan, J. A., Spector, S. A., & Richman, D. D. (1990). Quality of life in a placebo-controlled trial of zidovudine in patients with AIDS and AIDS-related complex. *Journal of Acquired Immune Deficiency Syndrome, 3*, 683–690.

Wu, A. W., Rubin, H. R., & Matthews, W. C. (1990, June). *Functional status and well-being in a placebo-controlled trial of zidovudine in early ARC.* Poster presented at the sixth International Conference on AIDS, THB19, San Francisco.

Wu, A. W., Rubin, H. R., Matthews, W. C., Ware, J. E., Brysk, L.T., Hardy, W. D., Bozette, S. A., Spector, S. A., & Richman, D. R. (1991). A health status questionnaire using 30 items from the medical outcomes study: Preliminary validation in persons with early HIV infection. *Medical Care, 29*, 786–798.

Ziller, R. C. (1974). Self-other orientation and quality of life. *Social Indicators Research, 1*, 301–327.

15 Quality of Life Research in Patients With Diabetes Mellitus

Alan M. Jacobson
Mary de Groot
Jacqueline Samson
Joslin Diabetes Center,
McLean Hospital and Harvard Medical School

All illnesses pose challenges to the adaptive capacity of individual patients and their families. They involve a common set of constraints, including decreased physical and role functioning, forced separations, and physical pain . However, each illness has its own specific variations or twists on these challenges and demands (Jacobson & Hauser, 1983). As such, any discussion of quality of life research pertaining to a particular illness should include a discussion of the pathophysiology of that illness and the ways that the condition and its treatment invades the real lives of patients and their families. Therefore, this presentation of quality of life research begins with a presentation of the clinical features of diabetes mellitus and its treatment. We then examine findings from studies that address quality of life issues in diabetes mellitus.

DIABETES MELLITUS

Diabetes mellitus is a common chronic condition that affects approximately 10 million people in the United States. The two most frequently diagnosed forms of the illness, Type I and Type II diabetes, have different causes, but similar clinical manifestations and courses. Type I diabetes, also frequently called insulin-dependent diabetes mellitus (IDDM), or juvenile diabetes, typically affects children and young adults with a peak age of incidence around puberty (Gill, 1992a). Although it aggregates in families, the genetics of this disorder have not been clearly delineated (Hitman & Marshall, 1992). Studies since the 1980s have indicated that the most common cause of Type I diabetes is an auto-immune attack on the pancreatic beta cell (i.e., the cell in the Islets of Langerhans that produces insulin). This is highly specific and eventually destroys all insulin-producing cells over a period of months to years (Chisholm & Kraegen, 1992). This process is set in motion by as yet unrecognized factors. The clinical presentation of the illness occurs when insulin producing capacity has dropped to a point below the metabolic requirements for insulin. Acute manifestations of the illness often occur at times of physiologic stress such as concurrent infection, puberty, or surgery, thereby leading to a sudden presentation of the common symptoms of poorly controlled diabetes. These include: frequent urination, dehydration, excessive thirst, and weight loss. Without replacement of insulin, the individual enters into a catabolic or starvation state and dies as a result of the complex array of metabolic alterations associated with this process (Gill, 1992a).

Replacement of insulin should return the metabolic condition of the individual to normal. However, the regulation of glucose metabolism by insulin cannot be perfectly replicated with current technologies. For example in the nondiabetic individual, insulin and other hormones regulate glucose levels in the blood within a narrow band (80–130 mg/dl) using an exquisitely sensitive feedback system. Insulin is released into the portal venous system to act initially on the liver. Current replacement techniques typically use one to several subcutaneous injections per day and/or continuous subcutaneous infusion. Thus, insulin therapies by entering the systemic, rather than the portal circulation, do not mimic the important effects of pancreatrically produced insulin on the liver's glucose regulation mechanisms. Furthermore, the relative infrequency of injections and home glucose testing means that patients with Type I diabetes may be subject to unexpected high or low blood glucose levels (hyperglycemia and hypoglycemia). Hypoglycemic episodes can lead to uncomfortable symptoms, loss of consciousness, coma, and seizures, and place the patient at high risk for accidental injury (e.g., when driving a car). Alternatively, hyperglycemia can lead to a partial starvation state, termed *diabetic ketoacidosis*, with altered pH and dehydration (Gill, 1992a). Thus, the patient with Type I diabetes must carefully regulate insulin, exercise, and diet to maintain a reasonable approximation of the nondiabetic metabolic state. Because patients are encouraged to care for themselves, careful education of the patient and, especially among child patients, of the family, is needed so that complex self-care activities can be undertaken properly. The treatment regimen for patients on insulin necessitates regularity and frequent attention. Thus, patients may feel like they have been imprisoned and may long for the day that they can stop their shots and testing. Furthermore, patients with Type I diabetes may experience themselves as living near a cliff that they can suddenly tumble off if they take too much or too little insulin or do not time doses or meals properly.

Type II diabetes typically occurs in older individuals and is approximately 10 times more common. It also has apparent familial associations with unknown genetic causation (Gill, 1992b). Type II diabetes occurs most frequently in patients who are obese. Presumptively, Type II diabetes in most patients is preceded by a long period of hyperinsulinemia that is thought to occur secondary to *insulin resistance* (i.e., a relative inability of cells to utilize insulin). Insulin resistance occurs commonly in obese individuals. After prolonged periods of insulin resistance and hyperinsulinemia, patients at risk for Type II diabetes appear to experience a loss of pancreatic beta cell mass leading to decreased insulin production and eventually, therefore, a clinical presentation of diabetes (Chisholm & Kraegen, 1992). Because this process of reduced insulin production capacity is gradual and often does not lead to a complete loss of insulin, patients with Type II diabetes can initially be treated with dietary restriction to decrease the metabolic pressures on insulin production. (Weight loss decreases insulin resistance.) Because oral agents act to increase pancreatic insulin release as well as lower insulin resistance, they can be used to supplement dietary therapy. Eventually insulin injections may be needed to augment the insulin-producing capability of the pancreatic beta cells that remain. Because of a prior history of obesity, the Type II patient is often faced with special demands to change diet.

Both types of diabetes are associated with similar medical complications that appear to be caused by chronic hyperglycemia and secondary changes in blood lipid levels (Gill, 1992a, 1992b). These include such manifestations of generalized microvascular damage as retinopathy and nephropathy. Although diabetic retinopathy can be treated with laser surgery, it can cause visual impairment and even legal blindness. Nephropathy may progress to renal failure necessitating chronic dialysis or a kidney transplant. Diabetes may also cause peripheral and autonomic nerve damage that can lead to chronic pain, chronic diarrhea, and gastric emptying problems. Peripheral nerve damage may lead to loss of joint sensation, which in turn can occasion chronic debilitating joint injuries. Impotence in males is also a common sequela of the neuropathy associated with diabetes. Diabetic patients are also at high risk for major vessel disease leading to myocardial infarction, stroke, foot ulcers, and gangrenous changes in the extremities. Unless careful glucose control is maintained during the pregnancies of diabetic women, newborns are at high risk for congenital abnormalities.

In summary, diabetes mellitus involves intensive change in common, habitual patterns of living as well as the threat of subsequent physically damaging and life-endangering complications. Patients and their families are very aware of the complications, often years before they occur, so for many (in particular parents and youngsters) the illness is experienced like a time bomb waiting to explode (Jacobson & Hauser, 1983).

QUALITY OF LIFE DEFINED

Quality of life may be defined as the individual's subjective perception of well-being as it relates to health status. Quality of life assessment is best thought of as being multidimensional and includes such areas as physical functioning, role functioning, pain, emotional status, satisfaction with treatment, and concerns about the future. Two approaches to quality of life assessment have evolved: generic and illness-specific measurement. Generic or nonspecific assessments of quality of life as exemplified by the Medical Outcome Survey (Ware & Sherbourne, 1992), the Quality of Well Being Instrument (QWB; Bush & Kaplan, 1982), or the Sickness Impact Profile (Bergner, Bobbitt, Carter, & Gibson, 1981). Some are multidimensional assessment tools designed to evaluate a broad array of functioning applicable to patients with all illnesses (e.g., Sickness Impact Profile and the Medical Outcome Survey). Even such multidimensional measures differ in the areas of function evaluated. Other measures (e.g. the QWB Scale) provide a single utility index of overall quality of life. These generic measures are most useful for cross-illness comparisons and in the case of the QWB Scale, which provides a single utility index, for economic analyses of treatments and illnesses. Some investigators have suggested that generic measures may be less sensitive to changes in functioning than illness-specific measures (Guyatt, Bombardier, & Tugwell, 1986). Certainly, their usefulness varies depending on the stage and type of illness. For example, the Sickness Impact Profile, with its heavy emphasis on capacity to perform physical functions, may be most useful for more physically infirm individuals, but inappropriate for patients early in the course of diabetes where physical capacities should essentially remain normal and where quality of life is most likely to be differentiated in terms of the lifestyle impacts of the illness.

Illness-specific measures offer the opportunity of focusing assessments on subtle distinctions as well as on specific problems posed by an individual illness. For example, an arthritis survey could address different forms and levels of joint pain, whereas a survey of diabetes might focus more extensively on diet-related concerns. Even off-the-shelf approaches to illness-specific quality of life assessment may be inadequate for addressing concerns of specific clinical trials or programs. Thus, a three-level approach that incorporates generic measures, illness-specific measures, and finally study-specific questions may be most appropriate in many studies that address quality of life (Jacobson, de Groot, & Samson, 1994a).

PSYCHOSOCIAL STUDIES OF DIABETES

Since 1969 a large number of studies have examined the psychosocial impacts of diabetes mellitus. To a great extent, these studies have been propelled by clinician and investigator recognition of the profound demands of the diabetic self-care regimen and multiple complications. Most of these studies have not incorporated quality of life measurement. Thus, these psychosocial studies provide a background for considering the few studies that have explicitly evaluated quality of life. It is beyond the scope of this chapter to provide an extensive review of these studies; therefore, the reader is directed to other reviews that provide fuller information (Jacobson, Hauser, Anderson, & Polonsky, 1994; Lustman, Griffith, Gavard, & Clouse, 1992; Rodin & Daneman, 1992; Rubin & Peyrot, 1992; Surwit, Schneider, & Feinglos, 1992).

Impact on Children

Psychosocial studies of diabetes have primarily been directed toward the impact of Type I diabetes on children, adolescents, and their families. Very few studies have addressed the psychosocial effects of Type II diabetes or of Type I diabetes on adults. These psychosocial studies of children have examined a wide variety of constructs. They include but are not exclusive to cognitive functioning, school performance, self-esteem, behavioral problems, psychiatric illness, and overall adjustment (Jacobson, Hauser, et al., 1994). Recent studies of cognitive functioning and school performance suggest that children and adolescents with diabetes are at an increased risk for mild cognitive impairments (Holmes, 1990; Ryan, Vega, & Drash, 1985). School performance problems may be more pronounced in boys as compared to girls (Holmes, Dunlap, Chen, & Cornwall, 1992). Furthermore, decreases in cognitive functioning appear to be most frequently found in patients with onset of diabetes prior to the age of five (Ryan et al., 1985). The etiology of these subtle impairments is not yet understood. Because of the increased risk of hypoglycemia in young children as well as the presence of a still-developing brain, one hypothesis has linked hypoglycemia to decreased mental efficiency in these children. It is certainly clear that profound and severe hypoglycemia can lead to coma and profound subsequent defects in cognitive functioning. One systematic study has linked these two phenomena, but this hypothesis remains controversial (Langan, Deary, Hepburn, & Frier, 1991). Current studies are now underway to disentangle the effect of hypoglycemia and treatment intensity on cognitive function among adolescents and adults with Type I diabetes (Diabetes Control and Complications Trial [DCCT], 1986; Ryan et al., 1991).

Psychological and personality inquiries have suggested that children and adolescents with diabetes show striking resilience in terms of their self-esteem, behavioral problems, and overall adjustment (Jacobson, Hauser, et al., 1994). One study by Kellerman, Zeltzer, Ellenberg, Dash, and Rigler (1980), for example, found no difference between diabetic patients and healthy controls in terms of anxiety levels and other measures of adjustment. One study by Jacobson et al. (1986), in a longitudinal study of children with diabetes, found little differences in psychosocial functioning over a 7-year follow-up period. However, there is controversy about the possible effects of diabetes on the development of psychiatric disorders in children and adults (Lustman, Griffith, Clouse, & Cryer, 1986; Rodin & Daneman, 1992; Samson, Jacobson, & de Groot, 1994; Wells, Golding, & Burnam, 1988). Research suggests that there may be an increased risk of depression in patients with longer term diabetes (Lustman et al., 1986) and an increased risk among adolescent and young adult women for bulimia (Rodin & Daneman, 1992). However, these conclusions must be tempered by limitations in the design and conflicts in the findings of many studies (e.g., Rodin & Daneman, 1992; Robinson, Fuller, & Edmeades, 1988). Furthermore, there is no evidence that diabetes leads to specific alterations in personality (Dunn & Turtle, 1981) and greater emotional dependency (Jacobson et al., 1986). Thus, the majority of psychosocial studies indicate that children with diabetes are not inevitably impaired by the demands of having this chronic illness. The greater than expected prevalence rates for depression and bulimia suggest that there may be certain psychosocial affects that accumulate as diabetes progresses.

Psychosocial Effects of Intensive Insulin Treatment

One recent area of inquiry deserves special attention. There is increasing evidence that treatment strategies that lead to normalized blood glucose levels, intensive insulin treatment, may delay the onset and progression of diabetes complications (Reichard et al., 1991). Thus, such intensive treatment approaches are increasingly recommended to patients and their families. Intensive insulin treatment involves a minimum of three insulin injections per day, frequent home glucose testing, very careful diet intake, and maintaining glucose levels close to the levels of nondiabetic individuals. Such regimens are very demanding and increase the risk of serious hypoglycemia (DCCT, 1991). Because intensive insulin treatment is so involving, some have speculated that it may have negative psychosocial consequences (DCCT, 1988). Some small short-term follow-up studies of adults with Type I diabetes have been performed. Subjects in these studies have been carefully selected research volunteers. Findings do not indicate problematic effects on self-esteem or psychological symptoms (Hirsch, Farkas-Hirsch, & Skyler, 1990; Nathan, 1988). Patients seem to feel in more control of their diabetes. The recently completed DCCT examined the effects of such an intensive treatment on quality of life over a 5- to 10-year follow-up: The study showed that intensive treatment did not lower quality of life of the participants. (DCCT, 1986, 1988, 1993).

SPECIFIC QUALITY OF LIFE STUDIES

Because clinical studies of diabetes have just begun to incorporate quality of life assessments, there is no consistent body of information about this aspect of diabetes or its treatment. We present the findings from those few studies that have examined the quality of life of patients with diabetes. Then, we turn for the remainder of the chapter to one area that has gained recent attention: the development of diabetes-oriented quality of life measures. Specifically, we focus our attention on the most widely used of these measures: the Diabetes Quality of Life Measure (DQOL). Our goal in the rest of the chapter is to introduce the measure and present some material regarding its reliability, validity, and sensitivity to change.

A few studies have now presented quality of life data on diabetic patients. In one national survey, patients with diabetes were not differentiated by type of illness, duration, or level of complications (Stewart, Greenfield, & Hays, 1989). This study suggested that although patients with diabetes had experienced a decrease in quality of life as compared to healthy individuals, these decreases were not as great as found in other patient groups such as those with coronary vascular disease. This is consistent with one psychiatric community study that showed that rates of depression in diabetes, although slightly higher than those in a healthy community sample, were lower than rates found in patients with chronic obstructive lung disease and coronary vascular disease (Wells et al., 1988). Jacobson, de Groot, & Samson (1994a) evaluated patients having Type I and Type II diabetes with a range in the number and severity of complications using the Medical Outcome Survey. (See Fig.15.1 for assessment of Type I patients.) They showed that quality of life decreased in relation to an increase in complications. Patients without complications showed minimal decrements in physical and social functioning, but still consistently rated themselves lower than healthy adults (Stewart et al., 1989). Comparison with results of the Medical Outcome Survey (see Fig. 15.1) suggest that patients with diabetes studied in this national survey were likely to have few complications. Thus, results of the Medical Outcome Study may understate the potential quality of life effects of diabetes. However, it is possible that such patients in all illness groups were underrepresented because of this study design.

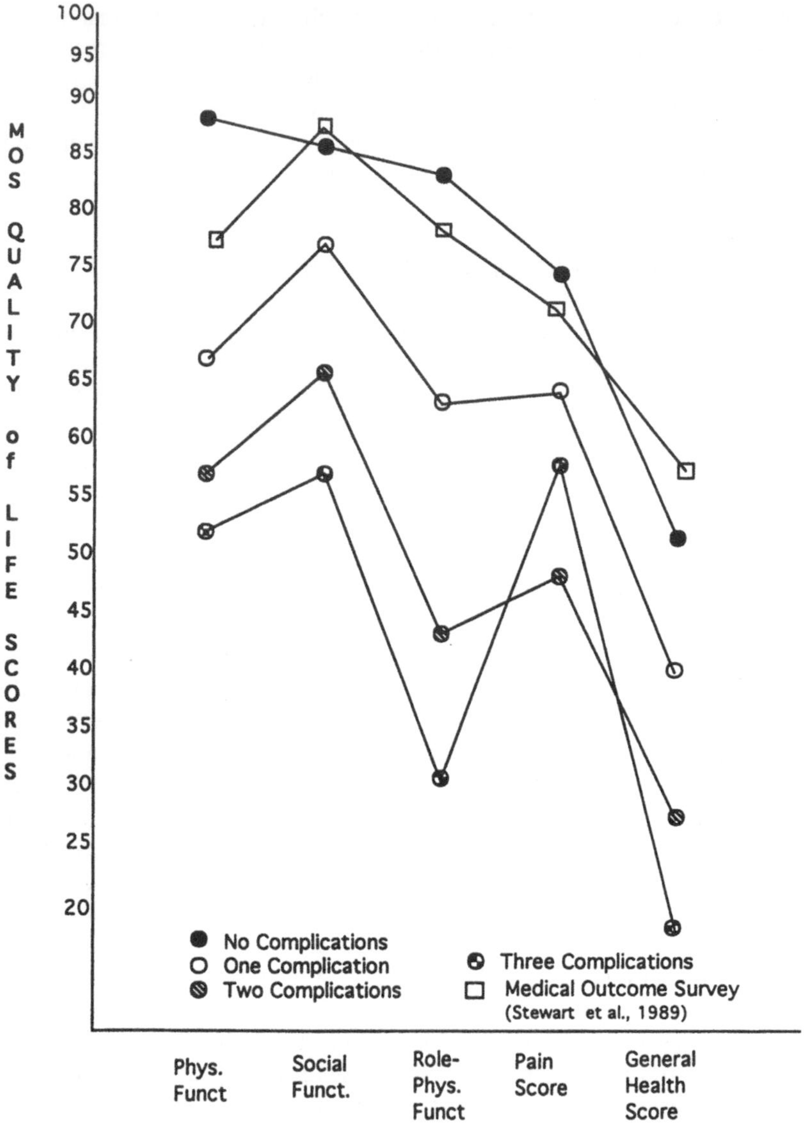

FIG. 15.1 Medical Outcome Survey scores for patients with number of diabetes complications: Type I diabetes mellitus (adapted from Jacobson, de Groot, & Samson, 1994a).

THE DIABETES QUALITY OF LIFE MEASURE

Diabetes-specific quality of life assessments have been developed since the 1980s with the specific goal of evaluating clinical treatments. As noted earlier, some investigators have suggested that such measures are more sensitive indicators of certain treatments. With that in mind, the DCCT Research Group developed the (DQOL) for use in a controlled, randomized, clinical trial comparing the efficacy of two different treatment regimens on the appearance and progression of chronic complications of Type I diabetes (DCCT, 1988). Specifically, the DQOL was designed to evaluate the relative burden of an intensive diabetes treatment regimen, with the goal of maintaining blood glucose levels as close as possible to those of people without diabetes, in comparison to standard diabetes therapy. Because intensive treatment would carry additional demands (e.g., extensive re-education, multiple daily injections of insulin or use of the insulin pump, frequent blood glucose monitoring, and greater need for cautious adjustment of food, exercise, and insulin doses), it was anticipated that it might affect the quality of life of patients. If quality of life was adversely influenced by intensive treatment then the willingness of patients and health-care providers to use intensive treatment could be affected. Thus, understanding the effects of the DCCT treatment regimens on quality of life was thought to be potentially useful for clinical application of the trial's findings.

Prior to the development of the DQOL, there were no available diabetes-specific or diabetes-oriented quality of life measures. Therefore, the DQOL had to be constructed for use within the trial. However, its structure purposely allowed for a broader application to other patients with Type I and even Type II diabetes. Thus, the scale items cover a range of issues directly relevant to diabetes and its treatment (DCCT, 1988).

Description of the Measure

The appendix presents the items of the DQOL. It is conceptualized as measuring the patient's personal experience of diabetes care and treatment. Four separate areas are addressed by the measure: satisfaction with treatment, impact of treatment, worry about the future effects of diabetes, and worry about social/vocational issues (DCCT, 1988). There is also a single overall well-being scale that is derived from national surveys of quality of well-being and can, therefore, be used to compare subjects to a wide variety of patients (Howie & Drury, 1978). In addition to these 46 core items and the well-being scale, the DQOL includes 16 items to assess adolescent populations who are in school or living at home with parents.

Responses to questions are made with a 5-point Likert scale. Satisfaction is rated from *very satisfied (1) to very dissatisfied* (5). Impact and Worry Scales are rated from *no impact or never worried* (1) to *always affected or always worried* (5). The single item assessing general quality of life is rated on a 4-point scale to maintain continuity with past use (Howie & Drury, 1978). Sixteen additional items assessing schooling, experience, and family relationships for patients living with their parents can be used to provide specific information about the life experiences of adolescent patients.

The DQOL is scored based on the approach of the Medical Outcome Survey (Ware & Sherbourne, 1992) so that each scale and the total is rated with 0 representing the lowest possible quality of life and 100 representing the highest possible quality of life (Jacobson, de Groot, & Samson, 1994a; Jacobson & the DCCT Research Group, in press).

Reliability and Construct Validity

Two studies (Jacobson, de Groot, & Samson, 1994a; DCCT, 1988) have examined the psychometric properties of the DQOL among patients with Type I and Type II diabetes. The scales show a high degree of internal consistency with Cronbach alphas in the .47 to .92 range (DCCT, 1988; Jacobson, de Groot & Samson, 1994a). Furthermore, the test–retest reliability based on retest results approximately 1 week after the original test were quite reasonable with correlations in the .78 to .92 range (DCCT, 1988). The first formal assessments of the validity of the DQOL by the DCCT Research Group (DCCT, 1988) examined the relationship of DQOL scores to three related measures of psychological symptoms, well-being, and adjustment to illness. There were moderately strong, consistent correlations of the total DQOL score with all three measures (DCCT, 1988). The pattern of correlations suggested that the Worry Scales indexed issues related most to psychological distress and symptomatology. The authors concluded that the satisfaction and impact scales serve as broad gauges of diabetes-related quality of life, whereas the Worry Scales address concerns more specific to patient perceptions of their diabetes-related psychological distress (DCCT, 1988).

Jacobson, de Groot & Samson (1994a) presented further information about construct validity of the DQOL by examining its relationship to a generic quality of life measure, the Medical Outcome Survey. The correlations between the Medical Outcome Survey and the DQOL were examined separately for adults with Type I and Type II diabetes. Overall, the patterns of correlation showed that the satisfaction and impact scores had the strongest relationships overall with the health functional status scales of the Medical Outcome Survey.

Discriminant Validity

The study by Jacobson, de Groot & Samson, 1994a, also provided information about the discriminant validity of the DQOL. In this study, patients with varying severity and numbers of complications were compared in terms of their diabetes quality of life. As shown in Fig. 15.2, number of

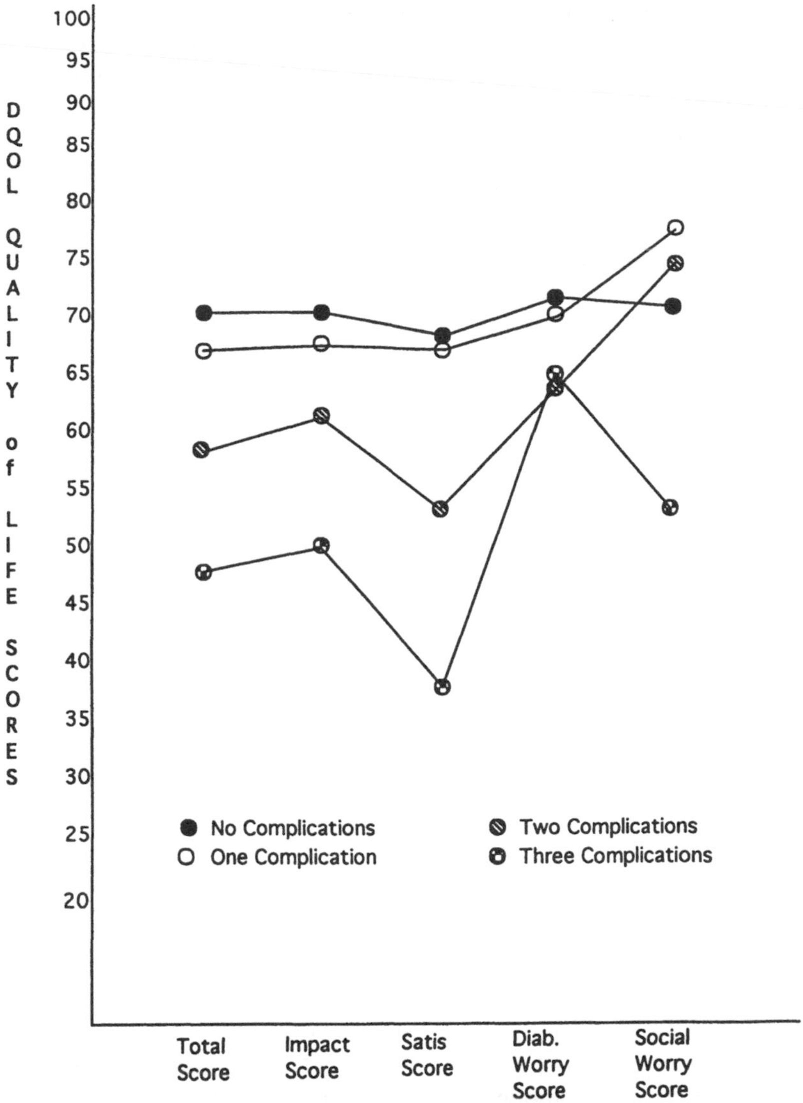

FIG. 15.2. Diabetes-related Quality of Life scores for patients with number of diabetes complications: Type I diabetes mellitus (adapted from Jacobson, de Groot & Samson, 1994a).

complications were associated with lower levels of satisfaction and greater impact of diabetes. This relationship held even after taking into account other relevant demographic data, such as age and marital status (Jacobson, de Groot & Samson, 1994a). In general, the worry scales were less sensitive to complications than the Satisfaction and Impact Scales, again suggesting that the Worry Scales measure a somewhat different aspect of quality of life than the other DQOL scales. The Worry Scales were incorporated in the DQOL because clinicians and investigators involved in the development of the measure realized that children, adolescents, and young adults with a chronic illness often were concerned about future effects of illness. Because worries reflect anticipated effects, it is entirely possible that patients react differently when evaluating them as opposed to current satisfaction and impact of illness and its treatment. Further research is needed to examine the conditions under which patient worries are increased and/or decreased. These analyses suggest that the advent of complications do not in themselves change the level of patient worries.

In this same study, discriminant validity was also examined by comparing patients with Type II diabetes using three different treatment regimens: insulin, oral agents, and diet alone. Patients who used insulin reported less satisfaction and greater impact of diabetes than patients taking and receiving an oral agent or diet. Strikingly, a different pattern was found regarding patient worries: Patients taking oral agents appeared to have more worries about their diabetes than patients who were taking insulin or only on a diet. This may reflect the anticipatory concerns of patients knowing that their diabetes has demanded more intensive treatment than diet and that they are on the road to insulin treatment, something that patients connect with having a more serious illness. This would be expected to lead to further worries. Together with the findings about the effect of complications on worry and correlations of the Worry scales with psychological distress measures, these results seem to suggest that worries about diabetes detect different aspects of patient experience. As such, further information is needed to characterize the Worry Scales. These data suggest that the Worry scales may be useful in understanding the impact of changes in regimens early in the course of illness when treatment approaches are undergoing change. It is important to recall that the social and diabetes worry scales, because they are designed for use with adolescents, are less relevant for adults who are settled in their lives.

A study by Lloyd, Matthews, and Wing (1992) provides further evidence for the discriminant validity of the DQOL. In this study, patients with differing numbers of complications were compared, and the results were similar to those reported by Jacobson, de Groot & Sampson (1994). Those patients having more complications had worse quality of life.

The study by Jacobson et al. (1994b) also demonstrated the combined and separate influences of comorbid psychiatric illness and progressive diabetes in patient quality of life. Patients having a current or past history of a psychiatric illness were more likely to experience poor quality of life than those without psychiatric illness (see Fig. 15.3). This effect of psychiatric illness on quality of life was independent of the effect of complications. The linkage of quality of life to psychiatric illness underlines

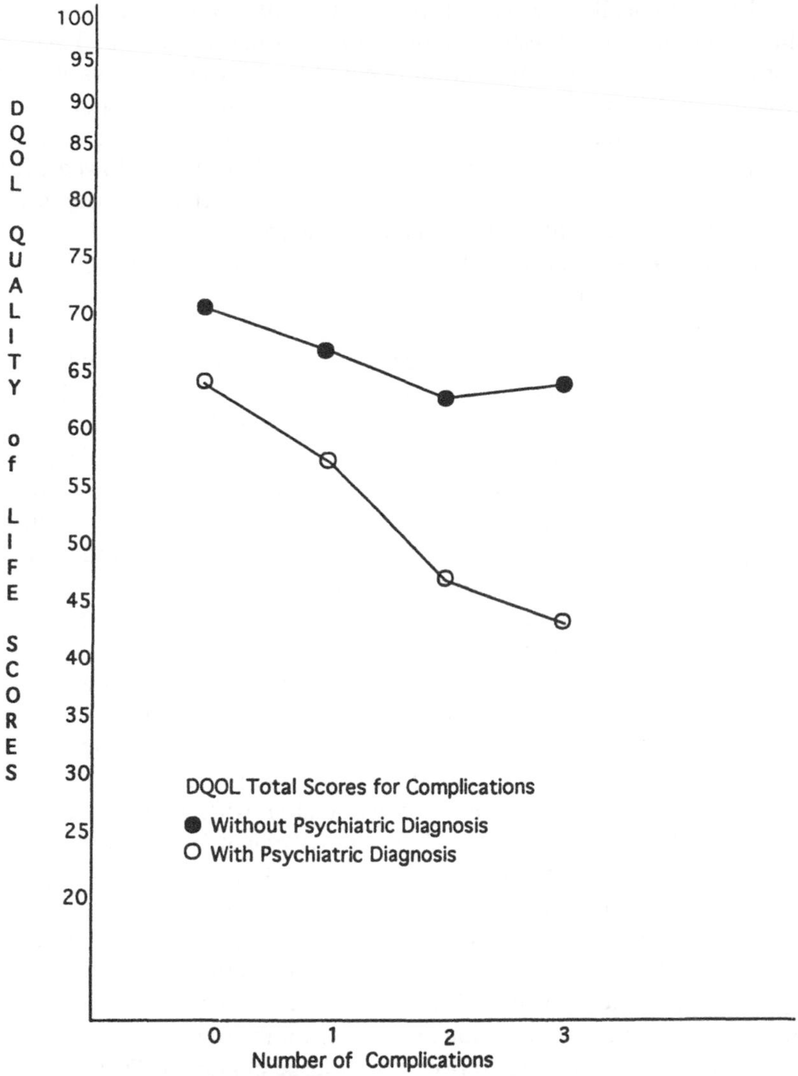

FIG. 15.3. Effect of complications and lifetime psychiatric diagnosis on quality of life (adapted from Jacobson, de Groot & Samson, 1994b).

the complex problems of comorbid psychiatric conditions on the burden of chronic medical illness (Wells et al., 1989).

Sensitivity to Change

All quality of life measures eventually must be evaluated in terms of their ability to capture important clinical changes in patient functioning. How ever, this is typically the last property of a quality of life scale to be evaluated because it necessarily involves longitudinal follow-up. There are two studies that provide information relevant to this question. Nathan and colleagues (1991) evaluated patients who had end-stage renal disease brought on by long-term diabetes. Patients were given either a kidney transplant or a combined pancreas/kidney transplant and followed over a 1-year period. At baseline, there were no significant between-group differences on the quality of life scales. The investigators found that there was a distinct improvement in the quality of life as measured by the DQOL total score and all subscales among patients who had received the combined kidney/pancreas transplant, whereas there was no improvement in quality of life for those patients who received the kidney transplant alone. Assessments using a generic quality of life measure showed no differences between the treatment groups before or after intervention. The only clinical differences in the two groups were in terms of improved glycemic control and the lifestyle change reflecting the freedom from daily self-care of diabetes in the patients receiving the pancreas transplant. Thus, it appears that improvement in quality of life appeared to reflect the freedom from diabetes self-care activities rather than differences in morbidity.

In a second study, the quality of life of patients who received an implantable pump was compared to usual insulin treatment (Selam, Micossi, & Dunn, 1992). This pump required periodic attention and did not relieve the patient from the need for regular daily glucose monitoring. Furthermore, patients had to continue to program the pump to give themselves insulin. Finally, the pump reservoir had to be filled with insulin on a monthly basis. The pump was associated with a decrease in the frequency of hypoglycemia and a slight improvement in overall metabolic control. Evaluations of the patients with the DQOL showed an improvement in the satisfaction subscale of the DQOL but no other changes.

These two studies provide an indication of the sensitivity of the DQOL to change. In the first instance, the treatment led to a substantial alteration in the patient's lifestyle as it related to diabetes. In essence, for a time, these patients were relieved from the metabolic disequilibrium of diabetes and its treatment demands. This was reflected in a large change in DQOL ratings even though the patients still had substantial complications of long-term diabetes. In the second study, the method of treatment led to a very modest change in lifestyle plus improvement in hypoglycemic frequency. This is reflected in a smaller improvement in quality of life detected only in the satisfaction scale.

IMPLICATIONS FOR FURTHER RESEARCH

As a chronic illness that involves threatened morbidity, together with treatments that are also demanding, diabetes is an ideal chronic illness for application of quality of life assessment. For example, the DCCT Research Group (1988) included an evaluation of patient quality of life because of the possibility that intensive insulin therapy with its attendant increased risk of hypoglycemia, weight gain, and lifestyle changes could pose a distinct threat to quality of life even while delaying the development or progression of complications. Because patient decisions about treatment are often made on basis of the quality of life implications of the treatment balanced against current symptoms of the illness, it is entirely possible that patients will prefer treatments that are easier even when the treatments hold promise for decreasing later medical problems. Based on the notion that a bird in the hand is worth two in the bush, patients not feeling the symptomatic benefit of a treatment, as in hypertension or the intensive treatment of diabetes, are likely to use the current impact of the treatment regimen as a basis for decisions about its use. For this reason quality of life assessment is particularly valuable in the evaluation of new approaches to diabetes treatment. Indeed the study by Nathan and colleagues (1991) demonstrates that removal of the apparatus of traditional diabetes treatment, insulin testing and careful diet, yields a definite improvement in quality of life even in patients with otherwise severe medical problems. This underlines the fact that the regimen demands themselves serve as major impediments to diabetic patients' sense of well-being. This also suggests that treatments that hold out improved ease of use even without alteration in the course of the medical condition will yield meaningful benefit based on the subjective experience of diabetic patients.

SUMMARY

In summary, quality of life assessment has only recently been applied to studies of patients with diabetes. The findings from these studies, highlighted in Table 15.1, indicate the effect of diabetes on quality of life, the potential effects of alternative treatment strategies on patient well-being, and the psychometric properties of two increasingly used quality of life measures. To date, research supports the reliability and validity of both the DQOL and Medical Outcome Survey in patients with Type I and Type II diabetes. These studies also suggest that these measures may be complimentary because of differences in focus and sensitivity to external factors such as disease severity and treatment strategies. Because of the profound lifestyle trade-offs involved in current therapies for diabetes, quality of life evaluation is likely to play an important role in future studies that evaluate the costs versus benefits of alternative therapies for both Type I and Type II diabetes.

ACKNOWLEDGMENTS

We wish to acknowledge James Rosenzweig, MD for his assistance in revising the medical description of diabetes mellitus and Noelle Cappella for

TABLE 15.1
Summary of Findings from Quality of Life Studies of Patients with Diabetes Mellitus

Authors	*Samples Studied*	*Measures*	*Findings/Comments*
DCCT Research Group, 1988	Type I patients without complications	DQOL[a]	Test re-test reliability, internal consistency, and construct validity of measure supported.
Stewart et al., 1989	Unspecified types of diabetes	MOS[b]	Quality of life in diabetics decreased less than in patients with coronary artery disease or chronic obstructive lung disease.
Wells et al., 1989	Unspecified types of diabetes	MOS	Depression has comparable impact on quality of life to physical illness.
Nathan et al., 1991	Type I patients with renal complications	DQOL	Diabetes-specific quality of life improves with pancreatic/renal transplant but not renal transplant alone.
Lloyd et al., 1992	Type I patients with wide range of complications	DQOL	DQOL measure sensitive to severity of complications.
Selam et al., 1992	Type I patients	DQOL	Diabetes-specific quality of life improves modestly using a programmable, implantable insulin pump that requires considerable patient activity.
Jacobson, de Groot, & Samson, 1994a	Type I and Type II patients with a wide range of complications	DQOL MOS	Evidence for reliability and discriminant validity of generic and diabetes-specific measures in well-characterized heterogeneous patient samples.
Jacobson, de Groot, & Samson, 1994b	Type I and Type II patients with a wide range of complications	DQOL MOS	Psychiatric illness influences quality of life independent of medical status.

[a]DQOL = Diabetes Quality of Life Measure
[b]MOS SF-36 = Medical Outcome Survey

typing the manuscript. The work was supported in part by a donation from Herbert Graetz and NIH grants #DK27845 and #DK42315.

APPENDIX: DIABETES QUALITY OF LIFE MEASURE

Please read each statement carefully. Please indicate how satisfied or dissatisfied you currently are with the aspect of your life described in the statement. Circle the number that best describes how you feel. There are no right or wrong answers to these questions. We are interested in your opinion.

	Very Satisfied	*Moderately Satisfied*	*Neither*	*Moderately Dissatisfied*	*Very Dissatisfied*
A1. How satisfied are you with the amount of time it takes to manage your diabetes?	1	2	3	4	5
A2. How satisfied are you with the amount of time you spend getting checkups?	1	2	3	4	5
A3. How satisfied are you with your current treatment?	1	2	3	4	5
A5. How satisfied are you with the flexibility you have in your diet?	1	2	3	4	5
A6. How satisfied are you with the burden your diabetes is placing on your family?	1	2	3	4	5
A7. How satisfied are you with your knowledge about your diabetes?	1	2	3	4	5
A8. How satisfied are you with your sleep?	1	2	3	4	5
A9.How satisfied are you with your social relationships and friendships?	1	2	3	4	5
A10. How satisfied are you with your sex life?	1	2	3	4	5
A11. How satisfied are you with your work, school, and household activities?	1	2	3	4	5
A12. How satisfied are you with the appearance of your body?	1	2	3	4	5
A13. How satisfied are you with the time you spend exercising?	1	2	3	4	5
A14. How satisfied are you with your leisure time?	1	2	3	4	5
A15. How satisfied are you with your life in general?	1	2	3	4	5

Please indicate how often the following events happen to you. Circle the appropriate number.

	Never	*Very Seldom*	*Sometimes*	*Often*	*All the Time*
B1. How often do you feel pain associated with the treatment for your diabetes?	1	2	3	4	5
B2. How often are you embarrassed by having to deal with your diabetes in public?	1	2	3	4	5
B3. How often do you have low blood sugar?	1	2	3	4	5
B4. How often do you feel physically ill?	1	2	3	4	5
B5. How often does your diabetes interfere with your family life?	1	2	3	4	5
B6. How often do you have a bad night's sleep?	1	2	3	4	5
B7. How often do you find your diabetes limiting your social relationships and friendships?	1	2	3	4	5
B8. How often do you feel good about yourself?	1	2	3	4	5
B9. How often do you feel restricted by your diet?	1	2	3	4	5
B10. How often does your diabetes interfere with your sex life?	1	2	3	4	5
B11. How often does your diabetes keep you from driving a car or using a machine (e.g., a typewriter)?	1	2	3	4	5
B12. How often does your diabetes interfere with your exercising?	1	2	3	4	5
B13. How often do you miss work, school, or household duties because of your diabetes?	1	2	3	4	5
B14. How often do you find yourself explaining what it means to have diabetes?	1	2	3	4	5
B15. How often do you find that your diabetes interrupts your leisure-time activities?	1	2	3	4	5
B16. How often do you tell others about your diabetes?	1	2	3	4	5
B17. How often are you teased because you have diabetes?	1	2	3	4	5
B18. How often do you feel that because of your diabetes you go to the bathroom more than others?	1	2	3	4	5

B19. How often do you find that you eat something you shouldn't rather than tell someone that you have diabetes?	1	2	3	4	5
B20. How often do you hide from others the fact that you are having an insulin reaction?	1	2	3	4	5

Please indicate how often the following events happen to you. Please circle the number that best describes your feelings. If the question is not relevant to you, circle non-applicable.

	Never	*Seldom*	*Sometimes*	*Often*	*Always*	*Does Not Apply*
C1. How often do you worry about whether you will get married?	1	2	3	4	5	0
C2. How often do you worry about whether you will have children?	1	2	3	4	5	0
C3. How often do you worry about whether you will not get a job you want?	1	2	3	4	5	0
C4. How often do you worry about whether you will be denied insurance?	1	2	3	4	5	0
C5. How often do you worry about whether you will be able to complete your education?	1	2	3	4	5	0
C6. How often do you worry about whether you will miss work?	1	2	3	4	5	0
C7. How often do you worry whether you will be able to take a vacation or a trip?	1	2	3	4	5	0
D1. How often do you worry about whether you will pass out?	1	2	3	4	5	0
D2. How often do you worry that your body looks differently because you have diabetes?	1	2	3	4	5	0
D3. How often do you worry that you will get complications from your diabetes?	1	2	3	4	5	0
D4. How often do you worry about whether someone will not go out with you because you have diabetes?	1	2	3	4	5	0

E1. Compared to other people your age, would you say your health is:

1. Excellent
2. Good
3. Fair
4. Poor

(Circle One)

REFERENCES

Bergner, M., Bobbitt, R. A., Carter, W. B., & Gibson, B. S. (1981). The Sickness Impact Profile: Development and final revision of a health status measure. *Medical Care, 19,* 787–805.

Bush, J. M, . & Kaplan, R. M. (1982). Health-related quality of life measurement. *Health Psychology, 1,* 61–80.

Chisholm, D. J. & Kraegen, E. W. (1992). The pathogenesis of non-insulin-dependent diabetes mellitus: The role of insulin resistance. In J.C. Pickup & G. Williams (Eds.), *Textbook of Diabetes* (pp. 192–197). Oxford: Blackwell Scientific Publications.

Diabetes Control and Complications Trial Research Group. (1986). Diabetes control and complications trial (DCCT): Design and methodological considerations for the feasibility phase. *Diabetes, 35,* 530–545.

Diabetes Control and Complications Trial Research Group. (1988). Reliability and validity of a diabetes quality of life measure for the diabetes control and complication trial (DCCT). *Diabetes Care, 11,* 725–732.

Diabetes Control and Complications Trial Research Group. (1991). Epidemiology of severe hypoglycemia in the diabetes control and complications trial. *American Journal of Medicine, 90,* 450–459.

Diabetes Control and Complications Trial Research Group. (1993). The effect of intensive treatment of diabetes on the development and progress of long-term complications in insulin-dependent diabetes mellitis. *New England Journal of Medicine, 329,* 977–986.

Dunn, S. M., & Turtle, J. R. (1981). The myth of the diabetic personality. *Diabetes Care, 4,* 640–646.

Gill, G. V. (1992a). Insulin-dependent diabetes dellitus. In J.C. Pickup & G. Williams (Eds.), *Textbook of diabetes* (pp. 17–23). Oxford: Blackwell Scientific Publications.

Gill, G. V. (1992b). Non-insulin-dependent diabetes mellitus. In J. C. Pickup & G. Williams (Eds.), *Textbook of diabetes* (pp. 24–29). Oxford: Blackwell Scientific Publications.

Guyatt, G., Bombardier, C., & Tugwell, P. (1986). Measuring disease-specific quality of life in clinical trials. *Canadian Medical Association Journal, 134* , 889–895.

Hirsch, I. B., Farkas-Hirsch, R., & Skyler, J.S. (1990). Intensive insulin therapy for Type I diabetes mellitus. *Diabetes Care, 13,* 1265–1283.

Hitman, G. A., Marshall, B. (1992). Genetics of Insulin-dependent diabetes mellitus. In J. C. Pickup & G. Williams (Eds.), *Textbook of diabetes (pp. 113–121), Oxford: Blackwell Scientific Publications.*

Holmes, C. S. (1990). Neuropsychological sequelae of acute and chronic blood glucose disruption in adults with IDDM. In C.S . Holmes (Ed.), *Neuropsychological and behavioral aspects of diabetes* (pp. 122–154). New York: Springer-Verlag.

Holmes, C. S., Dunlap, W. P., Chen, R. S., & Cornwall, J. M. (1992). Gender differences in the learning status of diabetic children. *Journal of Consulting and Clinical Psychology, 60,* 698–704.

Howie, L. J. & Drury, T. F. (1978). *Current estimate from the health interview survey: United States 1997.* Hyattsville, MD: National Center for Health Statistics.

Jacobson, A. M., & The DCCT Research Group. (in press). The diabetes quality of life measure. In C. Bradley (Ed.), *Handbook of psychology and diabetes.* London: Harwood Academic Publishers.

Jacobson, A. M., de Groot, M., & Samson, J. (1994a). Quality of life in patients with Type I and Type II diabetes mellitus. *Diabetes Care, 17,* 167–274.

Jacobson, A. M., de Groot, M,. & Samson, J.A. (1994b). *Psychiatric disorders and quality of life in diabetes mellitus.* Manuscript suvmitted for review.

Jacobson, A. M., & Hauser, S. T. (1983). Behavioral and psychological aspects of diabetes. In

M. Ellenberg & H. Rifkin (Eds.), *Diabetes Mellitus: Theory and practice* (pp. 1037–1052). New York: Medical Exam, Inc.

Jacobson, A. M., Hauser, S. T., Anderson, B. J., & Polonsky, W. (1994). Psychosocial aspects of diabetes. In C. Kahn & G. Weir (Eds.), *Joslin's diabetes mellitus* (13th Ed., pp. 431–450). Philadelphia: Lea Febiger.

Jacobson, A. M., Hauser, S. T., Wertlieb, D., Wolfsdorf, J. I., Orleans, J. & Vieyra, M. (1986). Psychological adjustment of children with recently diagnosed diabetes mellitus. *Diabetes Care,9, 323–329.*

Kellerman, J., Zeltzer, L., Ellenberg, L., Dash, J. & Rigler, D. (1980). Psychological effects of illness in adolescents. I. Anxiety, self-esteem, and perceptionof control. *Journal of Pediatrics, 27,* 126–131.

Langan, S. J., Deary, I. J., Hepburn, D. A., & Frier, B.M. (1991). Cumulative cognitive impairment following recurrent severe hypoglycemia in adult patients with insulin-treated in diabetes mellitus. *Diabetologia, 34,* 337–344.

Lloyd, C. E., Matthews, K. A., & Wing, R. R. (1992). Psychosocial factors and complications of IDDM. *Diabetes Care, 15,* 166–172.

Lustman, P. J., Griffith, L. S., Clouse, R.E., & Cryer, P. E. (1986). Psychiatric illness in diabetes mellitus. *Journal of Nervous and Mental Disorders, 174,* 736–742.

Lustman, P. J., Griffith, L .S., Gavard, J. A., & Clouse, R. E. (1992). Depression in adults with diabetes. *Diabetes Care,.15,* 1631–1639.

Nathan, D. M. (1988). Modern management of insulin dependent diabetes mellitus. *Medical Clinics of North America, 72,* 1365–1378.

Nathan, D. M., Fogel, H., Norman, D., Russell, P. S, Tolkoff-Rubin, N., Delmonico, F. L., Auchincloss, H., Camuso, J., & Cosimi, A.B (1991). Long-term metabolic and quality of life results with pancreatic/renal transplantation in insulin-dependent diabetes mellitus. *Transplantation, 52,* 85–91.

Reichard, P., Berglund, B., Britz, A., Cars, I., Nilsson, B. Y., & Rosenquist, U. (1991). Intensified conventional insulin treatment retards the microvascular complications of insulin-dependent diabetes mellitus (IDDM): The Stockholm Diabetes Intervention Study (SDIS) after 5 years. *Journal of Internal Medicine, 230,* 101–108.

Robinson, N., Fuller, J. H., & Edmeades, S. P. (1988). Depression and diabetes. *Diabetic Medicine, 5,* 268–274.

Rodin, G. M., & Daneman, D. (1992). Eating disorders and insulin-dependent diabetes mellitus: A problematic association. *Diabetes Care, 15,* 1402–1412.

Rubin, R. R., & Peyrot, M. (1992). Psychosocial problems and interventions in diabetes: A review of the literature. *Diabetes Care, 15,* 1640–1657.

Ryan, C., Adams, K., Heaton, R., Grant, I., Jacobson, A., & The DCCT Research Group. (1991). Neurobehavioral assessment of medical patients in clinical trials: The DCCT experience. In E. Mohr & P. Brouwers (Eds.), *Handbook of clinical trials: The neurobehavioral approach.* (pp. 217–242). Brwyn, PA: Swets & Zeitlinger.

Ryan, C. M., Vega, A., & Drash, A. (1985). Cognitive deficits in adolescents who developed diabetes early in life. *Pediatrics, 75,* 921–927.

Samson, J. A., Jacobson, A. M., de Groot, M. (1994). Psychiatric illness and diabetes mellitus. Manuscript submitted for review.

Selam, J. L., Micossi, P., & Dunn, F. L. (1992). Clinical trial of programmable implantable insulin pump for Type I diabetes. *Diabetes Care, 15,* 877–884.

Stewart, A. L., Greenfield, S., & Hays, R. D. (1989). Functional status and well-being of patients with chronic conditions. *Journal of the American Medical Association, 262,*907–913.

Surwit, R. S., Schneider, M. S., & Feinglos, M. N. (1992). Stress and diabetes mellitus. *Diabetes Care, 15,* 1413–1422.

Ware, J. H., & Sherbourne, C. D. (1992). The MOS 36-Item Short Form Health Survey

(SF-36). I. Conceptual framework and item selection. *Medical Care, 30,* 473–483.
Wells, K. B., Golding, J. M., & Burnam, M. A. (1988). Psychiatric disorder in a sample of the general population with and without chronic medical conditions. *American Journal of Psychiatry, 145,* 976–981.
Wells, K. B., Stewart, A., Hays, R. D., Burnam, A., Rogers, W., Daniels, M., Berry, S., Greenfield, S., & Ware, J. (1989). Functioning and well-being of depressed patients. *Journal of the American Medical Association, 262,* 914–919.

Author Index

A

B

D

E

F

G

H

S

Y

Z

Subject Index

A

B

C

Q

V

W

Y

Z